Teen Health Series

TOBACCO AND E-CIGARETTE INFORMATION FOR TEENS FIFTH EDITION

Teen Health Series

TOBACCO AND E-CIGARETTE INFORMATION FOR TEENS FIFTH EDITION

Health Insights on the Risks of Cigarette Smoking, Smokeless Tobacco, and Other Nicotine Products

Including Essential Information on Nicotine Addiction, Nicotine Delivery Systems, Secondhand Smoke, Health Consequences of Tobacco Use, E-cigarettes, Associated Cancers, and Strategies for Quitting Smoking

OMNIGRAPHICS
An imprint of Infobase

* * *

OMNIGRAPHICS
An imprint of Infobase
8 The Green
Suite 19225
Dover, DE 19901
www.infobase.com
James Chambers, *Editorial Director*

* * *

ISBN 978-0-7808-2106-4
E-ISBN 978-0-7808-2107-1

Library of Congress Cataloging-in-Publication Data

Names: Chambers, James, editor. | Omnigraphics, Inc.

Title: Tobacco and E-cigarette information for teens / edited by James Chambers. Other titles: Tobacco information for teens.

Description: Fifth edition. | Wilmington, DE: Omnigraphics, an imprint of Infobase, [2024] | Series: Teen health series | Includes index. | Audience: Ages 13 | Audience: Grades 7-9 | Summary: "Provides health tips about the risks of using cigarettes, e-cigarettes, smokeless tobacco, and nicotine products, along with facts about nicotine addiction, delivery systems, secondhand smoke, health consequences, associated cancers, smoking cessation, and statistics. Includes index and resources for additional help and information"-- Provided by publisher.

Identifiers: LCCN 2023045569 (print) | LCCN 2023045570 (ebook) | ISBN 9780780821064 | ISBN 9780780821071 (eISBN)

Subjects: LCSH: Tobacco use--Health aspects. | Smoking--Health aspects. | Nicotine--Health aspects. | Smoking cessation. | Teenagers--Tobacco use--Prevention.

Classification: LCC RA1242.T6 T615 2024 (print) | LCC RA1242.T6 (ebook) | DDC 613.850835--dc23/eng/20231103

LC record available at https://lccn.loc.gov/2023045569
LC ebook record available at https://lccn.loc.gov/2023045570

Printed in the United States

TABLE OF CONTENTS

Part 3 | Nicotine Delivery Systems

Part 4 | Common Cancers Linked to Tobacco Use

Part 5 | Other Health Concerns Related to Tobacco Use

Part 6 | Tobacco-Use Cessation

Part 7 | If You Need More Help or Information

PREFACE

About This Book

Tobacco use biggest avoidable cause of sickness and death in the United States. According to the Centers for Disease Control and Prevention (CDC), about 28.3 million U.S. adults smoke cigarettes and an estimated 3.08 million U.S. middle and high school students use some form of tobacco. Every day, roughly 1,600 U.S. youth under 18 years old try their first cigarette. Nearly half a million Americans die prematurely each year due to smoking or being around secondhand smoke, and another 16 million live with a serious illness caused by smoking.

Tobacco and E-cigarettes Information for Teens, Fifth Edition offers the latest details on the health consequences linked to smoking and other tobacco uses. It explains various ways nicotine is used, including different types of cigarettes, cigars, hookah pipes, smokeless and heated tobacco products, and secondhand smoke. The book discusses cancers associated with tobacco use, focusing on the organs most commonly affected. Another section covers additional health concerns related to tobacco use, discussing common smoking-related diseases affecting the heart, lungs, digestive system, eyes, and pregnancy. For teens aiming to quit smoking, or to assist a friend or family member, the book provides information on preparation, quitting tools and products, and details about nicotine replacement therapy. The book concludes with directories of resources to learn more about the health effects of tobacco use and smoking cessation.

How to Use This Book

This book is divided into parts and chapters. Parts focus on broad areas of interest; chapters are devoted to single topics within a part.

Part 1: Understanding Adolescent Tobacco Use explains the important facts about the use of tobacco and nicotine products. It provides information on global smoking trends and nicotine addiction. It also explores marketing strategies along with approaches for preventing tobacco use.

Part 2: Electronic Cigarettes or Vaping focuses on different types of e-cigarettes and provides guidance on quitting their use. This part also offers insights into various vaping methods.

Part 3: Nicotine Delivery Systems outlines various types of nicotine usage. It discusses e-cigarettes and the risks faced by secondhand smokers. It explains various methods through which nicotine is consumed, including different types of cigarettes, cigars, hookah pipes, and smokeless and heated tobacco products.

Part 4: Common Cancers Linked to Tobacco Use explores different cancers arising from tobacco use and emphasizes how smoking is the primary cause of cancer in the United States. It also outlines cancer treatment methods and prevention strategies.

Part 5: Other Health Concerns Related to Tobacco Use provides information on prevalent common smoking-related diseases affecting the heart, lungs, digestive system, eyes, and pregnancy. It covers various treatment options available for other health-related conditions.

Part 6: Tobacco-Use Cessation offers guidance for teens aiming to quit smoking or assist a friend or family member in quitting. It provides information on ways to prepare for and quit smoking, tools and products to aid during the quitting process, and details about nicotine replacement therapy. The part also includes tips for managing the effects of nicotine withdrawal.

Part 7: If You Need More Help or Information lists government and private organizations offering information on the health effects of tobacco use and quitting smoking.

Bibliographic Note

This volume contains documents and excerpts from publications issued by the following U.S. government agencies: Centers for Disease Control and Prevention (CDC); Federal Trade Commission (FTC); MedlinePlus; National Cancer Institute (NCI); National Heart, Lung, and Blood Institute (NHLBI); National Institute of Dental and Craniofacial Research (NIDCR); National Institute of Diabetes and Digestive and Kidney Diseases (NIDDK); National Institute of Neurological Disorders and Stroke (NINDS); National Institute on Drug Abuse (NIDA); Office of Disease Prevention and Health Promotion (ODPHP); Smokefree.gov; Smokefree Teen; Smokefree Women; U.S. Department of Health and Human Services (HHS); U.S. Department of Veterans Affairs (VA); and U.S. Food and Drug Administration (FDA).

It also contains original material produced by Infobase and reviewed by medical consultants.

The photograph on the front cover is © Zyn Chakrapong/Shutterstock.

Medical Review

Infobase contracts with a team of qualified, senior medical professionals who serve as medical consultants for the *Teen Health Series*. As necessary, medical consultants review reprinted and originally written material for currency and accuracy. Medical consultation services are provided to the *Teen Health Series* editors by:

Dr. Vijayalakshmi, MBBS, DGO, MD
Dr. Senthil Selvan, MBBS, DCH, MD
Dr. K. Sivanandham, MBBS, DCH, MS (Research), PhD

About the *Teen Health Series*

At the request of librarians serving today's teens and young adults, the *Teen Health Series* was developed as a specially focused set of volumes within *Health Reference Series*. Each volume deals comprehensively with a topic selected according to the needs and interests of people in middle school and high school. Teens seeking preventive guidance, information about disease warning signs, medical statistics, and risk factors for health problems will find answers to their questions in the *Teen Health Series*. The *Series*, however, is not intended to serve as a tool for diagnosing illness, in prescribing treatments, or as a substitute for the physician-patient relationship. All people concerned about medical symptoms or the possibility of disease are encouraged to seek professional care from an appropriate healthcare provider.

If there is a topic you would like to see addressed in a future volume of the *Teen Health Series*, please write to: custserv@infobaselearning.com.

A Note about Spelling and Style

Teen Health Series editors use *Stedman's Medical Dictionary* as an authority for questions related to the spelling of medical terms and *The Chicago Manual of Style* for questions related to grammatical structures, punctuation, and other editorial concerns. Consistent adherence is not always possible, however, because the individual volumes within the *Series* include many documents from a wide variety of different producers and copyright holders, and the editor's primary goal is to present material from each source as accurately as is possible following the terms specified by each document's producer. This sometimes means that information in different chapters may follow other guidelines and alternate spelling authorities. For example, occasionally a copyright holder may require that eponymous terms be shown in possessive forms (Crohn's disease vs. Crohn disease) or that British spelling norms be retained (leukaemia vs. leukemia).

PART 1 | UNDERSTANDING ADOLESCENT TOBACCO USE

CHAPTER 1
TOBACCO USE IN ADOLESCENCE

Smoking is dangerous to the health of both young people and older people who have been smoking longer. The chemicals from cigarette smoke damage the human body regardless of age.

Health Effects

Smoking by youth and young adults can cause serious and potentially deadly health issues immediately and into adulthood. Young people who smoke are in danger of:

- addiction to nicotine
- reduced lung function
- reduced lung growth
- early cardiovascular damage

Exposure to nicotine can have lasting effects on adolescent brain development. Cigarette smoking also causes children and teens to be short of breath and to have less stamina, both of which can affect athletic performance and other physically active pursuits.

Industry Marketing

Images that make smoking seem attractive and appealing are everywhere—in the movies, on television (TV), in video games, on the Internet, and in advertising at retail stores. Cigarette advertising and marketing cause youth and young adults to start smoking; nicotine addiction keeps them smoking into adulthood.

Although direct marketing to children is now prohibited, the tobacco industry is still developing, packaging, and advertising their products in ways that appeal to children. They promote new tobacco products such as:

- snus, a dry snuff in a small tea bag-like pouch that enables kids to consume tobacco products at school or in other tobacco-free environments
- dissolvable tobacco in sticks, lozenges, and strips
- fruit- and candy-flavored smokeless and dissolvable tobacco products

Except for menthol, cigarettes can no longer contain flavoring that appeals to children; however, tobacco companies can still include fruit and candy flavors in cigarette-sized cigars. In fact, as many high school boys now smoke cigars as those who smoke cigarettes. It is important to note that cigars that are small, cheap, flavored, and shaped and sized like cigarettes contain the same deadly poisons as cigarettes and are just as addictive.

Electronic Cigarettes

Many tobacco companies now produce and sell electronic nicotine delivery systems (ENDS), such as electronic cigarettes (e-cigarettes), vape pens, and e-hookahs. These devices deliver nicotine through an aerosol that is inhaled into the lungs the same way cigarette smoke is. So far, there are no studies on the health effects of long-term use of e-cigarettes and other ENDS or whether the use of ENDS leads to cigarette smoking by youth. However, nicotine is known to be addictive, toxic to developing fetuses, and harmful to adolescent brain development, so no youth should use e-cigarettes or any other tobacco product. Although cigarettes can no longer be advertised on TV, radio, or billboards or in magazines that appeal to youth, ENDS can be advertised anywhere.

Secondhand Smoke Exposure

Children between the ages of 3 and 18 in the United States are exposed to cigarette smoke regularly, either at home or in places such as restaurants that still allow smoking. Compared to children who are not exposed, children exposed to secondhand smoke:

- have more ear infections
- have more respiratory infections
- have more asthma attacks
- miss more days of school

Prevention and Cessation

No matter what age a person is, smoking is dangerous to health and can be hard to give up. Nicotine addiction is very powerful and happens quickly. It is easier to avoid starting to use tobacco in the first place than it is to quit later on. Encourage parents to talk to their kids about reasons to avoid tobacco use and to protect their children from secondhand smoke exposure.[1]

Usage of Tobacco in Adolescents

Most people who use tobacco started during adolescence and those who begin at a younger age are more likely to develop nicotine dependence and have trouble quitting. According to the 2022 Monitoring the Future (MTF) Survey, 4 percent of 12th

---

[1] "Smoking and Youth," Centers for Disease Control and Prevention (CDC), October 14, 2014. Available online. URL: www.cdc.gov/tobacco/sgr/50th-anniversary/pdfs/fs_smoking_youth_508.pdf. Accessed September 19, 2023.

graders, 1.7 percent of 10th graders, and 0.8 percent of 8th graders used cigarettes in the past month. An analysis of the 2022 National Youth Tobacco Survey (NYTS) found that 11.3 percent of middle and high school students reported using a tobacco product in the past 30 days, with higher rates among young people experiencing high levels of psychological distress. Young people whose guardians earned lower wages and young people from marginalized communities, such as lesbian, gay, and bisexual (LGB) young people and transgender young people, reported higher smoking rates. Other research has found that light and intermittent smoking among adolescents is associated with the same level of difficulty quitting as daily smoking.

Any exposure to nicotine among youth is a concern. The adolescent brain is still developing, and nicotine has effects on the brain's reward system and brain regions involved in emotional and cognitive functions. Research suggests that the nicotine-related changes to these areas of the brain during adolescence may perpetuate continued tobacco use into adulthood. These changes also contribute to a higher rate of other substance use disorders (SUDs) among people who use tobacco during adolescence, sometimes referred to as a "gateway" effect.

Mental health, beliefs about smoking, perception of schoolmates' smoking, and other substance use are additional factors that can influence an adolescent's risk for smoking and nicotine dependence. Emotional problems—including depression and recent negative life events—are associated with tobacco use among adolescents. Smoking among peers and within social groups is a major environmental factor that influences adolescent smoking; social smoking is a more important motivator for adolescents compared to adult smokers.

It is common for adolescent smoking to follow an intergenerational pattern, which has genetic, epigenetic, and environmental influences. Data from parents and adolescents suggest that current parental nicotine dependence is strongly linked with adolescent smoking and dependence. Other factors such as parents' education, marital status, and parenting behavior also influence teen smoking.[2]

[2] "How Many Adolescents Use Tobacco?" National Institute on Drug Abuse (NIDA), May 2022. Available online. URL: https://nida.nih.gov/publications/research-reports/tobacco-nicotine-e-cigarettes/how-many-adolescents-use-tobacco. Accessed September 19, 2023.

CHAPTER 2

TRENDS IN YOUTH TOBACCO CONSUMPTION

Youth use of tobacco products in any form is unsafe.

Preventing tobacco product use among youth is critical to reducing tobacco use among the nation's youth.

- Tobacco product use is started and established primarily during adolescence.
- Nearly 9 out of 10 adults who smoke cigarettes daily first try smoking by the age of 18.
- Flavorings in tobacco products can make them more appealing to youth.
    - In 2021, 80.2 percent of high school students and 74.6 percent of middle school students who used tobacco products in the past 30 days reported using a flavored tobacco product during that time.
    - In 2023, 90.3 percent of high school students (see Table 2.1) and 87.1 percent of middle school students (see Table 2.2) who used e-cigarettes in the past 30 days reported using a flavored e-cigarette during that time.

Estimates of Current Tobacco Use among Youth

Electronic Cigarettes

- E-cigarettes have been the most commonly used tobacco product among youth since 2014.
- In 2023, about 1 out of every 22 middle school students (4.6%) reported that they had used e-cigarettes in the past 30 days.
- In 2023, 1 of every 10 high school students (10.0%) reported that they had used e-cigarettes in the past 30 days.

Cigarettes

- In 2023, about 1 of every 100 middle school students (1.1%) reported that they had smoked cigarettes in the past 30 days.
- In 2023, nearly 2 of every 100 high school students (1.9%) reported that they had smoked cigarettes in the past 30 days.

Table 2.1. Current Tobacco Product Use* among High School Students in 2023

Tobacco Product	Overall (%)	Girls (%)	Boys (%)
Any tobacco product†	12.60	14.10	11.20
Electronic cigarettes	10.00	12.20	8.00
Cigarettes	1.90	1.50	2.30
Cigars	1.80	1.40	2.30
Smokeless tobacco	1.50	—	2.10
Hookah	1.10	1.40	0.90
Nicotine pouches	1.70	—	2.60
Heated tobacco products	1.00	0.70	1.40
Pipe tobacco	0.60	0.50	0.70

Notes:
** "Current use" is determined by respondents indicating that they have used a tobacco product on at least 1 day during the past 30 days.*
† In 2023, any tobacco product includes e-cigarettes, cigarettes, cigars, smokeless tobacco (composite), pipe tobacco, bidis (small brown cigarettes wrapped in a leaf), hookahs, heated tobacco products, nicotine pouches, and other oral nicotine products.

Table 2.2. Current Tobacco Product Use* among Middle School Students in 2023

Tobacco Product	Overall (%)	Girls (%)	Boys (%)
Any tobacco product†	6.60	7.50	5.70
Electronic cigarettes	4.60	5.60	3.50
Cigarettes	1.10	1.10	—
Cigars	1.10	1.20	1.00
Smokeless tobacco	0.70	0.60	—
Hookah	1.00	—	0.80
Nicotine pouches	—	—	—
Heated tobacco products	0.80	0.80	—
Pipe tobacco	0.40	—	—

Notes:
** "Current use" is determined by respondents indicating that they have used a tobacco product on at least 1 day during the past 30 days.*
† In 2023, any tobacco product includes e-cigarettes, cigarettes, cigars, smokeless tobacco (composite), pipe tobacco, bidis (small brown cigarettes wrapped in a leaf), hookahs, heated tobacco products, nicotine pouches, and other oral nicotine products.

Cigars

- In 2023, nearly 1 of every 100 middle school students (1.1%) reported that they had smoked cigars in the past 30 days.
- In 2023, nearly 2 of every 100 high school students (1.8%) reported that they had smoked cigars in the past 30 days.

Smokeless Tobacco

- In 2023, nearly 1 of every 100 middle school students (0.7%) reported that they had used smokeless tobacco in the past 30 days.
- In 2023, nearly 2 of every 100 high school students (1.5%) reported that they had used smokeless tobacco in the past 30 days.

Hookah

- In 2023, less than 1 of every 100 middle school students (1.0%) reported that they had smoked hookah in the past 30 days.
- In 2023, about 1 of every 100 high school students (1.1%) reported that they had smoked hookah in the past 30 days.

Heated Tobacco Products

- In 2023, less than 1 of every 100 middle school students (0.8%) and about 1 of every 100 high school students (1.0%) reported using heated tobacco products in the past 30 days.
- Heated tobacco products, also known as "heat-not-burn" products, deliver nicotine to the user by heating tobacco leaves rather than a nicotine-containing liquid like e-cigarettes.

Nicotine Pouches

- In 2023, about 1 of every 100 high school students (1.7%) reported using nicotine pouches in the past 30 days.
- Nicotine pouches are microfiber pouches with flavored nicotine powder that users dissolve in the mouth without spitting. Sales of nicotine pouches have increased rapidly in the United States.

All Tobacco Products Use

- In 2023, more than 6 of every 100 middle school students (6.6%) and about 1 of every 8 high school students (12.6%) reported current use of a tobacco product.
- In 2023, nearly 15 of every 100 middle school students (14.7%) and nearly 28 of every 100 high school students (27.9%) said they had ever tried a tobacco product.

Many Young People Use Multiple Tobacco Products

- In 2023, more than 2 of every 100 middle school students (2.5%) and about 1 of every 30 high school students (3.9%) reported current use of multiple tobacco products in the past 30 days.
- In 2023, about 6 of every 100 middle school students (6.1%) and more than 12 of every 100 high school students (12.7%) reported they had ever tried multiple tobacco products.

Youth who use multiple tobacco products are at higher risk for developing nicotine dependence and might be more likely to continue using tobacco into adulthood.

Factors Associated with Youth Tobacco Product Use

Factors associated with youth tobacco product use include the following:

- **Social and physical environments:**
  - The way mass media show tobacco product use as a normal activity can make young people want to try these products.
  - Youth are more likely to use tobacco products if they see people their age using these products.
  - High school athletes are more likely to use smokeless tobacco than those of the same age who are not athletes.
  - Young people may be more likely to use tobacco products if a parent uses these products.
- **Biological and genetic factors:**
  - There is evidence that youth may be sensitive to nicotine and that teens can feel dependent on nicotine sooner than adults.
  - Genetic factors may make quitting smoking harder for young people.
  - Smoking during pregnancy may increase the likelihood that the child will smoke cigarettes regularly in the future.
- **Mental health**. There is a strong relationship between youth smoking and depression, anxiety, and stress.
- **Personal views**. When young people expect positive things from smoking, such as coping with stress better or losing weight, they are more likely to smoke.
- **Other influences**. Influences that affect youth tobacco use include the following:
  - lower socioeconomic status, including lower income or education
  - not knowing how to say "no" to tobacco product use
  - lack of support or involvement from parents
  - accessibility, availability, and price of tobacco products
  - doing poorly in school
  - low self-image or self-esteem
  - seeing tobacco product advertising in stores, on television, on the Internet, in movies, or in magazines and newspapers

Reducing Youth Tobacco Product Use

National, state, and local program activities have been shown to reduce and prevent youth tobacco product use when implemented together. These activities include the following:

- higher costs for tobacco products (e.g., through increased taxes)
- prohibiting smoking in indoor areas of workplaces and public places
- raising the minimum age of sale for tobacco products to 21 years
- TV and radio commercials, posters, and other media messages aimed at kids and teens in order to counter tobacco product ads
- community programs and school and college policies that encourage tobacco-free places and lifestyles
- community programs that lower tobacco advertising and promotions and help make tobacco products less easily available

Some social and environmental factors are related to lower smoking levels among youth. Among these are:

- being part of a religious group or tradition
- racial/ethnic pride and strong racial identity
- higher academic achievement[1]

Current Cigarette Smoking among U.S. Adults Aged 18 and Older

Cigarette smoking remains the leading cause of preventable disease and death in the United States.

Cigarette smoking kills more than 480,000 Americans each year. Cigarette smoking costs the United States more than $600 billion in 2018, including more than $240 billion in health-care spending and nearly $372 billion in lost productivity.

In 2021, an estimated 11.5 percent (28.3 million) of U.S. adults currently smoked cigarettes. Current cigarette smoking was defined as smoking ≥100 cigarettes during a lifetime and now smoking cigarettes either every day or some days (see Table 2.3).[2]

Table 2.3. Percentage of Persons Aged 18 or Older Who Reported Cigarette Use "Every Day" or "Some Days" at the Time of Survey and Reported Smoking at Least 100 Cigarettes during Their Lifetime

Groups	Percentage (%)
By Sex	
Male	13.1
Female	10.1

[1] "Youth and Tobacco Use," Centers for Disease Control and Prevention (CDC), November 2, 2023. Available online. URL: www.cdc.gov/tobacco/data_statistics/fact_sheets/youth_data/tobacco_use/index.htm. Accessed November 24, 2023.

[2] "Burden of Cigarette Use in the United States," Centers for Disease Control and Prevention (CDC), May 4, 2023. Available online. URL: www.cdc.gov/tobacco/campaign/tips/resources/data/cigarette-smoking-in-united-states.html. Accessed September 26, 2023.

Table 2.3. Continued

Groups	Percentage (%)
By Age Group (Years)	
18–24	5.3
25–44	12.6
45–64	14.9
≥65	8.3
By Race/Ethnicity*	
White, non-Hispanic	12.9
Black, non-Hispanic	11.7
Asian, non-Hispanic	5.4
Hispanic	7.7
Other, non-Hispanic	14.9
By U.S. Census Region	
Northeast	10.40
Midwest	14.00
South	12.40
West	8.90
By Education (Adults Aged 25 or Older)	
0–12 years (no diploma)	20.1
General Educational Diploma (GED)	30.7
High school diploma	17.1
Some college, no degree	16.1
Associate degree (academic or technical/vocational)	13.7
Undergraduate degree (bachelor's)	5.3
Graduate degree (master's, doctoral, or professional)	3.2
By Marital Status	
Married/living with partner	10.4
Divorced/separated/widowed	16.8
Single/never married/not living with partner	10.9

Table 2.3. Continued

Groups	**Percentage (%)**
By Annual Household Income	
Low income	18.3
Middle income	12.3
High income	6.7
By Sexual Orientation	
Heterosexual/straight	11.4
Lesbian/gay/bisexual	15.3
By Health Insurance Coverage	
Private insurance	8.6
Medicaid	21.5
Medicare only (aged 65 or older)	8.4
Other public insurance	13.9
Uninsured	20.0
Having a Disability	
Yes	18.5
No	10.9
Regularly Having Feelings of Severe Psychological Distress[†]	
Yes	28.1
No	10.9
Being Ever Told by a Health-Care Provider That They Had Depression	
Yes	19.4
No	9.9

** 2021 Tobacco product estimates for American Indian/Alaska Native adults were not statistically reliable.*

[†] Serious psychological distress was assessed using the recorded question "Experienced serious psychological distress—K6 scale," which was recorded from the answers to the six-item Kessler scale.

CHAPTER 3

ADOLESCENTS AND TOBACCO: RISK AND PROTECTIVE FACTORS

What Are Some Health Problems Caused by Cigarette Smoking?

Smoking is the leading cause of premature, preventable death in this country. Cigarette smoking and exposure to tobacco smoke cause about 480,000 premature deaths each year in the United States. Of those premature deaths, about 36 percent are from cancer, 39 percent are from heart disease and stroke, and 24 percent are from lung disease. Mortality rates among smokers are about three times higher than among people who have never smoked.

Smoking harms nearly every bodily organ and organ system in the body and diminishes a person's overall health. Smoking causes cancers of the lung, esophagus, larynx, mouth, throat, kidney, bladder, liver, pancreas, stomach, cervix, colon, and rectum, as well as acute myeloid leukemia (AML).

Smoking also causes heart disease, stroke, aortic aneurysm (a balloon-like bulge in an artery in the chest), chronic obstructive pulmonary disease (COPD; chronic bronchitis and emphysema), diabetes, osteoporosis, rheumatoid arthritis (RA), age-related macular degeneration (AMD), and cataracts, and worsens asthma symptoms in adults. Smokers are at higher risk of developing pneumonia, tuberculosis (TB), and other airway infections. In addition, smoking causes inflammation and impairs immune function.

Since the 1960s, a smoker's risk of developing lung cancer or COPD has actually increased compared with nonsmokers, even though the number of cigarettes consumed per smoker has decreased. There have also been changes over time in the type of lung cancer smokers develop—a decline in squamous cell carcinomas (SCC) but a dramatic increase in adenocarcinomas. Both of these shifts may be due to changes in cigarette design and composition, in how tobacco leaves are cured, and in how deeply smokers inhale cigarette smoke and the toxicants it contains.

Smoking makes it harder for a woman to get pregnant. A pregnant smoker is at higher risk of miscarriage, having an ectopic pregnancy, having her baby born too early and with an abnormally low birth weight, and having her baby born with a cleft lip and/or cleft palate. A woman who smokes during or after pregnancy increases her infant's risk of death from sudden infant death syndrome (SIDS). Men who smoke are at greater risk of erectile dysfunction (ED).

The longer a smoker's duration of smoking, the greater their likelihood of experiencing harm from smoking, including earlier death. But, regardless of their age, smokers can substantially reduce their risk of disease, including cancer, by quitting.

What Are the Risks of Tobacco Smoke to Nonsmokers?

Secondhand smoke (also called "environmental tobacco smoke," "involuntary smoking," and "passive smoking") is the combination of "sidestream" smoke (the smoke given off by a burning tobacco product) and "mainstream" smoke (the smoke exhaled by a smoker).

The U.S. Environmental Protection Agency (EPA), the U.S. National Toxicology Program (NTP), the U.S. Surgeon General, and the International Agency for Research on Cancer (IARC) have classified secondhand smoke as a known human carcinogen (cancer-causing agent). Inhaling secondhand smoke causes lung cancer in nonsmoking adults. Approximately 7,300 lung cancer deaths occur each year among adult nonsmokers in the United States as a result of exposure to secondhand smoke. The U.S. Surgeon General estimates that living with a smoker increases a nonsmoker's chances of developing lung cancer by 20–30 percent.

Secondhand smoke causes disease and premature death in nonsmoking adults and children. Exposure to secondhand smoke irritates the airways and has immediate harmful effects on a person's heart and blood vessels. It increases the risk of heart disease by an estimated 25–30 percent. In the United States, exposure to secondhand smoke is estimated to cause about 34,000 deaths from heart disease each year. Exposure to secondhand smoke also increases the risk of stroke by 20–30 percent. Pregnant women exposed to secondhand smoke are at increased risk of having a baby with a small reduction in birth weight.

Children exposed to secondhand smoke are at an increased risk of SIDS, ear infections, colds, pneumonia, and bronchitis. Secondhand smoke exposure can also increase the frequency and severity of asthma symptoms among children who have asthma. Being exposed to secondhand smoke slows the growth of children's lungs and can cause them to cough, wheeze, and feel breathless.

Is Smoking Addictive?

Smoking is highly addictive. Nicotine is the drug, primarily responsible for a person's addiction to tobacco products, including cigarettes. The addiction to cigarettes and other tobacco products that nicotine causes is similar to the addiction produced by using drugs, such as heroin and cocaine. Nicotine is present naturally in the tobacco plant. However, tobacco companies intentionally design cigarettes to have enough nicotine to create and sustain addiction.

The amount of nicotine that gets into the body is determined by the way a person smokes a tobacco product and by the nicotine content and design of the product. Nicotine is absorbed into the bloodstream through the lining of the mouth and the lungs and travels to the brain in a matter of seconds. Taking more frequent and deeper puffs of tobacco smoke increases the amount of nicotine absorbed by the body.

Are Other Tobacco Products, Such as Smokeless Tobacco or Pipe Tobacco, Harmful and Addictive?

All forms of tobacco are harmful and addictive. There is no safe tobacco product.

In addition to cigarettes, other forms of tobacco include the following:

- **Smokeless tobacco**. This is a type of tobacco that is not burned. It includes chewing tobacco, oral tobacco, spit or spitting tobacco, dip, chew, snus, dissolvable tobacco, and snuff. Smokeless tobacco causes oral (mouth, tongue, cheek, and gum), esophageal, and pancreatic cancers and may also cause gum and heart disease.
- **Cigars**. These include premium cigars, little filtered cigars (LFCs), and cigarillos. LFCs resemble cigarettes, but both LFCs and cigarillos may have added flavors to increase appeal to youth and young adults. Most cigars are composed primarily of a single type of tobacco (air-cured and fermented), and have a tobacco leaf wrapper. Studies have found that cigar smoke contains higher levels of toxic chemicals than cigarette smoke, although unlike cigarette smoke, cigar smoke is often not inhaled. Cigar smoking causes cancer of the oral cavity, larynx, esophagus, and lung. It may also cause cancer of the pancreas. Moreover, daily cigar smokers, particularly those who inhale, are at increased risk for developing heart disease and other types of lung disease.
- **Pipes**. In pipe smoking, the tobacco is placed in a bowl that is connected to a stem with a mouthpiece at the other end. The smoke is usually not inhaled. Pipe smoking causes lung cancer and increases the risk of cancers of the mouth, throat, larynx, and esophagus.
- **Hookah or waterpipe (other names include argileh, ghelyoon, hubble bubble, shisha, boory, goza, and narghile)**. A hookah is a device used to smoke tobacco (often heavily flavored) by passing the smoke through a partially filled water bowl before being inhaled by the smoker. Although some people think hookah smoking is less harmful and addictive than cigarette smoking, research shows that hookah smoke is at least as toxic as cigarette smoke.

- **Bidis**. A bidi is a flavored cigarette made by rolling tobacco in a dried leaf from the tendu tree, which is native to India. Bidi use is associated with heart attacks and cancers of the mouth, throat, larynx, esophagus, and lung.
- **Kreteks**. A kretek is a cigarette made with a mixture of tobacco and cloves. Smoking kreteks is associated with lung cancer and other lung diseases.

Some people try to cut back on smoking cigarettes or work toward quitting smoking completely by using electronic cigarettes (e-cigarettes), smokeless tobacco, or other tobacco products in addition to regular cigarettes. This is called "dual use." Dual use is not an effective way to safeguard health.

Because smoking even a few cigarettes a day can be dangerous, quitting smoking completely is very important to protect your health. If you have never smoked or used other tobacco products, including e-cigarettes, do not start.

Source: "Dual Use of Tobacco Products," Centers for Disease Control and Prevention (CDC), May 5, 2022. Available online. URL: www.cdc.gov/tobacco/campaign/tips/diseases/dual-tobacco-use.html. Accessed September 25, 2023.

Is It Harmful to Smoke Just a Few Cigarettes a Day?

There is no safe level of smoking. Smoking even just one cigarette per day over a lifetime can cause smoking-related cancers (lung, bladder, and pancreas) and premature death.

What Are the Immediate Health Benefits of Quitting Smoking?

The immediate health benefits of quitting smoking are substantial:

- Heart rate and blood pressure, which are abnormally high while smoking, begin to return to normal.
- Within a few hours, the level of carbon monoxide in the blood begins to decline. (Carbon monoxide reduces the blood's ability to carry oxygen.)
- Within a few weeks, people who quit smoking have improved circulation, produce less phlegm, and do not cough or wheeze as often.
- Within several months of quitting, people can expect substantial improvements in lung function.
- Within a few years of quitting, people will have lower risks of cancer, heart disease, and other chronic diseases than if they had continued to smoke.

What Are the Long-Term Health Benefits of Quitting Smoking?

Quitting smoking reduces the risk of cancer and many other diseases, such as heart disease and COPD, caused by smoking.

Data from the U.S. National Health Interview Survey (NHIS) show that people who quit smoking, regardless of their age, are less likely to die from smoking-related illness than those who continue to smoke. Smokers who quit before the age of 40 reduce their chance of dying prematurely from smoking-related diseases by about 90 percent and those who quit by the ages of 45–54 reduce their chance of dying prematurely by about two-thirds.

Regardless of their age, people who quit smoking have substantial gains in life expectancy, compared with those who continue to smoke. Data from the NHIS also show that those who quit between the ages of 25 and 34 live about 10 years longer; those who quit between the ages of 35 and 44 live about 9 years longer; those who quit between the ages of 45 and 54 live about 6 years longer; and those who quit between the ages of 55 and 64 live about 4 years longer.

Also, a study that followed a large group of people aged 70 and older found that even smokers who quit smoking in their 60s had a lower risk of mortality during follow-up than smokers who continued smoking.

Does Quitting Smoking Lower the Risk of Getting and Dying from Cancer?

Quitting smoking reduces the risk of developing and dying from cancer and other diseases caused by smoking. Although it is never too late to benefit from quitting, the benefit is greatest among those who quit at a younger age.

The risk of premature death and the chances of developing and dying from a smoking-related cancer depend on many factors, including the number of years a person has smoked, the number of cigarettes smoked per day, and the age at which the person began smoking.

Is It Important for Someone Diagnosed with Cancer to Quit Smoking?

Quitting smoking improves the prognosis of cancer patients. For patients with some cancers, quitting smoking at the time of diagnosis may reduce the risk of dying by 30–40 percent. For those having surgery, chemotherapy, or other treatments, quitting smoking helps improve the body's ability to heal and respond to therapy. It also lowers the risk of pneumonia and respiratory failure. In addition, quitting smoking may lower the risk that the cancer will recur, that a second cancer will develop, or that the person will die from the cancer or other causes.[1]

[1] "Harms of Cigarette Smoking and Health Benefits of Quitting," National Cancer Institute (NCI), December 19, 2017. Available online. URL: www.cancer.gov/about-cancer/causes-prevention/risk/tobacco/cessation-fact-sheet#what-are-the-risks-of-tobacco-smoke-to-nonsmokers. Accessed September 25, 2023.

CHAPTER 4
CHEMICALS IN TOBACCO PRODUCTS AND YOUR HEALTH

You probably know that cigarette smoking kills you and contains chemicals—a mix of over 7,000 chemicals, in fact—that can cause diseases including cancer, cardiovascular disease (CVD), and chronic obstructive pulmonary disease (COPD). You may not know that other tobacco products, such as e-cigarettes, hookah, and smokeless tobacco, contain some of the same chemicals as cigarettes.

Nicotine: The Addictive Chemical in Tobacco

Nicotine is a highly addictive chemical found in the tobacco plant itself and is, therefore, present in all tobacco products. While nicotine is what addicts and keeps people using tobacco products, it is not what makes tobacco use so deadly. Tobacco and tobacco smoke contain thousands of chemicals. This mix of chemicals—not nicotine—is what causes serious disease and death in tobacco users.

Chemicals in Cigarettes: How Do They Get There?

You may believe that cigarettes are so deadly because chemicals are added to them in the manufacturing process. While some chemicals are added during this process, some chemicals in cigarettes—along with nicotine—are found in the tobacco plant itself. As the tobacco plant grows, it absorbs chemicals—such as cadmium, lead, and nitrates—from the soil and fertilizer. Cadmium is a carcinogen and is also found in batteries, while lead is a chemical that was once used in house paint. Cadmium and lead are both toxic metals. When the plant is harvested for manufacturing, these chemicals are present in the tobacco leaves.

As the tobacco leaves are cured, dangerous chemicals can form. These chemicals, called "tobacco-specific nitrosamines" (TSNAs), remain in the tobacco leaves after the curing process. During manufacturing, ammonia—a chemical found in household cleaning products—along with other chemicals may be added to increase nicotine absorption. Sugar and flavor additives may also be added during this stage to mask the harshness of the smoke. These additives form cancer-causing chemicals when they are burned.

Once a cigarette is lit, more chemicals are still formed in the burning process that were not present in the growing and manufacturing stages. These chemicals are then inhaled by smokers or those exposed to secondhand smoke. Lastly, dangerous chemicals that are detrimental to human health, wildlife, and water supplies can be released from cigarette butt waste into the environment.

Chemicals in Other Tobacco Products

Hookah

In addition to nicotine, other tobacco products, such as hookah, contain some of the same chemicals as cigarettes. Carbon monoxide, metals, and carcinogens can be found in hookah smoke, and hookah users are at risk for some of the same health effects as smokers as a result of these chemicals. Research shows that hookah smokers may absorb even more of the toxic chemicals found in cigarette smoke because of the length of hookah smoking sessions. A typical one-hour hookah session can produce as much smoke as several packs of cigarettes.

Smokeless Tobacco

Smokeless tobacco, although not combustible, contains a mix of 4,000 chemicals, including as many as 30 or more that are linked to cancer.

These chemicals include heavy metals cadmium, lead, and nickel; as well as arsenic, a chemical used in insecticides; formaldehyde, which is used in embalming fluid; and N-Nitrosonornicotine (NNN), among others. NNN is known to cause cancer in animals and has been linked to an increase in the risk of cancer among humans.

About 1,300 people in the United States are diagnosed with oral cancer each year because of smokeless tobacco use. Smokeless tobacco use also causes esophageal and pancreatic cancer.

E-cigarettes

As e-cigarettes have only recently come under the regulatory authority of the U.S. Food and Drug Administration (FDA), their effects on individual and population health are still being studied. Preliminary studies suggest switching completely to e-cigarettes could be less harmful than combustible cigarettes for adults who already have a nicotine addiction. Most e-cigarettes contain nicotine, the same highly addictive chemical in cigarettes that keeps people smoking even when they want to quit. Other chemicals found in cigarette smoke, such as formaldehyde, acrolein, and acetaldehyde, are also found in some e-cigarette aerosols. These chemicals can cause irreversible lung damage at certain concentrations. E-cigarettes can also contain flavorings such as diacetyl and acetoin. Diacetyl and acetoin are considered safe to eat but inhaling them can be harmful to the lungs.

Tobacco-Free: The Best Option for Health

Because all tobacco products contain the addictive chemical nicotine, no tobacco product can be considered safe. Using no tobacco products whatsoever is the best way to safeguard your health. But, if you are an adult with an established addiction, cessation will help protect you from the chemicals in tobacco products and tobacco smoke. Quitting smoking is often difficult and may take multiple attempts, but the longer a smoker is able to stay quit, the more of a chance the body gets to heal from the damage done from chemicals. Nicotine replacement therapies (NRTs) can be effective for cessation and can double your chances of quitting successfully. Although nicotine is an addictive chemical, it does not carry the same risks as some other chemicals found in tobacco products. Many FDA-approved NRTs, including gum, patches, and lozenges, are available without prescription and may be used in combination with each other. If you are an adult smoker and you are looking to quit, it is a good idea to talk to your doctor about your options.[1]

Chemicals in Cigarettes

It is a fact that cigarettes contain dangerous chemicals. But how do these chemicals get into cigarettes? Are most of the harmful chemicals added during the manufacturing process?

Fact. Some of the toxic chemicals in tobacco are present in the plant itself.

Chemicals in Every Cigarette Product

Harmful chemicals are in the tobacco plant. What happens during manufacturing? Is that when more dangerous chemicals are added?

Fact. Not all of the harmful chemicals created during cigarette manufacturing are man-made. Some of the carcinogens occur naturally as tobacco is cured.

Chemicals in Every Puff of Cigarette Smoke

How many harmful and potentially harmful chemicals are in a cigarette?

Fact. There are more than 7,000 chemicals in cigarette smoke. More than 70 of those chemicals are linked to cancer.

Source: "Chemicals in Cigarettes: From Plant to Product to Puff," U.S. Food and Drug Administration (FDA), June 3, 2020. Available online. URL: www.fda.gov/tobacco-products/products-ingredients-components/chemicals-cigarettes-plant-product-puff. Accessed September 29, 2023.

[1] "Chemicals in Tobacco Products and Your Health," U.S. Food and Drug Administration (FDA), May 1, 2020. Available online. URL: www.fda.gov/tobacco-products/health-effects-tobacco-use/chemicals-tobacco-products-and-your-health. Accessed September 29, 2023.

The U.S. Food and Drug Administration's Harmful and Potentially Harmful Constituents List

The chemicals and chemical compounds found in tobacco products or tobacco smoke that could cause harm to both smokers, or secondhand to nonsmokers, are called "harmful and potentially harmful constituents" (HPHCs). Manufacturers and importers are required to report the levels of HPHCs in their products to the FDA. A preliminary list of 93 HPHCs found in tobacco products and tobacco smoke linked to cancer, CVD, respiratory conditions, reproductive problems, and addiction are listed in Table 4.1.[2]

Table 4.1. Established List of Chemicals and Chemical Compounds Identified by the FDA as Harmful and Potentially Harmful Constituents in Tobacco Products and Tobacco Smoke

Constituent	Carcinogen (CA), Respiratory Toxicant (RT), Cardiovascular Toxicant (CT), Reproductive or Developmental Toxicant (RDT), Addictive (AD)
Acetaldehyde	CA, RT, AD
Acetamide	CA
Acetone	RT
Acrolein	RT, CT
Acrylamide	CA
Acrylonitrile	CA, RT
Aflatoxin B1	CA
4-Aminobiphenyl	CA
1-Aminonaphthalene	CA
2-Aminonaphthalene	CA
Ammonia	RT
Anabasine	AD
o-Anisidine	CA
Arsenic	CA, CT, RDT
A-α-C (2-Amino-9H-pyrido[2,3-b] indole)	CA
Benz[a]anthracene	CA, CT
Benz[j]aceanthrylene	CA

[2] "Harmful and Potentially Harmful Constituents in Tobacco Products and Tobacco Smoke: Established List," U.S. Food and Drug Administration (FDA), October 7, 2019. Available online. URL: www.fda.gov/tobacco-products/rules-regulations-and-guidance/harmful-and-potentially-harmful-constituents-tobacco-products-and-tobacco-smoke-established-list. Accessed November 24, 2023.

Table 4.1. Continued

Constituent	Carcinogen (CA), Respiratory Toxicant (RT), Cardiovascular Toxicant (CT), Reproductive or Developmental Toxicant (RDT), Addictive (AD)
Benzene	CA, CT, RDT
Benzo[b]fluoranthene	CA, CT
Benzo[k]fluoranthene	CA, CT
Benzo[b]furan	CA
Benzo[a]pyrene	CA
Benzo[c]phenanthrene	CA
Beryllium	CA
1,3-Butadiene	CA, RT, RDT
Cadmium	CA, RT, RDT
Caffeic acid	CA
Carbon monoxide	RDT
Catechol	CA
Chlorinated dioxins/furans	CA, RDT
Chromium	CA, RT, RDT
Chrysene	CA, CT
Cobalt	CA, CT
Coumarin	Banned in food
Cresols (o-, m-, and p-cresol)	CA, RT
Crotonaldehyde	CA
Cyclopenta[c,d]pyrene	CA
Dibenz[a,h]anthracene	CA
Dibenzo[a,e]pyrene	CA
Dibenzo[a,h]pyrene	CA
Dibenzo[a,i]pyrene	CA
Dibenzo[a,l]pyrene	CA
2,6-Dimethylaniline	CA
Ethyl carbamate (urethane)	CA, RDT
Ethylbenzene	CA
Ethylene oxide	CA, RT, RDT

Table 4.1. Continued

Constituent	Carcinogen (CA), Respiratory Toxicant (RT), Cardiovascular Toxicant (CT), Reproductive or Developmental Toxicant (RDT), Addictive (AD)
Formaldehyde	CA, RT
Furan	CA
Glu-P-1 (2-Amino-6-methyldipyrido[1,2-a:3',2'-d] imidazole)	CA
Glu-P-2 (2-Aminodipyrido[1,2-a:3',2'-d]imidazole)	CA
Hydrazine	CA, RT
Hydrogen cyanide	RT, CT
Indeno[1,2,3-cd]pyrene	CA
IQ (2-Amino-3-methylimidazo[4,5-f] quinoline)	CA
Isoprene	CA
Lead	CA, CT, RDT
MeA-α-C (2-Amino-3-methyl)-9H-pyrido[2,3-b]indole)	CA
Mercury	CA, RDT
Methyl ethyl ketone	RT
5-Methylchrysene	CA
4-(Methylnitrosamino)-1-(3-pyridyl)-1-butanone (NNK)	CA
Naphthalene	CA, RT
Nickel	CA, RT
Nicotine	RDT, AD
Nitrobenzene	CA, RT, RDT
Nitromethane	CA
2-Nitropropane	CA
N-Nitrosodiethanolamine (NDELA)	CA
N-Nitrosodiethylamine	CA
N-Nitrosodimethylamine (NDMA)	CA
N-Nitrosomethylethylamine	CA

Table 4.1. Continued

Constituent	Carcinogen (CA), Respiratory Toxicant (RT), Cardiovascular Toxicant (CT), Reproductive or Developmental Toxicant (RDT), Addictive (AD)
N-Nitrosomorpholine (NMOR)	CA
N-Nitrosonornicotine (NNN)	CA
N-Nitrosopiperidine (NPIP)	CA
N-Nitrosopyrrolidine (NPYR)	CA
N-Nitrososarcosine (NSAR)	CA
Nornicotine	AD
Phenol	RT, CT
PhIP (2-Amino-1-methyl-6-phenylimidazo[4,5-b]pyridine)	CA
Polonium-210	CA
Propionaldehyde	RT, CT
Propylene oxide	CA, RT
Quinoline	CA
Selenium	RT
Styrene	CA
o-Toluidine	CA
Toluene	RT, RDT
Trp-P-1 (3-Amino-1,4-dimethyl-5H-pyrido[4,3-b]indole)	CA
Trp-P-2 (1-Methyl-3-amino-5H-pyrido[4,3-b]indole)	CA
Uranium-235	CA, RT
Uranium-238	CA, RT
Vinyl acetate	CA, RT
Vinyl chloride	CA

CHAPTER 5
NICOTINE AND ADDICTION

What Is Nicotine?

Nicotine is the chemical found in tobacco products that is responsible for addiction. When you use tobacco, nicotine is quickly absorbed into your body and goes directly to your brain. Nicotine activates areas of the brain that make you feel satisfied and happy. Whether you smoke, vape, or dip, the nicotine you are putting in your body is dangerously addictive and can be harmful to your developing brain.

> You may think that you can use tobacco without becoming addicted. But, the truth is, most teens who use tobacco will get hooked. Three out of four teens who smoke cigarettes in high school will still be smoking as adults.
>
> *Source:* Smokefree Teen, "Nicotine and Addiction," U.S. Department of Health and Human Services (HHS), September 16, 2017. Available online. URL: https://teen.smokefree.gov/the-risks-of-tobacco/nicotine-addiction. Accessed October 3, 2023.

What Does Nicotine Addiction Look Like?

Nicotine addiction can look different from person to person. Even if you only use tobacco once in a while, you can be addicted and can have a hard time quitting.

Some signs of nicotine addiction include the following:

- cravings or feeling like you really need to use tobacco
- going out of your way to get tobacco
- feeling anxious or irritable if you want to use tobacco but cannot
- continuing to use tobacco because you find it hard to stop

When you are addicted to nicotine, you may experience symptoms of nicotine withdrawal after you stop using tobacco. Craving cigarettes, feeling sad or irritable, or having trouble sleeping are some common symptoms of withdrawal. These symptoms are usually strongest in the first week after quitting, but they are only temporary.

Why Is Nicotine Dangerous?

Nicotine can lead to addiction, which puts you at risk of becoming a lifelong smoker and exposing you to the many harmful chemicals in tobacco. These chemicals cause cancer and harm almost every organ in your body. Teens are especially sensitive to nicotine's addictive effects because their brains are still developing and this makes it easier to get hooked. Using nicotine at a young age can also rewire the brain to become more easily addicted to other drugs.

Nicotine can have other long-lasting effects on brain development, making it harder for you to concentrate, learn, and control impulses.[1]

Is Nicotine Addictive?

Most smokers use tobacco regularly because they are addicted to nicotine. Addiction is characterized by compulsive drug-seeking and use, even in the face of negative health consequences. The majority of smokers would like to stop smoking, and each year about half try to quit permanently. Yet only about 6 percent of smokers are able to quit in a given year. Most smokers will need to make multiple attempts before they are able to quit permanently. Medications such as varenicline, some antidepressants (e.g., bupropion), and nicotine replacement therapy can help in many cases.

A transient surge of endorphins in the reward circuits of the brain causes a slight, brief euphoria when nicotine is administered. This surge is much briefer than the "high" associated with other drugs. However, like other drugs of abuse, nicotine increases levels of the neurotransmitter dopamine in the reward circuits, which reinforces the behavior of taking the drug. Repeated exposure alters these circuits' sensitivity to dopamine and leads to changes in other brain circuits involved in learning, stress, and self-control. For many tobacco users, long-term brain changes induced by continued nicotine exposure result in addiction, which involves withdrawal symptoms when not smoking, and difficulty adhering to the resolution to quit.

The pharmacokinetic properties of nicotine, or the way it is processed by the body, contribute to its addictiveness. When cigarette smoke enters the lungs, nicotine is absorbed rapidly in the blood and delivered quickly to the brain so that nicotine levels peak within 10 seconds of inhalation. But the acute effects of nicotine also dissipate quickly, along with the associated feelings of reward; this rapid cycle causes the smoker to continue dosing to maintain the drug's pleasurable effects and prevent withdrawal symptoms.

Withdrawal occurs as a result of dependence when the body becomes used to having the drug in the system. Being without nicotine for too long can cause a regular

[1] Smokefree Teen, "Nicotine and Addiction," U.S. Department of Health and Human Services (HHS), September 16, 2017. Available online. URL: https://teen.smokefree.gov/the-risks-of-tobacco/nicotine-addiction. Accessed October 3, 2023.

user to experience irritability, craving, depression, anxiety, cognitive and attention deficits, sleep disturbances, and increased appetite. These withdrawal symptoms may begin within a few hours after the last cigarette, quickly driving people back to tobacco use.

When a person quits smoking, withdrawal symptoms peak within the first few days of the last cigarette smoked and usually subside within a few weeks. For some people, however, symptoms may persist for months, and the severity of withdrawal symptoms appears to be influenced by a person's genes.

In addition to its pleasurable effects, nicotine also temporarily boosts aspects of cognition, such as the ability to sustain attention and hold information in memory. However, long-term smoking is associated with cognitive decline and risk of Alzheimer disease, suggesting that short-term nicotine-related enhancement does not outweigh long-term consequences for cognitive functioning. In addition, people in withdrawal from nicotine experience neurocognitive deficits such as problems with attention or memory. These neurocognitive withdrawal symptoms are increasingly recognized as a contributor to continued smoking. A small research study also suggested that withdrawal may impair sleep for severely dependent smokers and that this may additionally contribute to relapse.

In addition to the drug's effect on multiple neurotransmitters and their receptors, many behavioral factors can affect the severity of withdrawal symptoms. For many people who smoke, the feel, smell, and sight of a cigarette and the ritual of obtaining, handling, lighting, and smoking a cigarette are all associated with the pleasurable effects of smoking and can make withdrawal or craving worse. Learning processes in the brain associate these cues with nicotine-induced dopamine surges in the reward system—similar to what occurs with other drug addictions. Nicotine replacement therapies such as gum, patches, and inhalers and other medications approved for the treatment of nicotine addiction may help alleviate the physiological aspects of withdrawal; however, cravings often persist because of the power of these cues. Behavioral therapies can help smokers identify environmental triggers of craving, so they can use strategies to avoid these triggers and manage the feelings that arise when triggers cannot be.[2]

The Power of Nicotine Addiction

Many smokers say they choose to continue smoking despite knowing the health risks. The reality is that smoking is not usually a choice. For most smokers, tobacco use is an addiction, and nicotine is the primary drug in tobacco that causes addiction. It only takes 10 seconds for the nicotine from one puff of smoke to reach the brain. This rapid delivery of nicotine from the lungs to the brain is one of the reasons that cigarettes are so addictive. And, once it gets there, nicotine causes cells in the brain to

[2] "Is Nicotine Addictive," National Institute on Drug Abuse (NIDA), May 2022. Available online. URL: https://nida.nih.gov/publications/research-reports/tobacco-nicotine-e-cigarettes/nicotine-addictive. Accessed October 3, 2023.

release dopamine. One of the effects of dopamine released in the brain is to create a heightened sense of alertness and contentment. Over time, the brain cells of smokers are changed to expect the regular bursts of extra dopamine that result from smoking. When a smoker tries to quit, these brain changes cause strong cravings for more nicotine.

Some cigarettes are more addictive than those from earlier decades. In part, this is a result of chemicals added to today's cigarettes that cause the nicotine to reach the brain more quickly. In addition, menthol reduces the harshness of the smoke and makes it easier to smoke—particularly for children and teens. Research suggests that children and adolescents may be sensitive to nicotine and can become addicted more easily than adults. The younger smokers are when they start, the more likely they are to become addicted, and the more likely that they will become heavily addicted.

In addition to causing addiction, nicotine that is rapidly delivered by cigarettes can affect the body in other ways. For example, a rapid increase in nicotine blood levels can raise the heart rate and blood pressure and narrow arteries around the heart. Fetal exposure to nicotine during pregnancy has long-lasting effects on brain development. At high-enough doses, nicotine is toxic, and nicotine poisoning can be very dangerous or even cause death. But the most common and most serious effect of nicotine is addiction. Nicotine addiction keeps people smoking longer, and the longer they smoke, the more damage they do to their bodies.[3]

[3] "Let's Make the Next Generation Tobacco-Free," U.S. Department of Health and Human Services (HHS), July 2015. Available online. URL: www.hhs.gov/sites/default/files/consequences-smoking-consumer-guide.pdf. Accessed October 3, 2023.

CHAPTER 6
THE EFFECTS OF TOBACCO ON HEALTH

What Are the Physical Health Consequences of Tobacco Use?

Cigarette smoking harms nearly every organ in the body, and smoking is the leading preventable cause of premature death in the United States. Although rates of smoking have declined, it is estimated that it leads to about 480,000 deaths yearly. Smokers aged 60 and older have a twofold increase in mortality compared with those who have never smoked, dying an estimated six years earlier. Quitting smoking results in immediate health benefits, and some or all of the reduced life expectancy can be recovered depending on the age a person quits.

Although nicotine itself does not cause cancer, at least 69 chemicals in tobacco smoke are carcinogenic, and cigarette smoking accounts for at least 30 percent of all cancer deaths. The overall rates of death from cancer are twice as high among smokers as nonsmokers, with heavy smokers having a four times greater risk of death from cancer than nonsmokers.

Foremost among the cancers caused by tobacco use is lung cancer. Cigarette smoking has been linked to about 80–90 percent of all cases of lung cancer, the leading cause of cancer death for both men and women, and it is responsible for roughly 80 percent of deaths from this disease. Smoking increases lung cancer risk five to tenfold, with a greater risk among heavy smokers. Smoking is also associated with cancers of the mouth, pharynx, larynx, esophagus, stomach, pancreas, cervix, kidney, and bladder, as well as acute myeloid. Cigarette smoking is not the only form of tobacco use associated with cancers. Smokeless tobacco has been linked to cancer of the pharynx, esophagus, stomach, and lung, as well as to colorectal cancer.

In addition to cancer, smoking causes lung diseases, such as chronic bronchitis and emphysema, and it has been found to exacerbate asthma symptoms in adults and children. Cigarette smoking is the most significant risk factor for chronic obstructive pulmonary disease (COPD). Survival statistics indicate that quitting smoking results in repair to much of the smoking-induced lung damage over time. However, once COPD develops, it is irreversible; COPD-related lung damage is not repaired with time.

Smoking also substantially increases the risk of heart disease, including stroke, heart attack, vascular disease, and aneurysm. Cardiovascular disease (CVD) is responsible for 40 percent of all smoking-related deaths. Smoking causes coronary heart disease (CHD), the leading cause of death in the United States. Smoking is also linked to many other major health conditions—including rheumatoid arthritis (RA), inflammation, and impaired immune function. Even young smokers aged 26–41 report reduced health-related quality of life (QOL) compared with nonsmoking peers, according to a cross-sectional population study. Recent animal research also identified a pathway between the pancreas and a part of the brain active in nicotine intake, potentially linking cigarette smoking to the risk of developing type 2 diabetes.[1]

How Smoking Affects Your Body

Smoking harms nearly every organ of the body. Some of these harmful and negative effects are immediate.

Brain

Nicotine from cigarettes is as addictive as heroin. Nicotine addiction is hard to beat because it changes your brain. The brain develops extra nicotine receptors to accommodate the large doses of nicotine from tobacco. When the brain stops getting the nicotine it is used to, the result is nicotine withdrawal. You may feel anxious, irritable, and have strong cravings for nicotine.

Head and Face

Ears

One effect of smoking is reduced oxygen supply to the cochlea, a snail-shaped organ in the inner ear. This may result in permanent damage to the cochlea and mild-to-moderate hearing loss.

Eyes

Smoking causes physical changes in the eyes that can threaten your eyesight. One of the effects of nicotine from cigarettes restricts the production of a chemical necessary for you to be able to see at night. Also, smoking increases your risk of developing cataracts and macular degeneration (both can lead to blindness).

Mouth

Smoking takes a toll on your mouth. Smokers have more oral health problems than nonsmokers, such as mouth sores, ulcers, and gum disease. You are more likely to

[1] "What Are the Physical Health Consequences of Tobacco Use?" National Institute on Drug Abuse (NIDA), May 2022. Available online. URL: https://nida.nih.gov/publications/research-reports/tobacco-nicotine-e-cigarettes/what-are-physical-health-consequences-tobacco-use. Accessed October 3, 2023.

have cavities and lose your teeth at a younger age. You are also more likely to get cancers of the mouth and throat.

Face

Smoking can cause your skin to be dry and lose elasticity, leading to wrinkles and stretch marks. Your skin tone may become dull and grayish. By your early 30s, wrinkles can begin to appear around your mouth and eyes, adding years to your face.

Heart

Stressed Heart

Smoking raises your blood pressure and puts stress on your heart. Over time, stress on the heart can weaken it, making it less able to pump blood to other parts of your body. Carbon monoxide from inhaled cigarette smoke also contributes to a lack of oxygen, making the heart work even harder. This increases the risk of heart disease, including heart attacks.

Sticky Blood

Smoking makes your blood thick and sticky. The stickier the blood, the harder your heart must work to move it around your body. Sticky blood is also more likely to form blood clots that block blood flow to your heart, brain, and legs. Over time, thick, sticky blood damages the delicate lining of your blood vessels. This damage can increase your risk for a heart attack or stroke.

Fatty Deposits

Smoking increases the cholesterol and unhealthy fats circulating in the blood, leading to unhealthy fatty deposits. Over time, cholesterol, fats, and other debris build up on the walls of your arteries. This buildup narrows the arteries and blocks normal blood flow to the heart, brain, and legs. Blocked blood flow to the heart or brain can cause a heart attack or stroke. Blockage in the blood vessels of your legs could result in the amputation of your toes or feet.

Lungs

Scarred Lungs

Smokers' lungs experience inflammation in the small airways and tissues of your lungs. This can make your chest feel tight or cause you to wheeze or feel short of breath. Continued inflammation builds up scar tissue, which leads to physical changes to your lungs and airways that can make breathing hard. Years of lung irritation can give you a chronic cough with mucus.

Emphysema

Smoking destroys the tiny air sacs, or alveoli, in the lungs that allow oxygen exchange. When you smoke, you are damaging some of those air sacs. Alveoli do not grow back, so when you destroy them, you have permanently destroyed part of your lungs. When enough alveoli are destroyed, the disease emphysema develops. Emphysema causes severe shortness of breath and can lead to death.

Cilia and Respiratory Infections

Your airways are lined with tiny brush-like hairs called "cilia." The cilia sweep out mucus and dirt, so your lungs stay clear. Smoking temporarily paralyzes and even kills cilia. This makes you more at risk for infection. Smokers get more colds and respiratory infections than nonsmokers.

Deoxyribonucleic Acid

Cancer

Your body is made up of cells that contain genetic material, or deoxyribonucleic acid (DNA), that acts as an instruction manual for cell growth and function. Every single puff of a cigarette causes damage to your DNA. When DNA is damaged, the instruction manual gets messed up, and the cell can begin growing out of control and create a cancer tumor. Your body tries to repair the damage that smoking does to your DNA, but over time, smoking can wear down this repair system and lead to cancer (such as lung cancer). One-third of all cancer deaths are caused by tobacco.

Stomach and Hormones

Belly

Need another reason why smoking is bad for you? Bigger belly. Smokers have bigger bellies and less muscle than nonsmokers. They are more likely to develop type 2 diabetes, even if they do not smoke every day. Smoking also makes it harder to control diabetes once you already have it. Diabetes is a serious disease that can lead to blindness, heart disease, kidney failure, and amputations.

Lower Estrogen Levels

Smoking lowers a woman's level of estrogen. Low estrogen levels can cause dry skin, thinning hair, and memory problems. Women who smoke have a harder time getting pregnant and having a healthy baby. Smoking can also lead to early menopause, which increases your risk of developing certain diseases (such as heart disease).[2]

Health Effects of Cigarette Smoking

Cigarette smoking causes many diseases and reduces the health of smokers in general.

Quitting smoking lowers your risk for smoking-related diseases and can add years to your life.

[2] Smokefree.gov, "Health Effects," U.S. Department of Health and Human Services (HHS), January 10, 2013. Available online. https://smokefree.gov/quit-smoking/why-you-should-quit/health-effects. Accessed October 3, 2023.

Smoking and Death

Cigarette smoking is the leading preventable cause of death in the United States.

- Smoking causes more deaths each year than the following causes combined:
  - human immunodeficiency virus (HIV)
  - illegal drug use
  - alcohol use
  - motor vehicle injuries
  - firearm-related incidents
- More than 10 times as many U.S. citizens have died prematurely from cigarette smoking than have died in all the wars fought by the United States.
- Smoking causes about 90 percent (or 9 out of 10) of all lung cancer deaths. More women die from lung cancer each year than from breast cancer.
- Smoking causes about 80 percent (or 8 out of 10) of all deaths from COPD.
- Cigarette smoking increases risk for death from all causes in men and women.
- The risk of dying from cigarette smoking has increased over the last 50 years in the United States.

Smoking and Increased Health Risks

Smokers are more likely than nonsmokers to develop heart disease, stroke, and lung cancer.

- Estimates show smoking increases the risk:
  - for CHD by two to four times
  - for stroke by two to four times
  - of men developing lung cancer by 25 times
  - of women developing lung cancer by 25.7 times
- Smoking causes diminished overall health, increased absenteeism from work, and increased health-care utilization and cost.

Smoking and Cardiovascular Disease

Smokers are at greater risk for diseases that affect the heart and blood vessels CVD.

- Smoking causes stroke and CHD which are among the leading causes of death in the United States.
- Even people who smoke fewer than five cigarettes a day can have early signs of CVD.
- Smoking damages blood vessels and can make them thicken and grow narrower. This makes your heart beat faster, and your blood pressure go up. Clots can also form.
- A stroke occurs when:
  - a clot blocks the blood flow to part of your brain
  - a blood vessel in or around your brain bursts
- Blockages caused by smoking can also reduce blood flow to your legs and skin.

Smoking and Respiratory Disease

Smoking can cause lung disease by damaging your airways and the small air sacs (alveoli) found in your lungs.

- Lung diseases caused by smoking include COPD, which includes emphysema and chronic bronchitis.
- Cigarette smoking causes most cases of lung cancer.
- If you have asthma, tobacco smoke can trigger an attack or make an attack worse.
- Smokers are 12–13 times more likely to die from COPD than nonsmokers.

Smoking and Cancer

Smoking can cause cancer almost anywhere in your body.

Smoking also increases the risk of dying from cancer and other diseases in cancer patients and survivors.

If nobody smoked, one of every three cancer deaths in the United States would not happen.

Quitting and Reduced Risks

- Quitting smoking cuts cardiovascular risks. Just one year after quitting smoking, your risk for a heart attack drops sharply.
- Within two to five years after quitting smoking, your risk for stroke may reduce to about that of a nonsmoker's.
- If you quit smoking, your risks for cancers of the mouth, throat, esophagus, and bladder drop by half within five years.
- Ten years after you quit smoking, your risk of dying from lung cancer drops by half.

Smoking and Other Health Risks

Smoking harms nearly every organ of the body and affects a person's overall health.

- Smoking can make it harder for a woman to become pregnant. It can also affect her baby's health before and after birth. Smoking increases risks for:
  - preterm (early) delivery
  - stillbirth (death of the baby before birth)
  - low birth weight
  - sudden infant death syndrome (known as "SIDS" or "crib death")
  - ectopic pregnancy
  - orofacial clefts in infants
- Smoking can also affect men's sperm, which can reduce fertility and also increase risks for birth defects and miscarriage.
- Smoking can affect bone health.
  - Women past childbearing years who smoke have weaker bones than women who never smoked. They are also at greater risk for broken bones.

- Smoking affects the health of your teeth and gums and can cause tooth loss.
- Smoking can increase your risk for cataracts (clouding of the eye's lens that makes it hard for you to see). It can also cause age-related macular degeneration (AMD). AMD is damage to a small spot near the center of the retina, the part of the eye needed for central vision.
- Smoking is a cause of type 2 diabetes mellitus and can make it harder to control. The risk of developing diabetes is 30–40 percent higher for active smokers than nonsmokers.
- Smoking causes general adverse effects on the body, including inflammation and decreased immune function.
- Smoking is a cause of rheumatoid arthritis (RA).[3]

Health Benefits of Quitting Smoking

Quitting smoking is one of the most important actions people can take to improve their health. This is true regardless of their age or how long they have been smoking.

Quitting smoking:

- improves health status and enhances quality of life (QOL)
- reduces the risk of premature death and can add as much as 10 years to life expectancy
- reduces the risk for many adverse health effects, including poor reproductive health outcomes, cardiovascular diseases (CVDs), chronic obstructive pulmonary disease (COPD), and cancer
- benefits people already diagnosed with coronary heart disease or COPD
- benefits the health of pregnant women and their fetuses and babies
- reduces the financial burden that smoking places on people who smoke, health-care systems, and society

While quitting earlier in life yields greater health benefits, quitting smoking is beneficial to health at any age. Even people who have smoked for many years or have smoked heavily will benefit from quitting.

Quitting smoking is the single best way to protect family members, coworkers, friends, and others from the health risks associated with breathing secondhand smoke.

Source: "Benefits of Quitting," Centers for Disease Control and Prevention (CDC), September 23, 2020. Available online. URL: www.cdc.gov/tobacco/quit_smoking/how_to_quit/benefits/index.htm. Accessed October 3, 2023.

[3] "Health Effects of Cigarette Smoking," Centers for Disease Control and Prevention (CDC), October 29, 2021. Available online. URL: www cdc.gov/tobacco/data_statistics/fact_sheets/health_effects/effects_cig_smoking/index.htm. Accessed October 3, 2023.

CHAPTER 7
ECONOMIC TRENDS IN TOBACCO

Tobacco-Related Spending

In 2019, the largest tobacco companies spent $8.2 billion on marketing cigarettes and smokeless tobacco in the United States. This amount translates to about $22.5 million each day, or nearly $1 million every hour.

- Cigarette advertising and promotional expenses totaled about $7.62 billion in 2019—a decrease from 2018. However, even though cigarette companies spent less overall on advertising and promotion in 2019 than in 2018, they spent a larger percentage (74.7%, or about $5.7 billion) of their 2019 advertising and promotion dollars on price discounts paid to cigarette retailers than they did the year before. These price discounts reduce the cost of cigarettes to consumers.
- Manufacturers spent a total of $576.1 million on smokeless tobacco advertising and promotion during 2019—a decrease from 2018. Smokeless tobacco products include dry snuff, moist snuff, plug/twist, loose-leaf chewing tobacco, snus, and dissolvable products.
- A number of electronic products, such as electronic cigarettes (e-cigarettes), electronic cigars (e-cigars), and electronic pipes (e-pipes), are on the market. However, current information on spending for marketing and promotion of these products is currently not available.
- From 2014 through 2020, e-cigarette sales in the United States generally increased as product prices decreased. Total e-cigarette sales increased by 122.2 percent during this time frame (i.e., from 7.7 million to 17.1 million units per four-week interval).
- Despite overall sales growth, e-cigarette sales fluctuated across time by product type. Specifically, from 2014 to 2019, sales of rechargeables, prefilled cartridges, and e-liquids grew relatively steadily over time. However, sales for disposables increased sharply from 10.3 percent of total sales in August 2019 to 19.8 percent in May 2020.

Tobacco Production in the United States

Although U.S. tobacco production has decreased significantly since the 1980s (from nearly 180,000 tobacco-growing farms to about 10,000 in 2012), the United States continues to be a leading producer of tobacco leaves.

- The United States is the fourth largest tobacco-producing country in the world, following China, India, and Brazil.
- Farms in the United States harvested more than 533 million pounds of tobacco in 2018.
- In 2018, two states—North Carolina and Kentucky—accounted for more than 70 percent of total tobacco cultivation.

Cigarette smoking remains the leading cause of preventable disease, disability, and death in the United States, accounting for more than 480,000 deaths every year, or about one in five deaths.

In 2021, nearly 12 of every 100 U.S. adults aged 18 or older (11.5%) currently* smoked cigarettes. This means an estimated 28.3 million adults in the United States currently smoke cigarettes. More than 16 million Americans live with a smoking-related disease.

Current smoking has declined from 20.9 percent (nearly 21 of every 100 adults) in 2005 to 11.5 percent (nearly 12 of every 100 adults) in 2021.

* *Current smokers are defined as people who reported smoking at least 100 cigarettes during their lifetime and who, at the time they participated in a survey about this topic, reported smoking every day or some days.*

Source: "Current Cigarette Smoking among Adults in the United States," Centers for Disease Control and Prevention (CDC), May 4, 2023. Available online. URL: www.cdc.gov/tobacco/data_statistics/fact_sheets/adult_data/cig_smoking/index.htm. Accessed September 26, 2023.

Tobacco Sales

Cigarette Sales

- During 2017, about 249 billion cigarettes were sold in the United States—a 3.5 percent decrease from the 258 billion sold in 2016.
  - Four companies—Philip Morris USA, Reynolds American Inc., ITG Brands, and Liggett—accounted for about 92 percent of U.S. cigarette sales.
  - Imports, primarily from Canada and South Korea, accounted for approximately 8.3 percent of U.S. cigarette inventories in 2016 and 7.9 percent in 2017.
- By state, the average retail price of a pack of 20 cigarettes (full-priced brands), including federal and state excise taxes, ranged from $4.62 in Missouri to a high of $10.67 in New York, as of November 2017.
- On average, federal and state excise taxes account for 44.3 percent of the retail price of cigarettes.

Other Tobacco Product Sales

- During 2012–2016, total U.S. cigar unit sales grew by 29 percent, which was largely driven by increasing sales of cigarillos.
- The total amount of smokeless tobacco sold by manufacturers to wholesalers and retailers in the United States was about 126 million pounds in 2019, a decrease from 128.41 million pounds sold in 2018.
    - From June 2018 to June 2019, three companies—Altria Group Inc., British American Tobacco, and Swedish Match—accounted for nearly 98 percent of U.S. dollar sales of smokeless tobacco, with combined sales of more than $6 billion.

Economic Cost Estimates Associated with Cigarette Smoking

Cigarette smoking costs the United States more than $600 billion in 2018, including the following:

- more than $240 billion in health-care spending
- nearly $185 billion in lost productivity from smoking-related illnesses and health conditions
- nearly $180 billion in lost productivity from smoking-related premature death
- $7 billion in lost productivity from premature death from secondhand smoke exposure

Effects of Increased Prices

Increasing the price of tobacco products is the single most effective way to reduce consumption.

- A 10 percent increase in price has been estimated to reduce overall cigarette consumption by 3–5 percent.
- Research on cigarette consumption suggests that:
    - both youth and young adults are two to three times more likely to respond to increases in price than adults
    - lower-income populations are more likely to increase quit attempts or smoke fewer cigarettes in response to price increases although the desire to quit and successful cessation may not be consistent across all racial/ethnic groups[1]

Cigarette Report for 2021

The expenditures on cigarette advertising in 2020–2021 are listed in Table 7.1.[2]

[1] "Economic Trends in Tobacco," Centers for Disease Control and Prevention (CDC), July 26, 2022. Available online. URL: www.cdc.gov/tobacco/data_statistics/fact_sheets/economics/econ_facts/index.htm. Accessed September 26, 2023.

[2] "Cigarette Report for 2021," Federal Trade Commission (FTC), 2023. Available online. URL: www.ftc.gov/system/files/ftc_gov/pdf/p114508cigarettereport2021.pdf. Accessed September 26, 2023.

Table 7.1. Cigarette Advertising and Promotional Expenditures for 2020–2021 (Dollars in Thousands)*

	2020	2021
Newspapers	N/A**	N/A**
Magazines	$11,332 (0.1%)	$4,328 (0.1%)
Outdoor	$1,815 (0.0%)	$2,161 (0.0%)
Point-of-sale	$47,117 (0.6%)	$49,074 (0.6%)
Direct mail	$12,303 (0.2%)	$19,110 (0.2%)
Price discounts—retailers	$6,065,320 (77.4%)	$6,011,776 (74.6%)
Price discounts—wholesalers	$875,976 (11.2%)	$917,321 (11.4%)
Promotional allowances—retailers	$181,052 (2.3%)	$235,356 (2.9%)
Promotional allowances—wholesalers	$343,281 (4.4%)	$487,129 (6.0%)
Promotional allowances—other	N/A**	N/A**
Sampling	$6 (0.0%)	$4 (0.0%)
Specialty item distribution—nonbranded	$41,262 (0.5%)	$43,519 (0.5%)
Consumer engagement—retail	$11,940 (0.2%)	N/A**
Consumer engagement—adult only	$11,535 (0.1%)	$9,984 (0.1%)
Public entertainment—adult only	$0 (0.0%)	N/A**
Public entertainment—general audience	$0 (0.0%)	$0 (0.0%)
Sponsorships	$0 (0.0%)	$0 (0.0%)
Endorsements and testimonials	$0 (0.0%)	$0 (0.0%)
Coupons	$156,509 (2.0%)	$152,335 (1.9%)
Retail value-added—bonus cigarettes	$0 (0.0%)	$0 (0.0%)
Retail value-added—noncigarette bonus	N/A**	N/A**
Company website	$8,379 (0.1%)	$7,781 (0.1%)
Internet—other	N/A**	$3,315 (0.0%)
Telephone	$0 (0.0%)	$0 (0.0%)
Audiovisual	$0 (0.0%)	$0 (0.0%)
Social media	N/A**	$0 (0.0%)
Other**	$78,682 (1.0%)	$109,721 (1.4%)
Total	$7,839,506	$8,059,919
Sports and sporting events	$0	$0

** Because of rounding, sums of percentages may not equal 100 percent.*
*** Expenditures denoted "N/A" are included in the "Other" category to avoid potential disclosure of individual company data.*

CHAPTER 8
BEWARE OF MARKETING STRATEGIES

Cigarette and smokeless tobacco companies spend billions of dollars each year to market their products.

- In 2019, the largest cigarette and smokeless tobacco companies spent $8.2 billion on advertising and promotional expenses in the United States alone.
  - The four major U.S. cigarette companies spent $7.62 billion on cigarette advertising and promotion in 2019.
  - The five major U.S. smokeless tobacco manufacturers spent $576.1 million on smokeless tobacco advertising and promotion in 2019. Smokeless tobacco products include dry snuff, moist snuff, plug/twist, loose-leaf chewing tobacco, snus, and dissolvable products.

The money cigarette and smokeless tobacco companies spent in 2019 on U.S. marketing amounted to:

- about $22.5 million each day
- about $25 for every person (adults and children) in the United States per year (according to 2019 population estimate of 328,239,523)
- about $240 per year for each U.S. adult smoker (based on 34.2 million adult smokers in 2018)

The following three categories totaled approximately $7.13 billion and accounted for 93.4 percent of all cigarette company marketing expenditures in 2019:

- price discounts paid to retailers and wholesalers to reduce the price of cigarettes to consumers—about $5.7 billion
- promotional allowances paid to cigarette retailers, such as payments for stocking, shelving, displaying, and merchandising particular brands—$174.9 million
- promotional allowances paid to cigarette wholesalers, such as payments for volume rebates, incentive payments, value-added services, and promotions—$336.6 million

Marketing to Specific Populations

Youth and Young Adults

Scientific evidence shows that tobacco company advertising and promotion influences young people to start using tobacco.

- Adolescents who are exposed to cigarette advertising often find the ads appealing.
- Tobacco ads make smoking appear to be appealing, which can increase adolescents' desire to smoke.

The three most heavily advertised brands—Marlboro, Newport, and Camel—were the preferred brands of cigarettes smoked by middle and high school students in 2016.

Cigarette brand preferences among U.S. middle school students:

- 38.3 percent preferred Marlboro
- 21.4 percent preferred Newport
- 13.4 percent preferred Camel

Cigarette brand preferences among U.S. high school students:

- 48.8 percent preferred Marlboro
- 16.6 percent preferred Newport
- 13.3 percent preferred Camel

Women

Women are also targeted by the tobacco industry, and tobacco companies continue to produce brands specifically for women. Marketing toward women is dominated by themes of social desirability, empowerment, and independence, which are conveyed by advertisements featuring slim, attractive, and athletic models.

Racial/Ethnic Communities

Advertisement and promotion of certain tobacco products appear to be targeted to members of racial/minority communities.

- Marketing to Hispanics and American Indians/Alaska Natives has included advertising and promotion of cigarette brands with names, such as Rio, Dorado, and American Spirit.
- The tobacco industry has targeted African-American communities in its advertisements and promotional efforts for menthol cigarettes. Strategies include the following:
  - campaigns that use urban culture and language to promote menthol cigarettes
  - tobacco-sponsored hip-hop bar nights with samples of specialty menthol cigarettes
  - targeted direct-mail promotions

- tobacco companies' marketing to Asian Americans has included the following:
    - sponsorship of Chinese and Vietnamese New Year festivals and other activities related to Asian/Pacific American Heritage Month
    - heavy billboard and in-store advertisements in predominantly urban Asian-American communities
    - financial and in-kind contributions to community organizations
    - support of Asian-American business associations[1]

Keeping Prices Down

Tobacco companies lower prices through coupons and other promotions so that consumers can afford to buy their products. Teens are especially sensitive to pricing.

In 2008, cigarette makers spent nearly $10 billion to market their products. Much of this spending—$6 out of every $7—was used to pay for price cuts through coupons, sales, and giveaways. Similarly, smokeless tobacco makers spent about $3 out of every $4 of their $547 million marketing budget to keep prices low.

Making Products Easy to Buy

A number of laws limit face-to-face and vending machine sales of tobacco products to young people. But there is less oversight online. While most websites say buyers must be at least 18 years old, research found that 15- and 16-year-olds were able to place orders successfully. Nearly 8 out of 10 of those young people received their orders, and only 1 out of 10 shipments required proof of age at the time of delivery of the tobacco product.

Designing Products That Appeal to Youth

Cigarettes that appeal to new smokers are often smoother and milder to improve taste and reduce the body's physical reaction to the smoke. While flavored cigarettes are now prohibited, the industry still puts fruit flavoring and other kid-friendly flavors in many of their cigars. This is especially true for cigarette-sized cigars, which are now available in many flavor varieties—such as grape and strawberry—that youth find appealing in other products. Many of these little cigars look exactly like cigarettes with a darker wrapper.

Many smokeless products are also flavored. These include chew and snuff—which come in a variety of forms—and new smokeless products, such as dissolvable tobacco. All of these products can cause serious health problems and lead to nicotine addiction and future smoking. Tobacco companies are still using different techniques to make

[1] "Tobacco Industry Marketing," Centers for Disease Control and Prevention (CDC), May 14, 2021. Available online. URL: www.cdc.gov/tobacco/data_statistics/fact_sheets/tobacco_industry/marketing/index.htm. Accessed September 27, 2023.

many cigarette brands taste less harsh—especially brands that young people often use when they start smoking.

Young people sometimes use smokeless tobacco products in places where cigarettes are banned, such as schools. Snus (dry snuff in a pouch), and dissolvable smokeless products in particular, provide a discreet way for young people to maintain their addiction to nicotine even when they cannot smoke. In fact, most youth users of these smokeless products also smoke cigarettes. The biggest danger of these products is that they may introduce kids to nicotine, putting them at risk for nicotine addiction.

Myth: Smoking Helps You Lose Weight

Many young people, especially girls and young women, believe that smoking can help them lose weight. But studies show that is not true—young people who smoke are not thinner than those who do not.

Cigarette marketing encourages the myth that smoking causes weight loss. And it targets women with brand names that suggest thinness, as well as with long, thin cigarettes.

Source: "Preventing Tobacco Use among Youth and Young Adults," Centers for Disease Control and Prevention (CDC), March 8, 2012. Available online. URL: www.cdc.gov/tobacco/data_statistics/sgr/2012/consumer_booklet/pdfs/consumer.pdf. Accessed September 27, 2023.

Creating a Package That Appeals to Youth

Packaging has a powerful visual effect. Users come to associate certain brands with certain qualities. Words on packages, such as "slims" and "thins," push the myth of weight loss. Before they were banned, some words ("low tar," "light," and "mild") falsely suggested safety. Studies show that color makes a difference too. Smokers tend to think that cigarettes in lighter-colored packs are "lighter" and safer than cigarettes in dark-colored packs—even when both packs contain the exact same cigarettes.

Retail Marketing

Tobacco companies use many marketing and advertising tools at stores that sell tobacco products. Even the locations where tobacco products are sold can have an effect on tobacco use by young people. For example, more cigarettes are sold in convenience stores than in any other type of store, and 70 percent of adolescents shop in convenience stores at least once a week—where they are more likely to be exposed to pro-smoking messages.

For many years, the tobacco industry has offered sellers financial rewards and discounts when they sell large volumes of their products. Some stores and gas stations place tobacco products on or near checkout counters—a visible spot that may trigger impulse buying.

They also run sales on tobacco products and place vivid, eye-catching ads in windows and outside their buildings. Ads inside the store are sometimes at eye level for preteen children, which research shows might influence them to try tobacco products later.

Using Media to Promote Products

The tobacco industry uses media to promote its products to young people. Here are some of the channels it uses.

Digital Media

Many cigarette companies use websites to promote their products. Some of these websites feature videos, games, coupons, and contests that may appeal to youth. Meanwhile, some young people are using social networking channels (Facebook, Twitter, discussion forums, message boards, and YouTube videos) to sing the praises of tobacco, especially to their peers.

Magazines

Tobacco ads are not allowed on TV or on billboards. But they may still be found in mainstream magazines targeted to adults, and many young people read these. These ads often suggest that using tobacco can make you sexy, popular, thin, and cool.

Policies and Programs: Which Work Best?

There are effective policies and programs that prevent young people from using tobacco. Policies and programs that contain several parts working together to make tobacco use more difficult and less accepted are the ones that work best.

Policies

Policies are very effective because they can change the environment so that choosing a tobacco-free life is encouraged and supported. Government and private entities have implemented a number of policies that are effective in preventing youth tobacco use.

Here are some policies proven to work best:

- Make tobacco products less affordable.
- Restrict tobacco marketing.
- Ban smoking in public places—such as workplaces, schools, day care centers, hospitals, restaurants, hotels, and parks.
- Require tobacco companies to label tobacco packages with large, graphic health warnings.

Programs

Many states and communities have programs to prevent tobacco use by young people. The most effective ones combine several elements, including evidence-based curricula in secondary schools, work with policies, and influence people at work, at home, in school, in health-care settings, and in public places.

Mass Media Campaigns

Mass media campaigns against tobacco use—most often TV ads—have proven very effective at helping prevent tobacco use by young people. Studies show that teens respond most to ads that trigger strong negative feelings, such as ads about how smoking and secondhand smoke harm health and ads that expose the tobacco industry's marketing strategies that target young people. Even ads that are designed for adult audiences help reduce tobacco use among young people.

Every three or four years, new groups of children and teens reach the age where they are vulnerable to influences encouraging them to smoke. To be effective, mass media campaigns must be repeated, so they will reach new vulnerable populations.

Parents: How You Can Help

You can help your children make healthy choices about tobacco use. Try the following tips:

Tell them:

- key facts about tobacco
- you do not want anyone—including them—to use tobacco in your house or car
- you expect they will never use tobacco or will stop using it

Help them:

- cope with their problems
- refuse tobacco
- quit if they are current users

Make sure you:

- know what they are doing and who their friends are
- network with other parents who can help you encourage children and teens to refuse tobacco
- encourage your children's schools to enforce tobacco-free policies for students, faculty, staff, and visitors both on campus and at all school-sponsored events off campus
- enforce movie age restrictions—and discourage teens from playing video games or using other media that feature smoking
- never give tobacco to children or teens
- set a good example by not using tobacco yourself[2]

[2] "A Report of the Surgeon General: Preventing Tobacco Use among Youth and Young Adults," Centers for Disease Control and Prevention (CDC), November 15, 2010. Available online. URL: www.cdc.gov/tobacco/data_statistics/sgr/2012/consumer_booklet/pdfs/consumer.pdf. Accessed September 27, 2023.

CHAPTER 9
TOBACCO MYTHS

Myth 1
Smoking is just a choice.

Fact
- The first time? Yes. After just a few cigarettes? No.
- Addiction to nicotine can happen quickly. It changes the chemical balance in your brain. Smoking may seem like it is just a choice or a habit. In fact, most people who use tobacco are addicted.
- Breaking nicotine addiction is harder for some people than others. Quitting can take several tries. But do not give up.
- If you need help to quit, ask your doctor about nicotine replacement, medicines, or coaching.

Myth 2
Filters make cigarettes safer.

Fact
- Filters do not protect you. They are designed to make smoke particles smaller. That makes nicotine easier to absorb. This increases addiction.
- Cigarettes have been engineered to speed up nicotine's path to your brain. Their design feeds addiction.
- Light or low-tar cigarettes may sound less dangerous. They are not. These misleading labels are no longer allowed.
- No cigarette is safe. Tobacco smoke contains more than 7,000 chemicals. At least 250 are toxic.

Myth 3

An occasional cigarette is no big deal.

Fact

- Smoking does not just cause diseases for heavy smokers or longtime smokers.
- The 2010 Surgeon General's Report shows how breathing tobacco smoke can cause immediate harm. Tobacco smoke can trigger sudden heart attacks and death, even in nonsmokers.
- Each cigarette you smoke hurts your lungs, your blood vessels, and cells throughout your body.
- Smoking a few cigarettes a week can cause a heart attack.
- Cutting back is not enough to protect you. You have to quit entirely.

Myth 4

It is too late to quit. The damage is already done.

Fact

- It is true that the longer you use tobacco, the more you hurt your body. But, at any age, the sooner you quit, the sooner your health can improve.
- The 2010 Surgeon General's Report shows how using tobacco causes disease almost everywhere in your body.
- Within 20 minutes after quitting, your body starts to heal.
- After two to five years, your risk for stroke is similar to that of a nonsmoker.
- In 10 years, your lung cancer risk is cut in half.

Myth 5

Secondhand smoke may bother people, but it is not dangerous.

Fact

- Tens of thousands of nonsmokers die every year from breathing others' secondhand smoke.
- Breathing the chemicals in tobacco smoke changes your blood's chemistry almost immediately. Deadly clots can form and block arteries in your heart or brain.
- When you smoke at work, at home, or at a restaurant, everyone there breathes poison.
- If you smoke in your car, rolling down a window does not protect your passengers.
- It is not healthy to breathe any amount of tobacco smoke.

Myth 6

The little bit of smoke that my kids get does not hurt them.

Fact

- Do not smoke or let others smoke around your children. They can get bronchitis, pneumonia, and ear infections from smoke.
- Even if you only smoke by an open window, some of the smoke stays in your house and poisons the air your children breathe.
- Children with asthma can have a serious, even deadly, asthma attack from breathing secondhand smoke.
- The best way to protect children is to quit smoking. If you or someone else in your household is not ready to quit, be sure to make your home and car 100 percent smoke-free.[1]

[1] "Is What You Know about Smoking Wrong?" Centers for Disease Control and Prevention (CDC), 2010. Available online. URL: www.cdc.gov/tobacco/sgr/2010/myths/pdfs/myths.pdf. Accessed September 26, 2023.

CHAPTER 10
PREVENTING TOBACCO USE

How Can We Prevent Tobacco Use?

The medical consequences of tobacco use—including secondhand exposure—make tobacco control and smoking prevention crucial parts of any public health strategy. Since the first Surgeon General's Report on Smoking and Health in 1964, states and communities have made efforts to reduce initiation of smoking, decrease exposure to smoke, and increase cessation. Researchers estimate that these tobacco control efforts are associated with averting an estimated 8 million premature deaths and extending the average life expectancy of men by 2.3 years and of women by 1.6 years. But there is a long way yet to go, roughly 5.6 million adolescents under the age of 18 are expected to die prematurely as a result of an illness related to smoking.

Prevention can take the form of policy-level measures, such as increased taxation of tobacco products, stricter laws (and enforcement of laws) regulating who can purchase tobacco products, how and where they can be purchased, where and when they can be used (i.e., smoke-free policies in restaurants, bars, and other public places), and restrictions on advertising and mandatory health warnings on packages. Over 100 studies have shown that higher taxes on cigarettes, for example, produce significant reductions in smoking, especially among youth and lower-income individuals. Smoke-free workplace laws and restrictions on advertising have also shown benefits.

Prevention can also take place at the school or community level. Merely educating potential smokers about the health risks has not proven effective. Successful evidence-based interventions aim to reduce or delay initiation of smoking, alcohol use, and illicit drug use, and otherwise improve outcomes for children and teens by reducing or mitigating modifiable risk factors and bolstering protective factors. Risk factors for smoking include having family members or peers who smoke, being in a lower socioeconomic status, living in a neighborhood with high density of tobacco outlets, not participating in team sports, being exposed to smoking in movies, and being sensation-seeking. Although older teens are more likely to smoke than younger teens, the earlier a person starts smoking or using any addictive substance, the more likely they are to develop an addiction. Males are also more likely to take up smoking in adolescence than females.

Some evidence-based interventions show lasting effects on reducing smoking initiation. For instance, communities utilizing the intervention-delivery system, Communities That Care (CTC), for students aged 10–14 show sustained reduction in male cigarette initiation up to nine years after the end of the intervention.[1]

Tobacco Control Interventions

What Are Effective Statewide Tobacco Interventions for Commercial Tobacco* Use?

Effective population-based commercial tobacco control interventions include tobacco price increases, high-impact anti-tobacco mass media campaigns, comprehensive smoke-free policies, and cessation access. The evidence shows that implementing and enforcing these strategies, both individually and as part of a comprehensive tobacco prevention and control effort, can reduce smoking initiation and use among adults and youths. Comprehensive commercial tobacco prevention and control efforts involve the coordinated implementation of population-based interventions to prevent tobacco initiation among youth and young adults, promote quitting among adults and youth, eliminate exposure to secondhand smoke, and identify and eliminate tobacco-related disparities among population groups. Tobacco products include cigarettes, e-cigarettes, cigars, pipes, hookah, smokeless tobacco, and other products. Programs combine and integrate multiple evidence-based strategies, including educational, regulatory, economic, and social strategies at local, state, or national levels.

Evidence-based interventions that are key components of a comprehensive commercial tobacco prevention and control effort include the following:

- mass-reach health communications campaigns that use multiple media formats; include hard-hitting or graphic images; are intended to change knowledge, beliefs, attitudes, and behaviors affecting tobacco use; and provide people who use tobacco with information on resources on how to quit
- increases in the unit price for tobacco products, which can decrease the number of people using tobacco, reduce the amount of tobacco consumed, and prevent young people from starting to use tobacco

* *"Commercial tobacco" means harmful products that are made and sold by tobacco companies. It does not include "traditional tobacco" used by Indigenous groups for religious or ceremonial purposes.*

[1] "How Can We Prevent Tobacco Use?" National Institute on Drug Abuse (NIDA), May 2022. Available online. URL: https://nida.nih.gov/publications/research-reports/tobacco-nicotine-e-cigarettes/how-can-we-prevent-tobacco-use. Accessed September 26, 2023.

- comprehensive smoke-free policies that prohibit smoking in all indoor areas of workplaces and public places, including restaurants and bars, to prevent involuntary exposure to secondhand smoke
- cessation access strategies, such as comprehensive insurance coverage for evidence-based cessation treatments; integration of tobacco screening and treatment into routine clinical care; and quitlines, which are highly cost-effective

What Is the Public Health Issue?

Tobacco use is the leading cause of preventable disease, disability, and death in the United States. Cigarette smoking harms nearly all organs of the body; it has been linked to heart disease, multiple cancers, lung diseases, and other illnesses. Smoking during pregnancy also causes harm to the fetus. In addition to adverse effects on individual- and population-level health, smoking imposes an immense financial burden on society, with over 480,000 premature deaths, over $170 billion in lost productivity costs, and over $225 billion in direct medical care expenditures in the United States each year. The use of smokeless tobacco, cigars, and pipes can also have deadly consequences, including lung, larynx, esophageal, and oral cancers. Moreover, the effects of tobacco use are not limited to the user. Secondhand smoke exposure can cause death and many serious diseases, including lung cancer, heart disease, and stroke among adults, and respiratory illness, ear infections, asthma attacks, and sudden infant death syndrome (SIDS) among children and infants. An estimated one in four nonsmokers (58 million people), including about two in five children, are exposed to secondhand smoke.

Electronic cigarettes (e-cigarettes) are not safe for youth, young adults, and pregnant women. Most e-cigarettes sold contain nicotine, which is highly addictive and can harm a developing fetus. Nicotine exposure can also harm adolescent and young adult brain development, which continues into the mid-20s. E-cigarette aerosol can contain harmful and potentially harmful chemicals. And youth e-cigarette use is associated with the use of other tobacco products, including cigarettes.

What Is the Evidence of the Health Outcome and Cost-Effectiveness?

A systematic review of proven population-based commercial tobacco control interventions found that these programs were associated with:

- reductions in the prevalence of tobacco use among adults and young people
- reductions in tobacco product consumption
- increased quitting

States that have made larger investments in comprehensive tobacco control efforts have seen larger declines in cigarettes sales than the United States as a whole, and the prevalence of cigarette smoking among adults and youth has declined faster as spending for tobacco control programs has increased. Comprehensive tobacco control efforts have also contributed to reductions in tobacco-related diseases and deaths and were effective across diverse racial, ethnic, educational, and socioeconomic groups. The review also found that these programs were cost-effective and that health-care savings were greater than the cost of the intervention.

Additional systematic reviews examining the effect of single interventions that may be implemented individually or included as part of a comprehensive commercial tobacco control program, such as mass media campaigns, price increases, and smoke-free policies, also found strong evidence of their efficacy and cost-effectiveness.

Mass-Reach Communications Campaigns

Mass media campaigns were associated with lower prevalence of tobacco use, increased cessation and use of available cessation services, and decreased initiation of tobacco use among young people:

- median decrease of 5.0 percentage points in the prevalence of tobacco use among adults
- median decrease of 3.4 percentage points in the prevalence of tobacco use among young people (ages of 11–24)
- median increase of 3.5 percentage points in cessation of tobacco use
- median relative increase of 132 percent in the number of calls to quitlines
- decrease of 6.7 percentage points in tobacco use initiation among young people (ages of 11–24)
- from 2012 to 2018, the Centers for Disease Control and Prevention (CDC) that estimates that more than 16.4 million people who smoke have attempted to quit and approximately 1 million have successfully quit because of exposure to the Tips From Former Smokers (www.cdc.gov/tobacco/campaign/tips/index.html) campaign
- the Tips campaign that was correlated with a 3.9 percent increase in quit attempts per quarter during 2012–2018

An economic review of the evidence found the following:

- The cost for mass-reach health communications campaigns was between $0.25 and $3.35 per person per year. The campaigns resulted in cost savings; averted health costs were greater than the cost of the campaign.
- Quitline promotion campaigns resulted in an estimated cost of $260 for each additional call to the Quitline.

Individual studies found the following:

- The return on investment (ROI) for the U.S. Food and Drug Administration (FDA) The Real Cost Campaign was $128 for every $1 spent.
- The ROI for the FinishIt campaign was $174 for every $1 spent. The cost-effectiveness measure for FinishIt was $1076 for every quality-adjusted life year (QALY) gained.

- During 2012–2018, the CDC's Tips From Former Smokers campaign helped prevent an estimated 129,000 early deaths and helped save an estimated $7.3 billion in smoking-related health-care costs.
- For every $3,800 spent on the Tips campaign between 2012 and 2018, it is estimated that one early death was prevented.

Increasing the Price of Tobacco Products

Increases in the price of tobacco products reduce the quantity demanded for tobacco, thereby prompting quit attempts, reducing consumption among those who do not quit, and preventing youth from starting. Increasing the unit price of tobacco by 20 percent would reduce overall consumption of tobacco products by 10.4 percent, prevalence of adult tobacco use by 3.6 percent, and initiation of tobacco use by young people by 8.6 percent.

An economic review of the evidence estimated that health-care cost savings from a 20 percent price increase for tobacco products ranged from -$0.14 to $90.02 per person per year (2011 dollars) in addition to averted productivity losses.

Comprehensive Smoke-Free Policies

Comprehensive smoke-free policies have been shown to substantially improve indoor air quality, reduce secondhand smoke exposure, change social norms regarding the acceptability of smoking, prevent smoking initiation by youth and young adults, help people who smoke quit, and reduce heart attack and asthma hospitalizations among people who do not smoke. Comprehensive smoke-free policies were associated with:

- decreased exposure to secondhand smoke
- decreased prevalence of tobacco smoking
- decreased tobacco consumption
- fewer deaths and hospitalizations from cardiovascular disease (CVD)
- decreased asthma attacks and hospitalizations
- decreased morbidity, hospitalizations, and deaths from respiratory diseases
- decreased risk of preterm birth
- a decrease in deaths from SIDS

An economic review of the evidence estimated that indoor smoke-free policies are cost-effective and do not reduce profits for hospitality businesses. The policies, which have implementation costs of $25 or less per person, lead to reduced mortality and health-care costs, and save QALYs. The policies have the potential to avert health-care costs of $150,000 to $4.8 million per 100,000 persons.[2]

[2] "Tobacco Control Interventions," Centers for Disease Control and Prevention (CDC), May 16, 2022. Available online. URL: www.cdc.gov/policy/hi5/tobaccointerventions/index.html. Accessed September 26, 2023.

PART 2 | ELECTRONIC CIGARETTES OR VAPING

CHAPTER 11
UNDERSTANDING ELECTRONIC CIGARETTES

What Are E-cigarettes?

- E-cigarettes are electronic devices that heat a liquid and produce an aerosol, or mix of small particles in the air.
- E-cigarettes come in many shapes and sizes. Most have a battery, a heating element, and a place to hold a liquid.
- Some e-cigarettes look like regular cigarettes, cigars, or pipes. Some look like USB flash drives, pens, and other everyday items. Larger devices such as tank systems, or "mods," do not look like other tobacco products.
- E-cigarettes are known by many different names. They are sometimes called "e-cigs," "e-hookahs," "mods," "vape pens," "vapes," "tank systems," and "electronic nicotine delivery systems (ENDS)."
- Using an e-cigarette is sometimes called "vaping."

How Do E-cigarettes Work?

- E-cigarettes produce an aerosol by heating a liquid that usually contains nicotine, flavorings, and other chemicals used to make the aerosol.
- The liquid used in e-cigarettes often contains nicotine and flavorings. This liquid is sometimes called "e-juice," "e-liquid," "vape juice," or "vape liquid."
- Users inhale e-cigarette aerosol into their lungs. Bystanders can also breathe in this aerosol when the user exhales it into the air.
- E-cigarette devices can be used to deliver marijuana and other drugs.

What Is JUUL?

- JUUL is a brand of e-cigarette that is shaped like a USB flash drive. Like other e-cigarettes, JUUL is a battery-powered device that heats a nicotine-containing liquid to produce an aerosol that is inhaled.
- All JUUL e-cigarettes have a high level of nicotine. According to the manufacturer, a single JUUL pod contains as much nicotine as a pack of 20 regular cigarettes.

- JUUL is one of a few e-cigarettes that use nicotine salts, which allow particularly high levels of nicotine to be inhaled more easily and with less irritation than the free-base nicotine that has traditionally been used in tobacco products, including e-cigarettes.
- News outlets and social media sites report widespread use of JUUL by students in schools, including classrooms and bathrooms.
- Approximately two-thirds of JUUL users aged 15–24 do not know that JUUL always contains nicotine.
- Although JUUL is currently the top-selling e-cigarette brand in the United States, other companies sell e-cigarettes that look like USB flash drives. Examples include the MarkTen Elite, a nicotine delivery device, and the PAX Era, a marijuana delivery device that looks like JUUL.
- Additional information about USB-shaped e-cigarettes and actions that parents, educators, and health-care providers can take to protect kids is available at the infographics of the Centers for Disease Control and Prevention (CDC) (www.cdc.gov/tobacco/infographics/youth/pdfs/e-cigarettes-usb-flash-508.pdf).

What Are the Other Risks of E-cigarettes for Kids, Teens, and Young Adults?

- Scientists are still learning about the long-term health effects of e-cigarettes.
- Some of the ingredients in e-cigarette aerosol could also be harmful to the lungs in the long term. For example, some E-cigarette flavorings may be safe to eat but not to inhale because the gut can process more substances than the lungs.
- Defective e-cigarette batteries have caused some fires and explosions, a few of which have resulted in serious injuries.
- Children and adults have been poisoned by swallowing, breathing, or absorbing e-cigarette liquid through their skin or eyes. Nationally, approximately 50 percent of calls to poison control centers for e-cigarettes are for kids five years of age or younger.

What Is in E-cigarette Aerosol?

- E-cigarette aerosol is not harmless "water vapor."
- The e-cigarette aerosol that users breathe from the device and exhale can contain harmful and potentially harmful substances, including the following:
  - nicotine
  - ultrafine particles that can be inhaled deep into the lungs
  - flavorings such as diacetyl, a chemical linked to a serious lung disease
  - volatile organic compounds
  - cancer-causing chemicals
  - heavy metals such as nickel, tin, and lead1

- The aerosol that users inhale and exhale from e-cigarettes can expose both themselves and bystanders to harmful substances.
- It is difficult for consumers to know what e-cigarette products contain. For example, some e-cigarettes marketed as containing zero percent nicotine have been found to contain nicotine.

Flavors and Marketing Make E-cigarettes Appealing to Youth

- E-cigarettes come in various flavors, including fruit, candy, mint, and menthol.
- A study from 2013–2014 showed that most youth who use e-cigarettes first start with a flavored variety, and flavors are the primary reason youth report using e-cigarettes.
- In 2022, most youth who reported using e-cigarettes used flavored varieties (84.9%). Among middle and high school students who currently used any type of flavored e-cigarette in 2022, the most commonly used flavors were fruit (69.1%); candy, desserts, or other sweets (38.3%); mint (29.4%); and menthol (26.6%).
- On January 2, 2020, the U.S. Food and Drug Administration (FDA) finalized an enforcement policy that prohibits the sale of prefilled cartridge e-cigarettes in any flavor other than tobacco or menthol, unless authorized by the FDA. The FDA has since taken additional steps to prohibit certain companies from selling youth-appealing, flavored disposable e-cigarettes and flavored e-liquids without authorization.
- Several states and communities have restricted the sale of flavored tobacco products, including menthol-flavored products.
- E-cigarettes are also advertised using the same themes and tactics that have been shown to increase youth initiation of other tobacco products, including cigarettes. In 2021, approximately 76 percent of students reported exposure to tobacco product marketing through traditional sources and approximately 74 percent of students who used social media had seen e-cigarette-related posts or content.
- Widespread advertising for e-cigarettes, including via media for which advertising for conventional tobacco products is prohibited (e.g., TV), and the lower costs of some e-cigarettes relative to regular cigarettes have contributed to use among youth.
- Many youth also reported using e-cigarettes because they are curious about these products.

Can Using E-cigarettes Lead to Future Cigarette Smoking among Kids, Teens, and Young Adults?

- Many young people who use e-cigarettes also smoke cigarettes. There is some evidence that young people who use e-cigarettes may be more likely to smoke cigarettes in the future.

- Specifically, a 2018 National Academy of Medicine (NAM) report found that there was some evidence that e-cigarette use increases the frequency and amount of cigarette smoking in the future.
- E-cigarettes can also be used to deliver other drugs, including marijuana; in 2016, approximately one-third of U.S. middle and high school students who have ever used an e-cigarette reported using marijuana in the device.
- But e-cigarette use among young people is still unsafe, even if they do not progress to future cigarette smoking.

Are E-cigarettes Safer than Cigarettes?

- E-cigarettes expose users to fewer harmful chemicals than burned cigarettes.
- But burned cigarettes are very dangerous, killing half of all people who smoke long term.
- The use of any tobacco product, including e-cigarettes, is unsafe for young people.

Are E-cigarettes Regulated at the Federal Level?

- In August 2016, the regulatory authority of the FDA was extended to cover e-cigarettes through the agency's "deeming rule."
- Through authority granted by the Family Smoking Prevention and Tobacco Control Act (FSPTCA), the FDA has authority to develop regulations that address the manufacturing, marketing, and sale of e-cigarettes.
- There are some strategies that the FDA does not have authority to implement, such as including e-cigarettes in smoke-free policies or increasing the minimum legal sales age for these products, unless directed to do so by Congress. However, the FSPTCA does not prevent states and communities from including e-cigarettes in smoke-free policies or from regulating the sale and distribution of e-cigarettes. These types of strategies can include further raising the minimum legal sales age, licensing retailers, implementing price policies, and restricting or prohibiting the sale of tobacco products.

Are There Any National Public Education Prevention Campaigns Focused on Youth and E-cigarettes?

- In 2018, the FDA expanded its successful youth tobacco prevention campaign, "The Real Cost," to reach the more than 10 million youth aged 12–17 who have used e-cigarettes or are open to trying them. The campaign educates youth about the potential risks of using e-cigarettes.
- The "Real Cost" reaches teens where they spend most of their time in school and online. The campaign is also placing e-cigarette prevention materials in high schools across the nation, both in school bathrooms and on educational digital platforms accessed by students during the school day.

The FDA Finalizes Enforcement Policy on Unauthorized Flavored Cartridge-Based E-cigarettes That Appeal to Children, including Fruit and Mint

Amid the epidemic levels of youth use of e-cigarettes and the popularity of certain products among children, the U.S. Food and Drug Administration (FDA) issued a policy prioritizing enforcement against certain unauthorized flavored e-cigarette products that appeal to kids, including fruit and mint flavors. Under this policy, companies that do not cease manufacture, distribution, and sale of unauthorized flavored cartridge-based e-cigarettes (other than tobacco or menthol) within 30 days risk FDA enforcement actions.

"The United States has never seen an epidemic of substance use arise as quickly as our current epidemic of youth use of e-cigarettes. The U.S. Department of Health and Human Services (HHS) is taking a comprehensive, aggressive approach to enforcing the law passed by Congress, under which no e-cigarettes are currently on the market legally," said HHS Secretary Alex Azar. "By prioritizing enforcement against the products that are most widely used by children, our action today seeks to strike the right public health balance by maintaining e-cigarettes as a potential off-ramp for adults using combustible tobacco while ensuring these products do not provide an on-ramp to nicotine addiction for our youth. We will not stand idly by as this crisis among America's youth grows and evolves, and we will continue monitoring the situation and take further actions as necessary."

"As we work to combat the troubling epidemic of youth e-cigarette use, the enforcement policy we are issuing today confirms our commitment to dramatically limit children's access to certain flavored e-cigarette products we know are so appealing to them—so-called cartridge-based products that are both easy to use and easily concealable. We will continue to use our full regulatory authority thoughtfully and thoroughly to tackle this alarming crisis that's affecting children, families, schools and communities," said FDA Commissioner Stephen M. Hahn, MD. "Coupled with the recently signed legislation increasing the minimum age of sale of tobacco to 21, we believe this policy balances the urgency with which we must address the public health threat of youth use of e-cigarette products with the potential role that e-cigarettes may play in helping adult smokers transition completely away from combustible tobacco to a potentially less risky form of nicotine delivery. While we expect that responsible members of industry will comply with premarket requirements, we're ready to take action against any unauthorized e-cigarette products as outlined in our priorities. We'll also closely monitor the use rates of all e-cigarette products and take additional steps to address youth use as necessary."

Source: "FDA Finalizes Enforcement Policy on Unauthorized Flavored Cartridge-Based E-cigarettes That Appeal to Children, including Fruit and Mint," U.S. Food and Drug Administration (FDA), January 2, 2020. Available online. URL: www.fda.gov/news-events/press-announcements/fda-finalizes-enforcement-policy-unauthorized-flavored-cartridge-based-e-cigarettes-appeal-children. Accessed September 27, 2023.

What Can You Do to Prevent Your Child from Using E-cigarettes or to Help Them Stop?

- Set a good example by being tobacco-free and ensure that your kid is not exposed to the secondhand emissions from any tobacco products, including e-cigarettes.
- If you use tobacco, it is never too late to quit. For free help, visit smokefree.gov or call 800-QUIT-NOW.
- Talk to your child or teen about why e-cigarettes are harmful for them. It is never too late.

- Get the Talk With Your Teen About E-cigarettes (https://e-cigarettes.surgeongeneral.gov/documents/SGR_ECig_ParentTipSheet_508.pdf) tip sheet for parents. Start the conversation early with children about why e-cigarettes are harmful for them.[1]

[1] "Quick Facts on the Risks of E-cigarettes for Kids, Teens, and Young Adults," Centers for Disease Control and Prevention (CDC), August 30, 2023. Available online. URL: www.cdc.gov/tobacco/basic_information/e-cigarettes/Quick-Facts-on-the-Risks-of-E-cigarettes-for-Kids-Teens-and-Young-Adults.html. Accessed September 27, 2023.

CHAPTER 12
LAWS AND REGULATIONS RELATED TO E-CIGARETTES

State Legislative Activity

Restrictions on Sales to Underage Persons

As of March 31, 2023, all 50 states, the District of Columbia, Guam, the Northern Mariana Islands, Palau, Puerto Rico, and the U.S. Virgin Islands have passed legislation prohibiting the sale of e-cigarettes to underage persons.

American Samoa and the Marshall Islands do not have any legislation prohibiting the sale of e-cigarettes to persons under a certain age.

Retail Licensure on E-cigarettes

As of March 31, 2023, 34 states (Alabama, Alaska, Arkansas, California, Colorado, Connecticut, Florida, Georgia, Hawaii, Idaho, Indiana, Iowa, Kansas, Louisiana, Maine, Maryland, Massachusetts, Minnesota, Montana, Nebraska, Nevada, New Hampshire, New Jersey, New Mexico, New York, North Dakota, Ohio, Oregon, Pennsylvania, Rhode Island, Texas, Utah, Vermont, and Washington), the District of Columbia, the Northern Mariana Islands, Palau, and the U.S. Virgin Islands have passed legislation that requires a retail license to sell e-cigarettes over the counter (OTC).

Smokefree Indoor Air Laws, including E-cigarettes

As of March 31, 2023, 17 states (California, Colorado, Connecticut, Delaware, Hawaii, Massachusetts, Minnesota, New Jersey, New Mexico, New York, North Dakota, Ohio, Oregon, Rhode Island, South Dakota, Utah, and Vermont), the District of Columbia, and Puerto Rico have passed comprehensive smoke-free indoor air laws that include e-cigarettes. These laws prohibit smoking and the use of e-cigarettes in indoor areas of private worksites, restaurants, and bars.

Effective October 1, 2018, Alaska implemented new legislation prohibiting smoking and the use of e-cigarettes in indoor areas of private worksites, restaurants, and bars. Also included in the legislation is an option for a municipality to opt out of these provisions through a voter referendum. Because municipalities in Alaska are able to exempt themselves from this legislation, it is not considered to be a comprehensive smoke-free indoor air policy that includes e-cigarettes.

E-cigarette Tax

As of March 31, 2023, 30 states (California, Colorado, Connecticut, Delaware, Georgia, Illinois, Indiana, Kansas, Kentucky, Louisiana, Maine, Maryland, Massachusetts, Minnesota, Nevada, New Hampshire, New Jersey, New Mexico, New York, North Carolina, Ohio, Oregon, Pennsylvania, Utah, Vermont, Virginia, Washington, West Virginia, Wisconsin, and Wyoming), the District of Columbia, Puerto Rico, and the U.S. Virgin Islands have passed legislation that requires a tax on e-cigarettes. Twelve states (Connecticut, Delaware, Kansas, Louisiana, New Jersey, North Carolina, Ohio, Utah, Virginia, Washington, West Virginia, and Wisconsin) tax e-cigarettes per milliliter of liquid or consumable material. Fifteen states (California, Colorado, Illinois, Indiana, Maine, Maryland, Massachusetts, Minnesota, Nevada, New York, Oregon, Pennsylvania, Utah, Vermont, and Wyoming), the District of Columbia, and the U.S. Virgin Islands tax e-cigarettes on a percentage of a specified cost. Georgia, Kentucky, New Hampshire, and New Mexico tax closed e-cigarette systems (prefilled cartridges) per milliliter of liquid and open e-cigarette systems (refillable cartridges) on a percentage of a specified cost. Puerto Rico taxes the e-cigarette device themselves if disposable, and the nicotine cartridge per milliliter of consumable liquid.[1]

Taxes on Tobacco Help Reduce the Number of Tobacco Users

In the United States, tobacco use is the leading cause of preventable disease, disability, and death. More than 480,000 people die prematurely in the United States annually, and another 16 million have a serious illness caused by smoking or exposure to secondhand smoke. Each year, smoking costs the United States more than $225 billion in direct medical costs and more than $156 billion in lost productivity. The Best Practices for Comprehensive Tobacco Control Programs of the Centers for Disease Control and Prevention (CDC) concludes that the more states spend on comprehensive tobacco control programs, the greater the reductions in smoking. However, in fiscal year 2021, states will receive $26.9 billion from tobacco taxes and cigarette company payments from the lawsuits they settled in 1998 but will only spend $656 million—less than 3 percent for tobacco control programs. In 2019, the tobacco industry spent $7.62 billion on advertising and promotion of cigarettes. This translates to more

[1] "State System E-cigarette Fact Sheet," Centers for Disease Control and Prevention (CDC), May 26, 2023. Available online. URL: www.cdc.gov/statesystem/factsheets/ecigarette/ECigarette.html. Accessed September 26, 2023.

than $21 million every day, or almost $1 million every hour. States reaching recommended levels of investment in tobacco control is an integral component of meeting the Healthy People 2030 objective to reduce current cigarette smoking among adults to 5 percent or less by the year 2030.

According to the U.S. Surgeon General, increasing the price of cigarettes through strategies such as excise tax increases are an effective policy intervention to prevent initiation of tobacco use, promote cessation, and reduce the prevalence and intensity of tobacco use among adolescents and young adults. The CDC found that an increase in excise taxes in Massachusetts, for example, when combined with an antismoking campaign, produced a 19.7 percent decline in cigarette consumption per capita four years after the tax increase was initiated. Young people are particularly sensitive to tobacco product price increases, and a study by the independent CDC Task Force on Community Preventive Services concluded that increasing the unit price for tobacco products is an effective method for reducing tobacco use among young adults and adolescents. The largest impact on cigarette demand for youths is the perceived price of cigarettes. Increasing excise taxes on tobacco products is especially effective in discouraging initiation among young people who have not developed an addiction to tobacco, thus protecting their health and increasing their likelihood of remaining tobacco-free.

States' Activity to Reduce Tobacco Use through Excise Taxes

Cigarettes

Through March 31, 2023, the state excise tax on cigarettes ranges from $0.17 per pack in Missouri to $4.35 per pack in Connecticut and New York. The federal tax remains at $1.01 per pack. Four states (Georgia, Missouri, North Carolina, and North Dakota) have an excise tax on cigarettes that is less than $0.50 per pack. Nine states (Alabama, Idaho, Indiana, Mississippi, Nebraska, South Carolina, Tennessee, Virginia, and Wyoming) have an excise tax on cigarettes from $0.50 to $0.99 per pack. Eight states (Arkansas, Florida, Iowa, Kansas, Kentucky, Louisiana, Texas, and West Virginia), the Marshall Islands, and the U.S. Virgin Islands have cigarette excise taxes from $1.00 to $1.49 per pack. Seven states (Colorado, Montana, Nevada, New Hampshire, Ohio, South Dakota, and Utah) have cigarette excise taxes from $1.50 to $1.99 per pack. In 2006, only six states had an excise tax rate of at least $2.00. Twelve states (Alaska, Arizona, California, Delaware, Illinois, Maine, Michigan, New Jersey, New Mexico, Oklahoma, Pennsylvania, and Wisconsin) have a cigarette excise tax from $2.00 to $2.99 per pack. Seven states (Hawaii, Maryland, Massachusetts, Minnesota, Oregon, Vermont, and Washington) and the Northern Mariana Islands have a cigarette excise tax from $3.00 to $3.99 per pack. Three states (Connecticut, New York, and Rhode Island), the District of Columbia, and Guam have a cigarette excise tax of $4.00 or greater. Palau and Puerto Rico have a cigarette excise tax of $5.00 or greater, and in American Samoa, the cigarette excise tax is $6.00.

Cigars

As of March 31, 2023, two states (Florida and Pennsylvania), the District of Columbia, and Palau do not tax cigars. The remaining states tax cigars either on a per-unit basis or by a percentage of the product price. Five states (Alabama, Arizona, Oklahoma, Texas, and Vermont), American Samoa, Guam, and Puerto Rico tax cigars based on a per-unit basis and vary greatly in range, from $0.01 to $2.00. The other 43 states, the Marshall Islands, the Northern Mariana Islands, and the U.S. Virgin Islands tax cigars as a percentage of the product price. Eight states (Arkansas, Connecticut, Iowa, Michigan, New Mexico, Oregon, Rhode Island, and Wisconsin) limit the maximum cigar tax to $0.50 per cigar. In North Carolina, the maximum cigar tax is $0.30 per cigar, and in Washington, the maximum cigar tax is $0.65 per cigar.

Little Cigars

States tax little cigars in one of the following ways: defined and taxed separately as "little cigars," defined as and taxed as "tobacco products," or defined as and taxed as "cigarettes." One state (Florida), the Marshall Islands, the Northern Mariana Islands, and Palau do not tax little cigars in any manner. Four states (Alabama, Arizona, Georgia, and Texas) tax little cigars separately with taxes ranging from $0.02 to $0.44 per pack. Sixteen states (California, Hawaii, Illinois, Iowa, Massachusetts, Minnesota, Nebraska, New Hampshire, New Mexico, New York, Oklahoma, Pennsylvania, Rhode Island, Utah, Vermont, and Washington), American Samoa, the District of Columbia, Guam, and Puerto Rico tax little cigars as cigarettes. The other 29 states and the U.S. Virgin Islands tax little cigars as tobacco products.

Roll-Your-Own Tobacco

Five states (Alabama, Arizona, Pennsylvania, Texas, and Vermont), American Samoa, Guam, and Palau tax roll-your-own tobacco on a per ounce basis ranging from $0.03 to $8.33. Two states (North Dakota and Rhode Island), the Marshall Islands, and Puerto Rico do not tax roll-your-own tobacco. The remaining states, the District of Columbia, the Northern Mariana Islands, and the U.S. Virgin Islands tax roll-your-own tobacco on a percentage of a specified cost.

Pipe Tobacco

The Marshall Islands and Puerto Rico do not tax pipe tobacco. Four states (Alabama, Arizona, Pennsylvania, and Texas), American Samoa, Guam, and Palau tax pipe tobacco on a per ounce basis ranging from $0.03 to $8.33. The remaining states, the District of Columbia, the Northern Mariana Islands, and the U.S. Virgin Islands tax pipe tobacco on a percentage of a specified cost.

Noncombustible Tobacco

Unlike the tax on cigarettes (calculated per pack), the tax on noncombustible tobacco (sometimes referred to as "smokeless tobacco") is usually measured either in a dollar amount per ounce or as a percentage of a price (such as the wholesale or manufacturer's price), and the calculations vary by state. There are five product types within the noncombustible tobacco category, and the states can tax all of the products equally under a broad definition, or separately, citing specific product types. For example, Montana taxes "smokeless tobacco" at 50 percent of the wholesale price with moist snuff taxed separately at $0.85 per ounce, whereas Minnesota's noncombustible tobacco tax is 95 percent of the Wholesale Sales Price across all product types. Twenty-one states and Puerto Rico have defined excise taxes on certain types of noncombustible tobacco, such as chewing tobacco and dry and moist snuff. American Samoa does not tax any form of noncombustible tobacco. The other 29 states, the District of Columbia, Guam, the Marshall Islands, the Northern Mariana Islands, Palau, and the U.S. Virgin Islands tax these products together generally.

Chewing Tobacco

Seven states (Alabama, Arizona, Kentucky, Maine, North Dakota, Pennsylvania, and Texas), Guam, and Puerto Rico tax chewing tobacco on a per-ounce basis, ranging from $0.01 to $3.31 per ounce. American Samoa, the Marshall Islands, and Palau do not tax chewing tobacco. The remaining states, the District of Columbia, the Northern Mariana Islands, and the U.S. Virgin Islands tax it on a percentage basis.

Dissolvable Tobacco

Twenty-five states, American Samoa, Guam, the Northern Mariana Islands, and Puerto Rico do not tax dissolvable tobacco. Three states (Pennsylvania, Texas, and Vermont), the Marshall Islands, and Palau tax dissolvables on a per ounce basis. The remaining states, the District of Columbia, and the U.S. Virgin Islands tax dissolvables on a percentage basis of a specified cost.

Dry Snuff Tobacco

Fourteen states (Alabama, Arizona, Connecticut, Iowa, Kentucky, Maine, Nebraska, New York, North Dakota, Pennsylvania, Rhode Island, Texas, Vermont, and Virginia), Guam, the Marshall Islands, Palau, and Puerto Rico tax dry snuff on a per-ounce basis ranging from $0.01 per ounce to $8.33 per ounce. American Samoa does not tax dry snuff. The rest of the states, the District of Columbia, the Northern Mariana Islands, and the U.S. Virgin Islands tax dry snuff on a percentage of a specified cost.

Moist Snuff Tobacco

Twenty-three states, Guam, the Marshall Islands, Palau, and Puerto Rico tax moist snuff on a per ounce basis ranging from $0.01 per ounce to $8.33 per ounce. American Samoa does not tax moist snuff. The remaining states, the District of Columbia, the Northern Mariana Islands, and the U.S. Virgin Islands tax moist snuff on a percentage of a specified cost.

Snus Tobacco

Four states (Alabama, Connecticut, New Hampshire, and North Dakota), American Samoa, the Northern Mariana Islands, and Puerto Rico do not tax snus. Six states (Arizona, Kentucky, Maine, Pennsylvania, Texas, and Vermont), Guam, the Marshall Islands, and Palau tax snus on a per ounce basis. The remaining states, the District of Columbia, and the U.S. Virgin Islands tax snus on a percentage of a specified cost.[2]

[2] "State System Excise Tax Fact Sheet," Centers for Disease Control and Prevention (CDC), May 26, 2023. Available online. URL: www.cdc.gov/statesystem/factsheets/excisetax/ExciseTax.html. Accessed September 26, 2023.

CHAPTER 13
VAPING CESSATION

Quitting vaping can be easier when you prepare in advance and have a plan. Find out what steps you can take to get ready to quit vaping.

Know Why You Are Quitting

There are many good reasons to stop vaping. Do you want to feel healthier? Save money? Knowing why you want to quit vaping can help you stay motivated and focused on your goal to become vape-free.

Think about the things in your life that are important to you. Does vaping get in the way of what is important? If you are not sure, try asking yourself the following questions:

- Is vaping affecting my health?
- Is vaping controlling my life?
- How does vaping affect the way I think and feel?
- How does vaping affect my relationships with my friends, parents, boyfriend/girlfriend, or other people important to me?
- How does vaping or thinking about vaping interfere with my schoolwork or grades?
- Are there activities that I used to enjoy that I do not enjoy anymore because of vaping?
- Am I spending a lot of money to keep vaping?
- What am I looking forward to the most after quitting?

Your answers to these questions can help you see how vaping is affecting your life, maybe in ways you had not thought about before. Make a list of all the reasons that you want to quit vaping and put it in a place where you will see it often. It might help keep the list on your phone. When you have the urge to vape, look at the list to remind yourself why you want to stop vaping. Frequently reminding yourself why you want to quit can keep you focused on quitting vaping.

Set Your Quit Date

The first step to giving up vaping is to choose a date to quit. Here are some tips to help you pick a quit date:

- **Give yourself time to get ready**. Getting ready can help you feel confident and give you the skills you will need to stay quit.
- **Do not put it off for too long**. Picking a date too far away gives you time to change your mind or become less interested in quitting. Choose a date that is no more than a week or two away.
- **Set yourself up for success**. Try not to pick a quit date that will be stressful, such as the day before a big test.

Have you picked your quit date? Circle it on your calendar or set an alert on your phone and make sure you have a plan for what you will do on the big day.

Know What Challenges to Expect

The first few weeks of quitting vaping are usually the hardest. Take it one day at a time. You may face some challenges along the way, but knowing what to expect and being prepared can help.

- **Learn your triggers**. Certain people, feelings, or situations can cause you to want to vape. It is important to know your triggers. It may be best to avoid situations that can trigger you to vape when you are in the early stages of your quit.
- **Prepare for cravings and withdrawal**. Think about how you will fight cravings and deal with withdrawal symptoms. Knowing what to expect and having strategies for handling thoughts about vaping or uncomfortable feelings will help you succeed and stay with your quit in those tough moments.
- **Resist temptations**. Avoid places and situations where others are vaping. If you cannot avoid being around vaping, plan for how you will handle these situations. Maybe that means you take a temporary break from friends you vape with and think about what you will say if somebody offers you a vape.

Imagine Your Vape-Free Self

It might be hard to imagine your life without e-cigarettes—especially if vaping is something you do a lot throughout the day. You might feel like a piece of yourself is missing when you first quit. It can take time to get used to the new vape-free you, but over time, this will become your new normal. Here are some strategies that can help:

- **Make the mental shift**. Start thinking of yourself as someone who does not vape. This will help separate you from vaping and give you the confidence to quit and stay quit.

- **Focus on the positive**. Make a list of all the positive things about yourself that do not involve vaping and put it somewhere you can see often, such as on your bedroom wall or phone. It will remind you that vaping does not define who you are.
- **Picture the future you**. Think about who you want to be in the future. Compare that with who you are now. Ask yourself: How are they different? How does vaping get in the way of what you want for the future? The answer to this can help motivate you to stick to your decision to quit.

Build Your Team

Surrounding yourself with supportive people can make it easier to quit vaping. Friends, family, coworkers, and others can be there to listen, boost your mood, and distract you from using your vape.

- **Ask for help**. You do not have to do it alone. If you feel comfortable, tell your friends and family that you are quitting vaping and that you will need their support. Here are some ways to ask for the support you need:
  - **Be specific**. Whether you need tough love or something softer, tell your friends and family what type of support you want and how often you want their help. For example, if you are feeling stressed or anxious after school, ask a friend to help keep you distracted.
  - **Say thank you**. Tell your support team you appreciate them. A thank-you can go a long way—and it does not take much time. Research also shows that being grateful can improve physical health, mental health, and self-esteem.
  - **Support others**. Support is a two-way street. Check in with your friends and ask them what you can do to help them. Or do something to brighten someone's day.
- **Talk to a doctor**. Talk to your doctor or another health-care professional about how to quit vaping. Ask how they might be able to help you. They can offer support and resources.
- **Talk to a tobacco cessation counselor**. Get free, personalized support from an expert. Call 800-QUIT-NOW (800-784-8669) or 877-44U-QUIT (877-448-7848) to talk with a tobacco cessation counselor. You can also chat online using the LiveHelp service of the National Cancer Institute (NCI).
- **Deal with people who do not get it**. Some important people in your life may not understand your decision to quit. It can be frustrating or discouraging when someone in your life is not as supportive as you would like. Try one of the following strategies:
  - **Distance yourself**. You may need to take a break from unsupportive people when you first quit. Let them know that you need to make quitting vaping your priority right now.

- **Recommit to quitting**. Remind yourself why you are quitting and why being vape-free is important to you.
- **Ask them to respect your decision**. Not everyone will know how to be supportive, and that is okay. Ask them not to vape around you or offer you to use their vape.
- **Lean on positive people**. Spend time with people who make you feel good about your decision and who want you to quit.[1]

[1] Smokefree Teen, "How to Quit Vaping," U.S. Department of Health and Human Services (HHS), July 18, 2019. Available online. URL: https://teen.smokefree.gov/quit-vaping/how-to-quit-vaping. Accessed October 4, 2023.

CHAPTER 14
DEALING WITH VAPING CESSATION

Your first day without vaping can be tough. Here are five steps you can take to handle your quit day.

Steps to Handle Your Quit Day

Step 1: Do Not Vape

On your quit day, the most important thing is that you do not vape—not even one hit. Having a plan for how you will deal with triggers and urges to vape can make your quit day easier. Take it one day at a time. Focus on getting through without vaping.

If you smoke cigarettes or use other tobacco products, now is a good time to quit those, too. We know it can seem challenging to quit smoking or using other tobacco products at the same time as quitting vaping, but becoming totally tobacco-free is the best thing you can do for your health. There are free tools to help you quit. Download the quitSTART app (https://teen.smokefree.gov/become-smokefree/quitstart-app), sign up for SmokefreeTXT (https://teen.smokefree.gov/become-smokefree/smoke-freeteen-signup), or chat with an expert online using LiveHelp of the National Cancer Institute (NCI).

Step 2: Stay Busy

You will probably think about vaping a lot, which is totally normal. Staying busy will help you keep your mind off vaping, withdrawal symptoms, and cravings. Try some of the following activities:

- Go for a walk, ride a bike, or do your favorite workout.
- Make a new playlist on your favorite music app.
- Have gum or sugar-free candy handy.
- Keep your hands busy with a pen or toothpick or play a game on your phone.
- Drink lots of water.

- Relax with deep breathing.
- Plan a fun activity with friends and family who do not use vapes or any other tobacco products.

Step 3: Avoid Vaping Triggers

Triggers are the people, places, things, and situations that set off your urge to vape. On your quit day, try to avoid triggers. Here are some tips to help you outsmart some common vaping triggers:

- Throw away your vapes, e-liquid bottles, pods, and chargers.
- Go to places where vaping is not allowed.
- Stay off social media accounts that remind you of vaping.
- Get plenty of rest and eat healthy. Feeling tired or run-down can trigger you to vape.
- Change your routine to avoid the places and things you might associate with vaping.

Step 4: Ask for Help

You do not have to do this alone. Tell your family and friends when your quit day is. Ask them for support on quit day and in the first few days and weeks after. They can help you get through the rough spots. Let them know exactly how they can support you. For example, ask a friend to help you celebrate your first day being vape-free.

You can also get free support from a tobacco cessation expert by calling 800-QUIT-NOW (800-784-8669) or 877-44U-QUIT (877-448-7848) or by chatting online using the NCI's LiveHelp chat service.

Step 5: Reward Yourself

At the end of the day, reward yourself for being vape-free for 24 hours. You deserve it. It does not have to be a big or expensive reward. Even taking extra time to do a favorite vape-free activity will make you feel good and help you be ready for day two of your quit attempt.[1]

[1] Smokefree Teen, "Your First Day without Vaping," U.S. Department of Health and Human Services (HHS), July 19, 2019. Available online. URL: https://teen.smokefree.gov/quit-vaping/your-first-day-without-vaping. Accessed October 4, 2023.

CHAPTER 15
UNDERSTANDING VAPING TRIGGERS

Triggers are the things that make you want to vape, such as dealing with a stressful situation or seeing someone else vape. Understanding your triggers and learning how to deal with them will help you quit vaping for good.

Know Your Triggers

When you first started vaping, it probably was not a big part of your life. But, over time, you have built up patterns and routines around vaping. When you quit vaping, it may seem like reminders of vaping are all around you. These reminders can make it hard to stay vape-free.

You may not be able to avoid all the things that remind you of vaping—especially if you vape during many different activities or frequently throughout the day. But knowing your triggers and having a plan will help you quit vaping for good. Here are some common triggers and strategies for how to deal with them.

Social Triggers

Social situations or events—even scrolling through social media—can trigger the desire to vape. For example, you may crave your vape when you:

- see someone else use a vape
- smell aerosol from a vape (sometimes called "vapor")
- hang out with friends who vape or use another tobacco product
- go to a party or other social event
- study with friends
- are offered a vape or a new flavor
- see vapes on social media

How to Deal with Social Triggers

Many people who have quit vaping find it helpful to make some changes to their social lives, at least for a little while. Once you have decided to quit, you may want to do the following:

- **Plan ahead**. Think about how you will handle social situations where others are vaping. Practice what you will say if somebody offers you a vape. Keep it simple and direct—"No thanks, I quit."
- **Avoid places where people vape**. Going to parties or hanging out at a friend's house where you know people will be vaping may make it harder to stay quit. Explain to your friends that you are not avoiding them but that you are avoiding situations that might make you want to vape.
- **Ask others not to vape around you**. If you are around people using vapes, ask them not to offer you to use theirs.
- **Take a break from social media**. Unfollow social media accounts with images and videos of vape tricks. Unsubscribe to emails that link to places that sell vapes, e-liquids, or pods.

Over time, it will get easier to handle social situations that make you want to vape. Try to stick with it and continue to ask friends and family for their support. You can quit vaping and still have a social life.

- **Lean on supportive people**. Tell your family and/or friends that you are quitting and ask for their help. Spend time with people who make you feel good about yourself and want you to achieve your vape-free goal.
- **Find other ways to connect and have fun**. Remember that vaping does not define you or your friendships. You and your friends have plenty of things in common besides vaping. It is helpful to remind yourself of what those things are.
- **Be ready for change**. If you want to quit and your friends do not, it could change some of your relationships. Being ready for those changes—some good, some bad—can help you when you stop vaping.

Source: Smokefree Teen, "Understand Your Vaping Triggers," U.S. Department of Health and Human Services (HHS), July 19, 2019. Available online. URL: https://teen.smokefree.gov/quit-vaping/understand-your-vaping-triggers. Accessed October 4, 2023.

Triggers in Your Everyday Life

Many people connect vaping with certain activities or parts of their daily routine. Plan ahead with ways to stay vape-free when you are:

- texting or playing on your phone
- going into the school bathroom
- seeing ads for vapes throughout the day
- studying or doing homework
- watching TV or playing video games
- walking or driving

How to Deal with Triggers in Your Everyday Life

Breaking the links between your daily routine and vaping can help you stay vape-free. Here are some tips:

- **Throw out your vapes, chargers, and pods**. Getting rid of daily reminders of vaping will help you resist temptations and make it harder to slip back into vaping.
- **Find a replacement behavior**. Do something else with your hands/mouth instead of using your vape, such as chewing sugar-free gum, eating sugar-free candy and mints, doodling, or playing a game on your phone.
- **Change your daily routine**. Switching things up can help you avoid triggers associated with your old routine. Take a different route to school, change where you eat lunch and/or who you eat with, or sign up for a new after-school activity.
- **Stay busy**. Go for a walk, study, exercise, or listen to a podcast. Try something new or do something you already love. Staying busy can take your mind off vaping.
- **Be careful of downtime**. You might be used to vaping during breaks or in between classes. Use this time to do something else—get a head start on your homework, read a book, or check sports stats.

If you smoke cigarettes or use other tobacco products besides vapes, now is a good time to quit those too. These products contain nicotine and are harmful to your health. There are free tools to help you quit. Download the quitSTART app, sign up for SmokefreeTXT, or chat with an expert online using the LiveHelp service of the National Cancer Institute (NCI; https://livehelp.cancer.gov/app/chat/chat_launch).

Emotional Triggers

Emotions can be powerful triggers for vaping. It is common to want to vape to escape a bad mood or to make a good mood better.

For example, you may notice an urge to vape when you are having negative emotions, such as:

- stressed or anxious
- lonely
- bored
- sad
- frustrated or upset after an argument

Positive emotions can also trigger the urge to vape, such as when you are feeling:

- happy
- excited
- relieved

Dealing with Emotional Triggers

You can learn to manage your feelings without reaching for your vape. Try the following tips:

- **Take a break**. Taking a "time-out" from an upsetting or stressful situation can help you calm down. Go for a walk, listen to music, or find a quiet spot and take some slow, deep breaths.
- **Move around**. Getting your body moving is a great way to handle emotions—both positive and negative. Dance, shoot some hoops, or find a workout class or video that gets you moving.
- **Care for yourself**. Eating a balanced diet, drinking lots of water, and getting enough sleep will help keep your mind and body feeling good.
- **Reward yourself**. Even small things such as watching a clip of your favorite show, listening to a favorite song or podcast, or giving yourself an extra 30 minutes of doing whatever makes you happy can boost your mood. This is also a great way to celebrate when you are feeling good.
- **Reach out to others**. Whether you are feeling good or bad, turn to the people who care about you. Your friends, parents, doctor, or other trusted adults can help you celebrate successes and bring you up when you are feeling down. You can also get free, personalized support from a tobacco cessation expert by calling 800-QUIT-NOW (800-784-8669) or 877-44U-QUIT (877-448-7848) or chatting with an expert online using the NCI's LiveHelp service.[1]

[1] Smokefree Teen, "Understand Your Vaping Triggers," U.S. Department of Health and Human Services (HHS), July 19, 2019. Available online. URL: https://teen.smokefree.gov/quit-vaping/understand-your-vaping-triggers. Accessed October 4, 2023.

CHAPTER 16

VAPING ADDICTION AND NICOTINE WITHDRAWAL

Most vapes contain nicotine, which is very addictive. Over time, your brain and body get used to having nicotine, which means you may have nicotine withdrawal symptoms when you quit vaping. Find out what you can do to help manage your withdrawal symptoms.

Nicotine Addiction

Nicotine is in most vapes and is very addictive. The more you vape, the more your brain and body get used to having nicotine, and the harder it is to go without it. When you go without vaping, the nicotine level in your bloodstream drops, which may cause unpleasant feelings, physical symptoms, and strong urges to vape. This is nicotine addiction.

If you answer yes to one or more of the following questions, you may be addicted to vaping:

- Do you continue to vape even though you want to quit or think it is hurting you in some way?
- Do you feel anxious or irritable when you want to use your vape but cannot?
- Do thoughts about vaping interrupt you when you are focused on other activities?
- Do you still vape after getting in trouble with your parents or school for vaping?
- Have you ever tried to quit vaping but could not?
- Do you feel like you have lost control over your vaping?

Knowing more about nicotine addiction—and recognizing that you may be addicted—will help you understand why your body feels like it does and why it sometimes feels like you cannot go a minute without thinking about vaping.

Nicotine Withdrawal Symptoms

When you quit vaping, your body and brain must get used to going without nicotine. This is called "nicotine withdrawal." The side effects of nicotine withdrawal can be uncomfortable and can trigger cravings for nicotine. Common nicotine withdrawal symptoms include the following:

- feeling irritable, restless, or jittery
- feeling sad or down
- feeling anxious
- feeling tired or groggy
- having trouble thinking clearly or concentrating
- having trouble sleeping
- feeling hungry
- having intense cravings for e-cigarettes[1]

Do Symptoms of Nicotine Withdrawal Improve after Quitting?

As long as a person stays quit, withdrawal symptoms will fade over time as the brain gets used to not having nicotine.

Does Quitting Vaping Improve Mental Health?

Scientists are still learning about the effects of quitting vaping on mental health. Quitting smoking cigarettes is associated with lower levels of anxiety, depression, and stress, as well as improved positive mood and quality of life (QOL).[2]

[1] Smokefree Teen, "Vaping Addiction and Nicotine Withdrawal," U.S. Department of Health and Human Services (HHS), July 19, 2019. Available online. URL: https://teen.smokefree.gov/quit-vaping/vaping-addiction-nicotine-withdrawal. Accessed September 28, 2023.

[2] "Quick Facts on the Risks of E-cigarettes for Kids, Teens, and Young Adults," Centers for Disease Control and Prevention (CDC), August 30, 2023. Available online. URL: www.cdc.gov/tobacco/basic_information/e-cigarettes/Quick-Facts-on-the-Risks-of-E-cigarettes-for-Kids-Teens-and-Young-Adults.html. Accessed September 28, 2023.

CHAPTER 17
ANXIETY, STRESS, AND VAPING

Stress and anxiety can trigger vape cravings and make it harder for you to quit for good. You may be tempted to reach for your vape when you have these feelings, but vaping is not an effective way to cope. There are healthy and effective ways to deal with stress and anxiety.

Stress and Anxiety

Stress is a normal part of life—everyday worries, responsibilities, and hassles all contribute to your overall stress level. Too much stress can make you feel overwhelmed and affect your mood. If you automatically reach for your vape when you are stressed out, you will need to have a plan for handling stress when you quit.

Anxiety is feeling worried, nervous, or panicky. Anxiety can be a reaction to stress, or it can be triggered by other things in your life. It is normal to experience anxiety from time to time, but anxiety can be a problem if it is frequent or interferes with your daily life.

Even if you rarely felt stressed or anxious before quitting vaping, you may feel increased stress, irritability, or anxiety after quitting. For some people, the experience of quitting can feel overwhelming. It might be hard to imagine yourself or your life without your vape. The good news is that these mood changes are usually temporary while your body adjusts to being without nicotine. The longer you go without nicotine, the better you will feel. When you are having a rough day, remember why quitting vaping will be better for you in the long run.

Tips for Managing Stress and Anxiety

You can manage feelings of stress and anxiety without reaching for your vape. Try these ideas—some may work better than others, so find the ones that work for you.

Stop and Breathe

Pause what you are doing and take a deep breath in through your nose and out through your mouth. Concentrate on the inhale and exhale of your breath. Interrupting the anxious feeling with conscious breathing can help you calm down and think clearly.

Learn Your Anxiety Triggers

Anxiety can happen without being triggered. But certain people, places, and situations can also trigger anxiety. Identify what makes you feel anxious or panicked and record it on your phone or in a journal. Do you see a pattern? Understanding your triggers is the first step in learning how to manage them.

Move Your Body

Getting your body moving is a great way to reduce stress and anxiety. When you exercise, your brain releases chemicals that make you feel good. Take a walk, hit the gym, or do some yoga.

Care for Yourself

Eating a balanced diet, drinking lots of water, and getting enough sleep will help your body keep your stress level down. Keep healthy snacks on hand and do not skip meals.

Be Present

Life can be overwhelming, especially when you get caught up in worrying about what is next. Instead, focus on what you can control and try to stay in the moment.

Decaffeinate

Caffeine can help you stay awake, but it can also make you feel tense, jittery, and stressed. That is not helpful when you are quitting vaping. Cutting back on or gradually eliminating caffeinated products—such as coffee, energy drinks, and some sodas—while you are quitting can reduce feelings of stress and anxiety.

Look Out for Signs of Serious Anxiety

Feeling anxious or irritable as you are quitting vaping is normal. But, if you are feeling extreme anxiety or mood changes, you may need help from a professional. You may feel like the symptoms are too extreme or will not go away. Watch for this, especially if you have ever had severe anxiety. If you feel like the anxiety is overwhelming, tell a supportive friend or family member and talk to your doctor.

If you need help now, do the following:

- Text the Crisis Text Line to talk with a trained crisis counselor via text message at any time of day or night by texting TALK to 741741. Counselors are trained to address any serious problems you may be having.
- Chat with a National Suicide Prevention Lifeline counselor (www.suicidepreventionlifeline.org/chat).
- Call the 24/7 National Suicide Prevention Lifeline at 800-273-TALK (800-273-8255) or 800-SUICIDE (800-784-2433) for free, private help or dial 911.

Source: Smokefree Teen, "Anxiety, Stress, and Vaping," U.S. Department of Health and Human Services (HHS), July 18, 2019. Available online. URL: https://teen.smokefree.gov/quit-vaping/anxiety-stress-vaping. Accessed October 4, 2023.

Reach Out to Loved Ones

You do not have to deal with stress alone. Focus on spending time with people who make you feel good about yourself and want to help you stay vape-free. Talk to your friends, family, teachers, school counselors, and other important people in your life who support you and your decision to stop vaping.

Accept Life's Ups and Downs

Life is full of twists and turns. You will always have some stress in your life. It helps understand that there will be good days and bad days.[1]

[1] Smokefree Teen, "Anxiety, Stress, and Vaping," U.S. Department of Health and Human Services (HHS), July 18, 2019. Available online. URL: https://teen.smokefree.gov/quit-vaping/anxiety-stress-vaping. Accessed October 4, 2023.

CHAPTER 18
DEPRESSION AND VAPING

You may be tempted to reach for your vape when you are feeling down, but vaping is not an effective way to cope with sadness or depression.

Sadness is a common emotion that can be triggered by ordinary life circumstances such as disappointments, challenges, or loss. Everyone has down days and times when they feel sad. If feelings of sadness are extreme, last for a long time, or interfere with your daily activities and/or relationships, you may be experiencing a depressed mood.

Even if you rarely felt sad before quitting vaping, you may feel increased sadness, irritability, or sluggishness after quitting. These mood changes are usually temporary while your body adjusts to being without nicotine. When you are having a rough day, remember why quitting vaping will be better for you in the long run.

You can learn to manage your feelings without reaching for your vape. Try these ideas—some may work better than others, so find the ones that work for you.

Get Active

Any kind of physical activity can help boost your mood, for example, taking a walk, going to the gym, or playing Frisbee with friends. If you need to, start small and build up over time. This can be hard to do because feeling down can drain your energy, but making the effort will pay off. It will help you feel better in the long run.

Stay Busy

Sadness and negative thoughts tend to creep up when you are bored and doing nothing. Create a schedule of activities that you do every day. Sticking to a daily routine can help you stay busy and avoid getting caught up in negative moods.

Do Something You Enjoy Each Day

Find ways to incorporate fun activities into your daily life. Small things—such as watching your favorite show or listening to music—add up and can help your mood. Choose an activity that you really enjoy but have not done in a while or try something new that you have always wanted to do.

Talk with Friends and Loved Ones

Getting support from the important people in your life can help your mood and make a big difference as you quit. They can be key to helping you feel better. Focus on spending time with people who make you feel good about yourself and want you to succeed in staying vape-free.

Do Good

Small acts of kindness, such as letting someone else go ahead of you in line, picking up litter, or giving someone a compliment, can boost your mood.

Look Out for Signs of Depression

It is normal to have ups and downs in your mood as you quit vaping. But, if you are feeling extreme sadness or mood changes, you may need help from a mental health professional. You may feel like the sadness is lasting too long or will not go away. Do not ignore these feelings, especially if a doctor has ever diagnosed you with depression. Take a quick quiz to find out if you have signs of depression. If you become depressed or are having extreme sadness, let a friend or family member know and think about talking to your doctor.[1]

[1] Smokefree Teen, "Depression and Vaping," U.S. Department of Health and Human Services (HHS), July 19, 2019. Available online. URL: https://teen.smokefree.gov/quit-vaping/depression-vaping. Accessed October 4, 2023.

CHAPTER 19
VAPING-RELATED LUNG INJURY OUTBREAK

Emergency department (ED) visits related to e-cigarette, or vaping, products continue to decline, after sharply increasing in August 2019 and peaking in September.

National and state data from patient reports and product sample testing show e-cigarette, or vaping, products containing tetrahydrocannabinol (THC), particularly from informal sources such as friends, family, or in-person or online dealers, are linked to most e-cigarette- or vaping-use-associated lung injury (EVALI) cases and play a major role in the outbreak.

Vitamin E acetate is strongly linked to the EVALI outbreak. Vitamin E acetate has been found in product samples tested by the U.S. Food and Drug Administration (FDA) and state laboratories and inpatient lung fluid samples tested by the Centers for Disease Control and Prevention (CDC) from geographically diverse states. Vitamin E acetate has not been found in the lung fluid of people who do not have EVALI.

Evidence is not sufficient to rule out the contribution of other chemicals of concern, including chemicals in either THC or non-THC products, in some of the reported EVALI cases.

Use of E-cigarette, or Vaping, Products

- Electronic cigarettes—or e-cigarettes—are also called "vapes," "e-hookahs," "vape pens," "tank systems," "mods," and "electronic nicotine delivery systems" (ENDS).
- Using an e-cigarette is commonly called "vaping."
- E-cigarettes work by heating a liquid to produce an aerosol that users inhale into their lungs.
- The liquid can contain nicotine, tetrahydrocannabinol (THC) and cannabinoid (CBD) oils, and other substances, flavorings, and additives. THC is the psychoactive mind-altering compound of marijuana that produces the "high."

Source: "Outbreak of Lung Injury Associated with the Use of E-cigarette, or Vaping, Products," Centers for Disease Control and Prevention (CDC), August 3, 2021. Available online. URL: www.cdc.gov/tobacco/basic_information/e-cigarettes/severe-lung-disease.html. Accessed September 26, 2023.

About the Outbreak

- As of February 18, 2020, a total of 2,807 hospitalized EVALI cases or deaths have been reported to the CDC from all 50 states, the District of Columbia, and two U.S. territories (Puerto Rico and the U.S. Virgin Islands).
  - Sixty-eight deaths have been confirmed in 29 states and the District of Columbia (as of February 18, 2020).
- ED visits related to e-cigarette, or vaping, products continue to decline, after sharply increasing in August 2019 and peaking in September.
  - National ED data and active case reporting from state health departments around the country show a sharp rise in symptoms or cases of EVALI in August 2019, a peak in September 2019, and a gradual, but persistent decline since then.
  - Reasons for the decline are likely multifactorial and may be related to the following:
    - increased public awareness of the risk associated with THC-containing e-cigarette, or vaping, product use as a result of the rapid public health response
    - removal of vitamin E acetate from some products
    - law enforcement actions related to illicit products
- Laboratory data show that vitamin E acetate, an additive in some THC-containing e-cigarette, or vaping, products, is strongly linked to the EVALI outbreak.
  - A study analyzed samples from 51 EVALI cases from 16 states and a comparison group of samples from 99 comparison individuals without EVALI for vitamin E acetate, plant oils, medium-chain triglyceride (MCT) oil, coconut oil, petroleum distillates, and diluent terpenes.
  - Vitamin E acetate was identified in bronchoalveolar lavage (BAL) fluid samples (fluid samples collected from the lungs) from 48 of the 51 EVALI patients but not in the BAL fluid from the healthy comparison group.
  - No other toxicants were found in BAL fluid from either group, except for coconut oil and limonene (one EVALI patient each).
- In August 2019, the CDC started collecting data from states on EVALI cases using a standardized case report form. The data were voluntarily collected and submitted by each state to the CDC on a routine basis. Due to the subsequent identification of the primary cause of EVALI and the considerable decline in EVALI cases and deaths since a peak in September 2019, the CDC stopped collecting these data from states as of February 2020.
  - However, the CDC continues to monitor EVALI-related trends using emergency department data from the BioSense/Electronic Surveillance System for the Early Notification of Community-based Epidemics (ESSENCE) platform of the National Syndromic Surveillance Program (NSSP). These data do not suggest a resurgence of EVALI at this time.

- The CDC encourages clinicians to continue to report possible cases of EVALI to their local or state health department for further investigation.[1]

Vitamin E Acetate

- Vitamin E acetate is used as an additive, most notably in THC-containing e-cigarette, or vaping, products.
- Vitamin E is a vitamin found in many foods, including vegetable oils, cereals, meat, fruits, and vegetables. It is also available as a dietary supplement and in many cosmetic products, such as skin creams.
- Vitamin E acetate usually does not cause harm when ingested as a vitamin supplement or applied to the skin. However, previous research suggests that when vitamin E acetate is inhaled, it may interfere with normal lung functioning. Vitamin E acetate is used as an additive, most notably in THC-containing e-cigarette, or vaping, products. Vitamin E is a vitamin found in many foods, including vegetable oils, cereals, meat, fruits, and vegetables. It is also available as a dietary supplement and in many cosmetic products, such as skin creams. Vitamin E acetate usually does not cause harm when ingested as a vitamin supplement or applied to the skin. However, previous research suggests that when vitamin E acetate is inhaled, it may interfere with normal lung functioning.

Source: "Outbreak of Lung Injury Associated with the Use of E-cigarette, or Vaping, Products," Centers for Disease Control and Prevention (CDC), August 3, 2021. Available online. URL: www.cdc.gov/tobacco/basic_information/e-cigarettes/severe-lung-disease.html. Accessed September 26, 2023.

Characteristics of a Nationwide Outbreak of E-cigarette- or Vaping-Use-Associated Lung Injury

Nationwide, 82 percent of patients hospitalized with EVALI reported the use of products that contain tetrahydrocannabinol (THC). Vitamin E acetate, an additive to THC-containing e-cigarette, or vaping, products, is strongly linked to the EVALI outbreak.

The number of EVALI cases reported to the CDC (see Table 19.1) peaked during the week of September 15, 2019; the weekly number of hospitalized patients has since steadily declined.

Clinicians and public health practitioners should remain vigilant for EVALI cases. The CDC recommends that persons not use THC-containing e-cigarette, or vaping, products, particularly from informal sources. Evidence is not sufficient to rule out the contribution of other chemicals of concern, including chemicals in either THC- or non-THC-containing products, in some reported EVALI cases.[2]

[1] "Outbreak of Lung Injury Associated with the Use of E-cigarette, or Vaping, Products," Centers for Disease Control and Prevention (CDC), August 3, 2021. Available online. URL: www.cdc.gov/tobacco/basic_information/e-cigarettes/severe-lung-disease.html. Accessed September 26, 2023.

[2] "Update: Characteristics of a Nationwide Outbreak of E-cigarette, or Vaping, Product Use–Associated Lung Injury—United States, August 2019–January 2020," Centers for Disease Control and Prevention (CDC), March 17, 2023. Available online. URL: www.cdc.gov/mmwr/volumes/69/wr/mm6903e2.htm?s_cid=mm6903e2_w. Accessed September 26, 2023.

Table 19.1. Demographic and Product Use Characteristics among Hospitalized Patients with E-cigarette- or Vaping-Use-Associated Lung Injury (EVALI) Reported to the CDC, United States, August 2019–January 2020*

Characteristic (No. with Available Information)	No. (%)[†] (N = 2,668)
Sex (2,606)	
Male	1,731 (66)
Female	875 (34)
Median age, years (range)	24 (13–85)
Age Group, Years (2,619)	
13–17	404 (15)
18–24	979 (37)
25–34	631 (24)
35–44	335 (13)
45–64	223 (9)
≥65	47 (2)
Race/Ethnicity[§] (1,856)	
White	1,360 (73)
Black	64 (3)
American Indian/Alaska Native	12 (1)
Asian/Native Hawaiian/Other Pacific Islander	38 (2)
Other	97 (5)
Hispanic	285 (15)
Case Status (2,668)	
Confirmed	1,401 (53)
Probable	1,267 (47)
Substances Used in E-cigarette, or Vaping, Products (2,022)[¶,]**	
Any THC-containing product	1,650 (82)
Any nicotine-containing product	1,162 (57)
Both THC- and nicotine-containing product use	834 (41)
Exclusive THC-containing product use	669 (33)
Exclusive nicotine-containing product use	274 (14)
No THC- or nicotine-containing product use reported	44 (2)

Abbreviation: *THC = tetrahydrocannabinol.*

** For cases reported to the CDC as of January 14, 2020.*

† Percentages might not sum to 100 percent because of rounding.

§ These were mutually exclusive groups. Whites, Blacks, American Indians/Alaska Natives, Asians/Native Hawaiians/Other Pacific Islanders, and Others were non-Hispanic. Hispanic persons could be of any race.

¶ Limited to persons who reported vaping or dabbing at least one substance in the past three months.

*** In the three months preceding symptom onset.*

PART 3 | NICOTINE DELIVERY SYSTEMS

CHAPTER 20
LIGHT CIGARETTES

What Is a Light Cigarette?

Tobacco manufacturers have been redesigning cigarettes since the 1950s. Certain redesigned cigarettes with the following features were marketed as "light" cigarettes:

- cellulose acetate filters (to trap tar)
- highly porous cigarette paper (to allow toxic chemicals to escape)
- ventilation holes in the filter tip (to dilute smoke with air)
- different blends of tobacco

When analyzed by a smoking machine, the smoke from a light cigarette has a lower yield of tar than the smoke from a regular cigarette. However, a machine cannot predict how much tar a smoker inhales. Also, studies have shown that changes in cigarette design have not lowered the risk of disease caused by cigarettes.

Are Light Cigarettes Less Hazardous Than Regular Cigarettes?

Many smokers chose low-tar, mild, light, or ultralight cigarettes because they thought these cigarettes would expose them to less tar and would be less harmful to their health than regular or full-flavor cigarettes. However, light cigarettes are no safer than regular cigarettes. Tar exposure from a light cigarette can be just as high as that from a regular cigarette if the smoker takes long, deep, or frequent puffs. The bottom line is that light cigarettes do not reduce the health risks of smoking.

Moreover, there is no such thing as a safe cigarette. The only guaranteed way to reduce the risk to your health, as well as the risk to others, is to stop smoking completely.

Because all tobacco products are harmful and cause cancer, the use of these products is strongly discouraged. There is no safe level of tobacco use. People who use any type of tobacco product should quit.

Do Light Cigarettes Cause Cancer?

People who smoke any kind of cigarette are at much greater risk of lung cancer than people who do not smoke. Smoking harms nearly every organ of the body and diminishes a person's overall health.

People who switch to light cigarettes from regular cigarettes are likely to have inhaled the same amount of toxic chemicals, and they remain at high risk of developing smoking-related cancers and other diseases. Smoking causes cancers of the lung, esophagus, larynx (voice box), mouth, throat, kidney, bladder, pancreas, stomach, and cervix, as well as acute myeloid leukemia.

Regardless of their age, smokers can substantially reduce their risk of disease, including cancer, by quitting.

Why Would Someone Smoking a Light Cigarette Take Bigger Puffs Than a Regular Cigarette?

Cigarette features that reduce the yield of machine-measured tar also reduce the yield of nicotine. Because smokers crave nicotine, they may inhale more deeply; take larger, more rapid, or more frequent puffs; or smoke extra cigarettes each day to get enough nicotine to satisfy their craving. As a result, smokers end up inhaling more tar, nicotine, and other harmful chemicals than the machine-based numbers suggest.

Tobacco industry documents show that companies were aware that smokers of light cigarettes compensated by taking bigger puffs. Industry documents also show that the companies were aware of the difference between machine-measured yields of tar and nicotine and what the smoker actually inhaled.[1]

Light Smoking

Light smoking is smoking regularly but not a lot of cigarettes at a time—maybe a few cigarettes a day. The term light does not mean this type of smoking is any less harmful. Light smoking has similar health risks to heavier smoking and can lead to addiction.

Source: Smokefree Teen, "Occasional & Social Smoking," U.S. Department of Health and Human Services (HHS), September 16, 2017. Available online. URL: https://teen.smokefree.gov/the-risks-of-tobacco/occasional-social-smoking. Accessed October 4, 2023.

[1] "'Light' Cigarettes and Cancer Risk," National Cancer Institute (NCI), October 28, 2010. Available online. URL: www.cancer.gov/about-cancer/causes-prevention/risk/tobacco/light-cigarettes-fact-sheet. Accessed October 4, 2023.

CHAPTER 21
MENTHOL CIGARETTES

Menthol is a chemical compound found naturally in peppermint and other similar plants. Menthol can also be produced in a lab.

Menthol can change the way the brain registers the sensations of taste and pain. In cigarettes, menthol creates a cooling sensation in the throat and airways, making the smoke feel less harsh and easier to inhale. Menthol is also used in other commercial tobacco products, such as e-cigarettes, cigars, hookah tobacco, smokeless tobacco, nicotine pouches, and heated tobacco products.

According to federal law, tobacco manufacturers cannot market cigarettes with "characterizing flavors," except for menthol- or tobacco-flavored cigarettes. Almost all the cigarettes sold in the United States contain some natural or lab-created menthol. However, there is usually more menthol in cigarettes marketed specifically as "menthol" compared to other cigarettes. In 2021, sales of menthol-flavored cigarettes made up 37 percent of all cigarette sales in the United States. This is the highest proportion since major tobacco companies were first required to report those data to the federal government in 1963 when menthol cigarettes made up 16 percent of all cigarette sales in the United States.

Menthol Tobacco Products Are a Public Health Problem

A Threat to Advancing Health Equity

Menthol cigarettes, including how and to whom they are marketed and sold, are a significant risk to public health and advancing health equity due to their role in initiation, progression to regular smoking and dependence, reduced cessation success, and contributing to health disparities.

The Tobacco Industry Marketing Menthol Products to Certain Populations

The tobacco industry targets menthol cigarette marketing to certain populations through advertisements, giveaways, lower prices, lifestyle branding, and event sponsorships. For example, tobacco companies have heavily marketed in Black-owned publications, through sponsorship of jazz concerts and certain civil rights groups, through advertisements showing people dressed in clothing popular with rap and hip-hop artists, and in neighborhoods with more Black residents. These aggressive marketing tactics likely have contributed to some groups of people having higher rates of use than others. Given how menthol interacts with nicotine, people who smoke menthol cigarettes are also more likely to continue smoking, which puts them at higher risk of getting tobacco-related diseases.

The tobacco industry uses similar strategies to market menthol cigars. For example, tobacco companies published advertisements in newspapers with a large proportion of readers who were Black persons. The industry has advertised menthol cigars on social media and has used hip-hop and rap artists, models, and music that are appealing to youth.

Menthol Cigarettes Putting Your Health at Risk Just as Much as Any Other Type of Cigarette

No tobacco product is safe, including those with menthol. Despite this, tobacco companies market menthol cigarettes as "smoother" than other cigarettes, and marketing messages imply that menthol cigarettes are a "healthier" alternative.

Menthol Increasing Initiation and Dependence in Youth and Young Adults

Menthol makes cigarettes more appealing and easier to smoke. In addition, menthol enhances the addictive effects of nicotine in the brain. The amount of nicotine, the addictive drug in tobacco products, in menthol cigarettes has increased in recent years.

Menthol in cigarettes makes it more likely that youth and young adults will try smoking and that those who start smoking will continue to smoke on a regular basis.

Tobacco companies have conducted extensive research on menthol. They adjust the amounts of menthol in cigarette brands to make each brand most appealing to the people they target. For example, the companies lowered the amount of menthol in some brands to make them more appealing to young people who smoke and those just starting to smoke. The companies increased the amount of menthol in other brands to make them more appealing to older people.

Menthol in other tobacco products can also lead to continued use of those products. For example, youth and young adults whose first cigar was flavored with mint or menthol were 72 percent more likely to use cigars a year or more later compared to youth and young adults who reported their first cigar was not flavored.

Menthol Making Quitting Smoking More Difficult

People who smoke menthol cigarettes are less likely to successfully quit than people who smoke nonmenthol cigarettes. For example, young adults and adults who smoke menthol cigarettes make more attempts to quit smoking than those who smoke nonmenthol cigarettes. However, the proportion of people who tried and succeeded in quitting nonmenthol cigarettes is greater than the proportion of people who have tried and succeeded in quitting menthol cigarettes. This could be partly due to the way in which menthol enhances the addictive effects of nicotine in the brain.[1]

Restricting Sales of Flavored Tobacco Products

Federal law prohibits cigarettes from being marketed with characterizing flavors, except tobacco or menthol. As of March 2023, over 170 U.S. communities have implemented laws prohibiting the sale of menthol and other flavored tobacco products. Massachusetts became the first U.S. state to prohibit the sale of menthol and other flavored tobacco products. Its law went into effect in 2020. In December 2022, a similar statewide law went into effect in California.

Studies of local U.S. policies have shown that restricting the sale of flavored tobacco products reduces the proportion of youth who try or use tobacco products. Evidence from other countries supports the public health benefits of removing menthol cigarettes from the marketplace. For example, after laws prohibiting the sale of menthol cigarettes were implemented in Canada, adults who smoked menthol cigarettes reported high rates of quit attempts and quit successes. Adults who had smoked menthol cigarettes daily before the law went into effect and tried quitting smoking were more likely to report having quit cigarettes than adults who had smoked nonmenthol cigarettes.

Source: "Addressing Menthol Tobacco Products," Centers for Disease Control and Prevention (CDC), August 23, 2023. Available online. URL: www.cdc.gov/tobacco/basic_information/menthol/addressing-menthol.html. Accessed September 27, 2023.

Other Flavors in Tobacco Products

In 2009, the U.S. Food and Drug Administration (FDA) banned cigarettes with characterizing flavors other than menthol (e.g., cherry, chocolate), which are known to appeal to youth and young adults. This ban was an important first step for responsible tobacco regulation to protect the American public, particularly children, from the dangers of cigarettes—the product most responsible for tobacco-related death and disease in the United States.

Currently, no flavors are banned from other tobacco products although research suggests flavors may also make these products more enticing to youth and young adults. Data from the FDA's Population Assessment of Tobacco and Health (PATH) study found that nearly 80 percent of youth aged 12–17 and nearly 75 percent of young adults aged 18–25 who were current tobacco users in 2014 reported that the first tobacco product they ever used was flavored. Alternatively, the FDA is aware of self-reported information suggesting that the availability of flavors in some noncombusted tobacco products such as e-cigarettes and other electronic nicotine delivery systems may help some adult users reduce cigarette use or switch to potentially less harmful products.[2]

[1] "Menthol Tobacco Products," Centers for Disease Control and Prevention (CDC), August 23, 2023. Available online. URL: www.cdc.gov/tobacco/basic_information/menthol/index.html. Accessed September 27, 2023.

[2] "Menthol and Other Flavors in Tobacco Products," U.S. Food and Drug Administration (FDA), April 29, 2021. Available online. URL: www.fda.gov/tobacco-products/products-ingredients-components/menthol-and-other-flavors-tobacco-products. Accessed September 27, 2023.

CHAPTER 22
CIGARS

A cigar is defined as a roll of tobacco wrapped in leaf tobacco or in a substance that contains tobacco.

Cigars differ from cigarettes in that cigarettes are a roll of tobacco wrapped in paper or in a substance that does not contain tobacco.

The three major types of cigars sold in the United States are large cigars, cigarillos, and little cigars.

In 2022, cigars were the second most commonly used tobacco product among U.S. middle and high school students. The availability of flavors in cigars that are prohibited in cigarettes (such as cherry), and the fact that they are commonly sold as a single stick, has raised concerns that these products may be especially appealing to youth.

In 2021, among middle and high school students who used cigars in the past 30 days, 44.4 percent reported using a flavored cigar during that time. See Table 22.1 for the unit sale share of cigar types.

Little cigars are the same size and shape as cigarettes, often include a filter, and are packaged in a similar way, but they are taxed differently than cigarettes. Rather than reduce consumption, people who smoke and are cost-conscious might switch from cigarettes to cheaper little cigars.

Table 22.1. Description and Unit Sale Share of Cigar Types

Type	Description	Share of Unit Sales (2016–2020)*
Large cigar	Cigar that typically contains at least one-half ounce of aged, fermented tobacco (i.e., as much as a pack of cigarettes) and usually takes one to two hours to smoke	2.70%
Cigarillo	A short (three to four inches) and narrow cigar that typically contains about 3 grams of tobacco and usually does not include a filter	94.20%
Little cigar	A small cigar that typically is about the same size as a cigarette and usually includes a filter	3.10%

** Percentage of U.S. market for cigar products*

Historically, cigar smoking in the United States has been a behavior of older men, but the industry's increased marketing of these products to the targeted groups increased the prevalence of use among adolescents.

Cigar use is higher among youth who use other tobacco products or other drugs (e.g., alcohol, marijuana, and inhalants) than among youth who do not use these products.

Cigars contain the same toxic and carcinogenic compounds found in cigarettes and are not a safe alternative to cigarettes.

Health Effects

- Regularly smoking cigars is associated with an increased risk for cancers of the lung, esophagus, larynx (voice box), and oral cavity (lip, tongue, mouth, and throat).
- Cigar smoking is linked to gum disease and tooth loss.
- Heavy cigar smoking and inhaling cigar smoke deeply may increase the risk of developing coronary heart disease.
- Heavy cigar smoking increases the risk of lung diseases, such as emphysema and chronic bronchitis.

Cigar Use

Adults*

The percentage of U.S. adults who currently smoked cigars† in 2021 is as follows:

- 3.5 percent of all adults
- 6.2 percent of adult men
- 1.0 percent of adult women
- 5.1 percent of non-Hispanic Black adults
- 3.7 percent of non-Hispanic White adults
- 2.5 percent of Hispanic adults
- 1.2 percent of non-Hispanic Asian adults

High School Students

The percentage of U.S. high school students who currently smoked cigars† in 2022 is as follows:

- 2.8 percent of all students in grades 9–12
- 2.1 percent of female students in grades 9–12
- 3.5 percent of male students in grades 9–12

** Adults are defined as persons aged 18 or older.*

† Current cigar use is defined as smoking cigars on 1 or more of the 30 days before participation in a survey about this topic.

Middle School Students

The percentage of U.S. middle school students who currently smoked cigars† in 2022 is as follows:

- 0.6 percent of all U.S. students in grades 6–8
- 0.6 percent of female students in grades 6–8
- 0.6 percent of male students in grades 6–8

Overall

- In 2021, an estimated 8.6 million adults aged 18 and older (3.5%) currently smoked cigars.

Marketing Information on Cigars

Marketing efforts promote cigars as symbols of a luxurious and successful lifestyle. The following strategies can contribute to the increased acceptability of cigar smoking:

- endorsements by male and female celebrities
- development of cigar-focused magazines (e.g., *Cigar Aficionado*)
- product placement in movies

In 2001, the Federal Trade Commission (FTC) mandated that cigar packaging and advertisements display one of the following five "SURGEON GENERAL'S WARNING" text-only labels on a rotating basis:

- Cigar Smoking Can Cause Cancers of the Mouth and Throat, Even If You Do Not Inhale.
- Cigar Smoking Can Cause Lung Cancer and Heart Disease.
- Tobacco Use Increases the Risk of Infertility, Stillbirth, and Low Birth Weight.
- Cigars Are Not a Safe Alternative to Cigarettes.
- Tobacco Smoke Increases the Risk of Lung Cancer and Heart Disease, Even in Nonsmokers.[1]

[1] "Cigars," Centers for Disease Control and Prevention (CDC), May 4, 2023. Available online. URL: www.cdc.gov/tobacco/data_statistics/fact_sheets/tobacco_industry/cigars/index.htm. Accessed September 27, 2023.

CHAPTER 23
HOOKAH PIPES

Hookahs are water pipes that are used to smoke specially made tobacco that comes in different flavors, such as apple, mint, cherry, chocolate, coconut, licorice, cappuccino, and watermelon.

Although many users think it is less harmful, hookah smoking has many of the same health risks as cigarette smoking.

Hookah is also called "narghile," "argileh," "shisha," "hubble-bubble," and "goza."

Hookahs vary in size, shape, and style.

A typical modern hookah has a head (with holes in the bottom), a metal body, a water bowl, and a flexible hose with a mouthpiece.

Hookah smoking is typically done in groups, with the same mouthpiece passed from person to person.

Hookah Use

- Hookah use began centuries ago in ancient Persia and India.
- In 2018, the Monitoring the Future survey found the following:
  - Nearly 1 in every 13 (7.8%) high school students in the United States had used a hookah to smoke tobacco during the previous year.
  - About one in every eight (12.3%) young adults aged 19–30 had used a hookah to smoke tobacco during the previous year.
- Among 12th graders, annual hookah use increased from nearly 1 in 6 students (17.1%) in 2010 to about 1 in 4 students (22.9%) in 2014 but, since that time, decreased sharply to nearly 1 in 13 students (7.8%) in 2018.
- Monitoring the Future also shows variations in hookah use by region and population density. In 2018, the highest prevalence of use was observed in the Northeast, where one in six (15.0%) young adults aged 19–30 years had used a hookah to smoke tobacco during the previous year, and in very large cities, where almost one in five (19.3%) young adults in this age group reported 2020 use.

- Other small studies of young adults have found a high prevalence of hookah use among college students in the United States. These studies show past-year use ranging from 22 to 40 percent.
- New forms of electronic hookah products, including steam stones and hookah pens, have been introduced.
  - These products are battery-powered and turn liquid containing nicotine, flavorings, and other chemicals into an aerosol, which is inhaled.
  - Limited information is currently available on the health risks of electronic tobacco products, including electronic hookahs.

Health Effects

Hookah Smoke and Cancer

- The charcoal used to heat the tobacco can raise health risks by producing high levels of carbon monoxide, metals, and cancer-causing chemicals.
- Even after it has passed through water, the smoke from a hookah has high levels of these toxic agents.
- Hookah tobacco and smoke contain several toxic agents known to cause lung, bladder, and oral cancers.
- Tobacco juices from hookahs irritate the mouth and increase the risk of developing oral cancers.

Other Health Effects of Hookah Smoke

- Hookah tobacco and smoke contain many toxic agents that can cause clogged arteries and heart disease.
- Babies born to people who smoked water pipes every day while pregnant weigh less at birth (at least 3½ ounces less) than babies born to those who do not smoke.
- Babies born to people who use hookah are also at increased risk for respiratory diseases.

Hookah Smoking Compared with Cigarette Smoking

- Although many users think it is less harmful, studies have shown that hookah smoke contains many of the same harmful components found in cigarette smoke, such as nicotine, tar, and heavy metals.
  - Water pipe smoking delivers nicotine—the same highly addictive drug found in other tobacco products.
  - The tobacco in hookahs is exposed to high heat from burning charcoal, and the smoke is at least as toxic as cigarette smoke.
  - The heat sources used to burn hookah tobacco release other dangerous substances, such as carbon monoxide. This may put hookah users at additional risk.

- Because of the way a hookah is used, people who smoke hookah may absorb more of the toxic substances also found in cigarette smoke than people who smoke cigarettes do.
    - In a typical one-hour hookah smoking session, users may inhale 100–200 times the amount of smoke they would inhale from a single cigarette. In a single water pipe session, users are exposed to up to 9 times the carbon monoxide and 1.7 times the nicotine of a single cigarette.
    - The amount of smoke inhaled during a typical hookah session is about 90,000 ml, compared with 500–600 ml inhaled when smoking a cigarette.
- People who smoke hookah may be at risk for some of the same diseases as cigarette smokers. These include the following:
    - oral cancer
    - lung cancer
    - stomach cancer
    - cancer of the esophagus
    - reduced lung function
    - decreased fertility

The U.S. Food and Drug Administration Regulation of Hookah Tobacco Products

In 2016, the U.S. Food and Drug Administration (FDA) finalized a rule extending regulatory authority to cover all tobacco products, including hookah tobacco. The FDA regulates the manufacture, import, packaging, labeling, advertising, promotion, sale, and distribution of hookah tobacco. This includes components and parts of tobacco products regulated by the 2016 rule but excludes accessories such as lighters, tongs, or external burners.

"Components" or "parts" include, among other things, software or an assembly of materials intended or reasonably expected to alter or affect the tobacco product's performance, composition, constituents, or characteristics or to be used with or for the human consumption of a tobacco product. Examples of components and parts that are regulated include, but are not limited to:

- hookah
- flavor enhancers
- hose cooling attachments
- water filtration base additives (including those that are flavored)
- charcoal made from wood, coconut shell, or other materials, as well as electric heating systems
- bowls, valves, hoses, and heads

Source: "Hookah Tobacco (Shisha or Waterpipe Tobacco)," U.S. Food and Drug Administration (FDA), September 6, 2023. Available online. URL: www.fda.gov/tobacco-products/products-ingredients-components/hookah-tobacco-shisha-or-waterpipe-tobacco. Accessed September 27, 2023.

Hookahs and Secondhand Smoke

- Secondhand smoke from hookahs can be a health risk for people who do not smoke. It contains smoke from the tobacco as well as smoke from the heat source (e.g., charcoal) used in the hookah.

Nontobacco Hookah Products

- Some sweetened and flavored nontobacco products are sold for use in hookahs.
- Labels and ads for these products often claim that users can enjoy the same taste without the harmful effects of tobacco.
- Studies of tobacco-based shisha and "herbal" shisha show that smoke from both preparations contains carbon monoxide and other toxic agents known to increase the risks for smoking-related cancers, heart disease, and lung disease.[1]

[1] "Hookahs," Centers for Disease Control and Prevention (CDC), April 22, 2021. Available online. URL: www.cdc.gov/tobacco/data_statistics/fact_sheets/tobacco_industry/hookahs/index.htm. Accessed September 27, 2023.

CHAPTER 24
SMOKELESS TOBACCO

Smokeless tobacco is associated with many health problems. Using smokeless tobacco:

- can lead to nicotine addiction
- causes cancer of the mouth, esophagus (the passage that connects the throat to the stomach), and the pancreas (a gland that helps with digestion and maintaining proper blood sugar levels)
- is associated with diseases of the mouth
- can increase risks for early delivery and stillbirth when used during pregnancy
- can cause nicotine poisoning in children
- may increase the risk for death from heart disease and stroke[1]

Using smokeless products can cause serious health problems. Protect your health; do not start. If you do use them, quit.

Source: "Smokeless Tobacco: Health Effects," Centers for Disease Control and Prevention (CDC), August 13, 2020. Available online. URL: www.cdc.gov/tobacco/data_statistics/fact_sheets/smokeless/health_effects/index.htm. Accessed September 27, 2023.

What Are Smokeless Tobacco Products, including Dip, Snuff, Snus, and Chewing Tobacco?

Most smokeless tobacco use involves placing the product between the gum and the cheek or lip. Smokeless tobacco is a noncombusted tobacco product.

There are two main types of smokeless tobacco that have been traditionally marketed in the United States: chewing tobacco and snuff, including snus.*

** If a snus or other smokeless tobacco product claims to be made with synthetic nicotine, it is subject to requirements for non-tobacco nicotine (NTN) products.*

[1] "Smokeless Tobacco: Health Effects," Centers for Disease Control and Prevention (CDC), August 13, 2020. Available online. URL: www.cdc.gov/tobacco/data_statistics/fact_sheets/smokeless/health_effects/index.htm. Accessed September 27, 2023.

- Chewing tobacco is cured tobacco in the form of loose leaf, plug, or twist.
- Dry snuff is loose finely cut or powdered dry tobacco that is typically sniffed through the nostrils.
- Moist snuff and snus are cut tobacco that can be loose or pouched and placed in the mouth. Dip is a common form of moist snuff.
- Some dissolvable tobacco products can be classified as smokeless tobacco products.[2]

Health Problems Caused by Smokeless Tobacco

Addiction to Smokeless Tobacco

- Smokeless tobacco contains nicotine, which is highly addictive.
- Because young people who use smokeless tobacco can become addicted to nicotine, they may be more likely to also become cigarette smokers.

Cancer

- Many smokeless tobacco products contain cancer-causing chemicals.
  - The most harmful chemicals are tobacco-specific nitrosamines, which form during the growing, curing, fermenting, and aging of tobacco. The amount of these chemicals varies by product.
  - The higher the levels of these chemicals, the greater the risk for cancer.
  - Other chemicals found in tobacco can also cause cancer. These include the following:
    - a radioactive element (polonium-210) found in tobacco fertilizer
    - chemicals formed when tobacco is cured with heat (polynuclear aromatic hydrocarbons—also known as "polycyclic aromatic hydrocarbons")
    - harmful metals (arsenic, beryllium, cadmium, chromium, cobalt, lead, nickel, and mercury)
  - Smokeless tobacco causes cancer of the mouth, esophagus, and pancreas.

Oral Disease

- Smokeless tobacco can cause white or gray patches inside the mouth (leukoplakia) that can lead to cancer.
- Smokeless tobacco can cause gum disease, tooth decay, and tooth loss.

Reproductive and Developmental Risks

- Using smokeless tobacco during pregnancy can increase the risk for early delivery and stillbirth.

[2] "Smokeless Tobacco Products, Including Dip, Snuff, Snus, and Chewing Tobacco," U.S. Food and Drug Administration (FDA), June 7, 2023. Available online. URL: www.fda.gov/tobacco-products/products-ingredients-components/smokeless-tobacco-products-including-dip-snuff-snus-and-chewing-tobacco. Accessed September 27, 2023.

- Nicotine in smokeless tobacco products that are used during pregnancy can affect how a baby's brain develops before birth.

Other Risks

- Using smokeless tobacco increases the risk for death from heart disease and stroke.
- Smokeless tobacco can cause nicotine poisoning in children.
- Additional research is needed to examine the long-term effects of newer smokeless tobacco products, such as dissolvables and U.S. snus.[3]

Are There Harmful Chemicals in Smokeless Tobacco?

There is no safe form of tobacco. At least 28 chemicals in smokeless tobacco have been found to cause cancer. The most harmful chemicals in smokeless tobacco are tobacco-specific nitrosamines, which are formed during the growing, curing, fermenting, and aging of tobacco. The level of tobacco-specific nitrosamines varies by product. Scientists have found that the nitrosamine level is directly related to the risk of cancer.

In addition to a variety of nitrosamines, other cancer-causing substances in smokeless tobacco include polonium-210 (a radioactive element found in tobacco fertilizer) and polynuclear aromatic hydrocarbons (also known as "polycyclic aromatic hydrocarbons").

Can a User Get Addicted to Smokeless Tobacco?

All tobacco products, including smokeless tobacco, contain nicotine, which is addictive. Users of smokeless tobacco and users of cigarettes have comparable levels of nicotine in their blood. In users of smokeless tobacco, nicotine is absorbed through the mouth tissues directly into the blood, where it goes to the brain. Even after the tobacco is removed from the mouth, nicotine continues to be absorbed into the bloodstream. Also, the nicotine stays in the blood longer for users of smokeless tobacco than for smokers.

The level of nicotine in the blood depends on the amount of nicotine in the smokeless tobacco product, the tobacco cut size, the product's pH (a measure of its acidity or basicity), and other factors.

A Centers for Disease Control and Prevention (CDC) study of the 40 most widely used popular brands of moist snuff showed that the amount of nicotine per gram of tobacco ranged from 4.4 to 25.0 mg. Other studies have shown that moist snuff had between 4.7 and 24.3 mg per gram of tobacco, dry snuff had between 10.5 and 24.8 mg per gram of tobacco, and chewing tobacco had between 3.4 and 39.7 mg per gram of tobacco.

[3] See footnote [1].

Is Using Smokeless Tobacco Less Hazardous Than Smoking Cigarettes?

Because all tobacco products are harmful and cause cancer, the use of all of these products should be strongly discouraged. There is no safe level of tobacco use. People who use any type of tobacco product should be urged to quit.

As long ago as 1986, the advisory committee to the Surgeon General concluded that the use of smokeless tobacco "is not a safe substitute for smoking cigarettes. It can cause cancer and a number of noncancerous oral conditions and can lead to nicotine addiction and dependence." Furthermore, a panel of experts convened by the National Institutes of Health (NIH) in 2006 stated that the "range of risks, including nicotine addiction, from smokeless tobacco products may vary extensively because of differing levels of nicotine, carcinogens, and other toxins in different products."

Should Smokeless Tobacco Be Used to Help a Person Quit Smoking?

There is no scientific evidence that using smokeless tobacco can help a person quit smoking. Because all tobacco products are harmful and cause cancer, the use of all tobacco products is strongly discouraged. There is no safe level of tobacco use. People who use any type of tobacco product should be urged to quit. For help with quitting, ask your doctor about individual or group counseling, telephone quitlines, or other methods.

How Can You Get Help Quitting Smokeless Tobacco?

The National Cancer Institute (NCI) offers free information about quitting smokeless tobacco:

- Call the NCI's Smoking Quitline at 877-44U-QUIT (877-448-7848). Talk with a smoking cessation counselor about quitting smokeless tobacco. You can call the quitline, within the United States, Monday through Friday, 9:00 a.m. to 9:00 p.m., Eastern time.
- Use LiveHelp (https://livehelp.cancer.gov/app/chat/chat_launch) online chat. You can have a confidential online text chat with an NCI smoking cessation counselor, Monday through Friday, 9:00 a.m. to 9:00 p.m., Eastern time.[4]

---

[4] "Smokeless Tobacco and Cancer," National Cancer Institute (NCI), October 25, 2010. Available online. URL: www.cancer.gov/about-cancer/causes-prevention/risk/tobacco/smokeless-fact-sheet. Accessed September 27, 2023.

CHAPTER 25
HEATED TOBACCO PRODUCTS

What Are Heated Tobacco Products?

- Sometimes marketed as "heat-not-burn" products, heated tobacco products come in many forms.
- Some heated tobacco products use electronic heating elements.
    - Some heat specially designed sticks, plugs, or capsules containing tobacco. This is how the electronically heated tobacco product authorized for sale in the United States works.
    - Some work by heating liquids that create an emission that then passes through a tobacco plug to absorb flavor and nicotine from the tobacco.
    - Some have a sealed part of the device that heats loose tobacco, either alone or together with flowers from the marijuana (cannabis) plant.
    - Some are used with flavorings.
    - Some allow users to control factors such as the temperature.
- Some heated tobacco products have a similar size and shape as regular cigarettes and have a carbon tip wrapped in glass fibers that the user heats with a lighter or match. Federal law allows this type of product to be sold in the United States.

Are Heated Tobacco Products the Same as Electronic Cigarettes?

- Heated tobacco products heat actual tobacco leaves. By contrast, e-cigarettes heat liquids that typically contain nicotine derived from tobacco, as well as flavorings and other ingredients.

What Are the Health Effects of Using Heated Tobacco Products?

- Heated tobacco products are still new in the United States, and scientists are still learning about their short- and long-term health effects.
- The use of any tobacco product—including heated tobacco products—is harmful, especially for youth, young adults, and pregnant women, as well as adults who do not currently use tobacco products.

- Regardless of whether they are heated by flame or electronically, heated tobacco products contain nicotine.
- Nicotine is highly addictive.
- Nicotine exposure can also harm the developing adolescent brain. The brain keeps developing until about age 25.
  - Using nicotine in adolescence can harm the parts of the brain that control attention, learning, mood, and impulse control.
  - Using nicotine in adolescence may also increase the risk for future addiction to other drugs.
- Nicotine is toxic to developing fetuses.

Is It Harmful to Breathe the Secondhand Emissions from Heated Tobacco Products?

- Heated tobacco products produce emissions that are not as safe as clean air.
- Studies of secondhand emissions from heated tobacco products suggest that the products expose both users and bystanders to some of the same chemicals found in cigarette smoke although at lower levels than cigarette smoke.
- Additional research is needed to understand the health effects of heated tobacco products and their emissions.

Who Is Using Heated Tobacco Products?

- These products are new in the United States. As of February 2022, the U.S. Food and Drug Administration (FDA) has authorized only I Quit Ordinary Smoking (IQOS) and Eclipse heated tobacco products for sale in this country. Sales of other heated tobacco products are growing worldwide.
- The Centers for Disease Control and Prevention (CDC) began tracking the use of heated tobacco products among U.S. adults in 2017. At that time, 0.7 percent of adults, including 2.7 percent of people who currently smoked regular cigarettes, reported they had ever used a heated tobacco product.
- Reported use of heated tobacco products went up in 2018 when 2.4 percent of adults, including 6.7 percent of people who currently smoked regular cigarettes, reported to the CDC that they had ever used a heated tobacco product.
- A different survey from 2019 found that the proportion of adults who use e-cigarettes and reported they have ever used a heated tobacco product was higher than the proportion of adults who smoke cigarettes and reported that they had ever used a heated tobacco product.
- In 2022, 1 percent of U.S. middle and high school students, combined, reported having used heated tobacco products in the past 30 days.

Are Heated Tobacco Products Less Harmful Than Regular Cigarettes?

- The emissions created from heated tobacco products generally contain lower levels of harmful ingredients than the smoke from regular cigarettes. However, that does not mean heated tobacco products are safe.
- Research suggests that heated tobacco products and their emissions contain many of the same harmful ingredients as regular cigarettes, as well as other harmful ingredients not present in regular cigarettes.
- Additional research is needed to determine whether adult cigarette smokers who completely switch to heated tobacco products might reduce their risks of tobacco-related disease. Studies from other countries suggest that most adults who use heated tobacco products have not quit using cigarettes. Surveys of young adults in the United States suggest that young adults also use heated tobacco products in combination with other tobacco products. The use of multiple tobacco products is associated with increased risk for nicotine dependence and adverse health effects.
- As of February 2022, the U.S. Food and Drug Administration (FDA) has authorized only one heated tobacco product system (I Quit Ordinary Smoking (IQOS) and three of its tobacco-containing Heatstick products) to be marketed as modified-risk tobacco products. These were the first tobacco products to receive "exposure modification" orders. These specific products may be marketed with claims that a person who uses regular cigarettes and fully switches to IQOS can reduce their exposure to harmful chemicals.

Similar claims may not be made about other heated tobacco products or about secondhand exposure to emissions from these products. In addition, the manufacturer of IQOS may not claim that using IQOS reduces the risk of disease, that the products are endorsed or approved by the FDA, or that the FDA deems the products to be safe for use by consumers.

Source: "Heated Tobacco Products," Centers for Disease Control and Prevention (CDC), November 10, 2022. Available online. URL: www.cdc.gov/tobacco/basic_information/heated-tobacco-products/index.html. Accessed September 28, 2023.

What Can People Do to Address the Use of Heated Tobacco Products?

- States, communities, tribes, and territories can implement evidence-based, population-level strategies that address the use of all forms of tobacco products, including heated tobacco products, such as:
  - incorporating all tobacco products, including heated tobacco products, into smoke-free and tobacco-free policies
  - licensing retailers who sell tobacco products, restricting young people's access to tobacco products in retail settings, and enforcing laws that penalize retailers who sell tobacco products to underage persons
  - implementing policies to raise the price of tobacco products
  - reducing access to flavored tobacco products
  - curbing advertising and marketing for tobacco products that are appealing to young people

    - developing educational initiatives that warn about the risks of tobacco product use, especially among young people
- Parents and teachers can:
    - learn about the different types of tobacco products and the risks of using tobacco products, including heated tobacco products
    - set a good example by being tobacco-free and maintaining a tobacco-free home
    - talk to children, teens, and young adults about why all forms of tobacco products are harmful to them
    - develop, implement, and enforce tobacco-free school policies and prevention programs that are free from tobacco industry influence and that address all types of tobacco products, including heated tobacco products[1]

[1] "Heated Tobacco Products," Centers for Disease Control and Prevention (CDC), November 10, 2022. Available online. URL: www.cdc.gov/tobacco/basic_information/heated-tobacco-products/index.html. Accessed September 28, 2023.

CHAPTER 26
SECONDHAND SMOKE

What Is Secondhand Smoke?

Secondhand smoke (sometimes called passive smoke, environmental tobacco smoke, or involuntary smoke) is a mixture of sidestream smoke (the smoke from the burning tip of a cigarette or other smoked tobacco product) and mainstream smoke (smoke exhaled by a smoker that is diluted by the surrounding air).

Major settings of exposure to secondhand smoke include workplaces, public places such as bars, restaurants and recreational settings, and homes. Workplaces and homes are especially important sources of exposure because of the length of time people spend in these settings. The home is a particularly important source of exposure for infants and young children. Children and nonsmoking adults can also be exposed to secondhand smoke in vehicles, where levels of exposure can be high. Exposure levels can also be high in enclosed public places where smoking is allowed, such as restaurants, bars, and casinos, resulting in substantial exposures for both workers and patrons.

How Is Secondhand Smoke Exposure Measured?

Secondhand smoke exposure can be measured by testing indoor air for respirable (breathable) suspended particles (particles small enough to reach the lower airways of the human lung) or individual chemicals such as nicotine or other harmful and potentially harmful constituents of tobacco smoke.

Exposure to secondhand smoke can also be evaluated by measuring the level of biomarkers such as cotinine (a byproduct of nicotine metabolism) in a nonsmoker's blood, saliva, or urine. Nicotine, cotinine, and other chemicals present in secondhand smoke have been found in the body fluids of nonsmokers exposed to secondhand smoke.

Do Electronic Cigarettes Emit Secondhand Smoke?

The use of electronic cigarettes results in exposure to secondhand aerosols (rather than secondhand smoke). Secondhand aerosols contain harmful and potentially harmful substances, including nicotine, heavy metals such as lead, volatile organic compounds, and cancer-causing agents.

What Is Being Done to Reduce Nonsmokers' Exposure to Secondhand Smoke?

On the federal level, several policies restricting smoking in public places have been implemented. Federal law prohibits smoking on airline flights, interstate buses, and most trains. Smoking is also prohibited in most federal buildings by Executive Order 13058 of 1997. The Pro-Children Act of 1994 prohibits smoking in facilities that routinely provide federally funded services to children. The Department of Housing and Urban Development published a final rule in December 2016, which was fully implemented in July 2018, that prohibits the use of cigarettes, cigars, pipes, and hookah (water pipes) in public housing authorities, including all living units, indoor common areas, and administrative offices, as well as outdoor areas within 25 feet of buildings.

Many state and local governments have enacted laws that prohibit smoking in workplaces and public places, including restaurants, bars, schools, hospitals, airports, bus terminals, parks, and beaches. These smoke-free policies have substantially decreased exposure to secondhand smoke in many U.S. workplaces. More than half of all states have implemented comprehensive smoke-free laws that prohibit smoking in indoor areas of workplaces, restaurants, and bars, and some states and communities have also enacted laws regulating smoking in multiunit housing and cars. The American Nonsmokers' Rights (ANR) Foundation provides a list of state and local smoke-free air policies (https://no-smoke.org/wp-content/uploads/pdf/WRBLawsMap.pdf).

To highlight the health risks from secondhand smoke, the National Cancer Institute (NCI) requires that meetings and conferences organized or primarily sponsored by the NCI be held in a state, county, city, or town that has adopted a comprehensive smoke-free policy unless specific circumstances justify an exception to this policy.

Healthy People 2020, a comprehensive nationwide health promotion and disease prevention framework established by the U.S. Department of Health and Human Services (HHS), includes several objectives addressing the goal of reducing illness, disability, and death caused by tobacco use and secondhand smoke exposure. For 2020, the Healthy People goal is to reduce the proportion of nonsmokers exposed to secondhand smoke by 10 percent. To assist with achieving this goal, Healthy People 2020 includes ideas for community interventions, such as encouraging the introduction of smoke-free policies in all workplaces and other public gathering places, such as public parks, sporting arenas, and beaches.

Because of these policies and other actions, the percentage of nonsmokers who are exposed to secondhand smoke declined from 52.5 percent during 1999–2000 to 25.3 percent during 2011–2014. Exposure to secondhand smoke declined among all population subgroups, but disparities still exist. During 2011–2014, 38 percent of children aged 3–11, 50 percent of non-Hispanic blacks, 48 percent of people living below the poverty level, and 39 percent of people living in rental housing were exposed to secondhand smoke.[1]

[1] "Secondhand Smoke and Cancer," National Cancer Institute (NCI), December 4, 2018. Available online. URL: www.cancer.gov/about-cancer/causes-prevention/risk/tobacco/second-hand-smoke-fact-sheet. Accessed September 28, 2023.

Health Problems Caused by Secondhand Smoke

- There is no safe level of exposure to secondhand smoke; even brief exposure can cause immediate harm.
- Health problems caused by secondhand smoke in adults who do not smoke include coronary heart disease, stroke, and lung cancer, as well as adverse reproductive health effects in women, including low birth weight.
- Secondhand smoke can cause sudden infant death syndrome (SIDS), respiratory infections, ear infections, and asthma attacks in infants and children.

How Can You Protect Yourself and Family from Secondhand Smoke Outside Your Home?

- If your child goes to day care or school, talk to the provider or school officials to make sure all the day-care or school facility has a tobacco-free policy. This type of policy can set a good example for young people and can also protect children from secondhand smoke and e-cigarette emissions. This includes the following:
  - tobacco-free school events
  - tobacco-free school policies that apply to buildings and grounds and include e-cigarettes
- If neither your state nor community has adopted laws preventing exposure to secondhand smoke in public areas, look for restaurants and other public places that do not allow smoking. "No Smoking" sections in restaurants that separate people who smoke from those who do not smoke do not protect you or your children from secondhand smoke.
- Talk to your employer about the benefits of a smoke-free policy in your workplace.
- Educate others about the benefits of smoke-free laws and policies in public places, workplaces, and housing.
- If you own or manage a business, adopt a smoke-free policy for employees and customers.

Source: "Preventing Exposure to Secondhand Smoke in the Home," Centers for Disease Control and Prevention (CDC), November 28, 2022. Available online. URL: www.cdc.gov/tobacco/secondhand-smoke/home.html. Accessed September 28, 2023.

What Health Problems Can Secondhand Smoke Cause?

- There is no safe level of exposure to secondhand smoke. People who do not smoke and those who are exposed to secondhand smoke, even for a short time, can suffer harmful health effects.
- In adults who do not smoke, secondhand smoke exposure can cause coronary heart disease, stroke, lung cancer, and other diseases. It can also result in premature death.
- Secondhand smoke can cause adverse reproductive health effects in women, including low birth weight.
- In children, secondhand smoke exposure can cause respiratory infections, ear infections, and asthma attacks. In babies, secondhand smoke can cause SIDS.

- Since 1964, about 2,500,000 people who did not smoke died from health problems caused by secondhand smoke exposure.
- The effects of secondhand smoke exposure on the body are immediate. Secondhand smoke exposure can produce harmful inflammatory and respiratory effects within 60 minutes of exposure that can last for at least three hours after exposure.

Secondhand Smoke Causes Heart Disease and Stroke

- For adults who do not smoke, exposure to secondhand smoke has immediate harmful effects on the heart and blood vessels and can cause coronary heart disease and stroke.
- Among adults who do not smoke, secondhand smoke causes nearly 34,000 premature deaths from heart disease each year in the United States.
- Adults who do not smoke and are exposed to secondhand smoke increase their risk of developing coronary heart disease by 25–30 percent.
- Adults who do not smoke and are exposed to secondhand smoke increase their risk of stroke by 20–30 percent.
- Exposure to secondhand smoke interferes with the normal functioning of the heart, blood, and vascular systems in ways that increase the risk of having a heart attack.
- Even brief exposure to secondhand smoke can damage the lining of blood vessels and cause blood platelets to become stickier. These changes can cause an increased risk of heart attack.
- People who already have heart disease are at especially high risk of suffering the harmful effects of breathing secondhand smoke and should take special precautions to avoid even brief exposures.

Secondhand Smoke Causes Lung Cancer

- Adults who do not smoke and are exposed to secondhand smoke increase their risk of developing lung cancer by 20–30 percent.
- Secondhand smoke causes more than 7,300 lung cancer deaths each year among U.S. adults who do not smoke.
- People who do not smoke but are exposed to secondhand smoke are inhaling many of the same cancer-causing substances and poisons that are inhaled by people who smoke.
- Even brief exposure to secondhand smoke can damage the body's cells in ways that set the cancer process in motion.
- As with active smoking, the longer the duration and the higher the level of exposure to secondhand smoke, the greater the risk of developing lung cancer.

Secondhand Smoke Causes Reproductive Health Problems in Pregnant People

- Women exposed to secondhand smoke during pregnancy are more likely to have newborns with lower birth weight, increasing the risk of health complications.

Secondhand Smoke Causes Sudden Infant Death Syndrome

- Infants exposed to secondhand smoke after birth are more likely to die from SIDS than infants who are not exposed to smoke from burning commercial tobacco products. SIDS is the sudden, unexplained, unexpected death of an infant in the first year of life.
- SIDS is the leading cause of death in otherwise healthy infants.
- Smoking by women during pregnancy increases the risk for SIDS.
- Chemicals in secondhand smoke appear to affect the brain in ways that interfere with its regulation of infants' breathing.
- Infants who die from SIDS have higher concentrations of nicotine in their lungs and higher levels of cotinine (a biological marker for secondhand smoke exposure) than infants who die from other causes.

Secondhand Smoke Can Trigger Asthma Attacks and Cause Other Health Problems in Children

- Children who are exposed to secondhand smoke are at an increased risk for acute respiratory infections, such as pneumonia and bronchitis, middle ear disease, more frequent and severe asthma, respiratory symptoms, and slowed lung growth.
- Wheezing, coughing, and shortness of breath are more common in children exposed to secondhand smoke.
- Children whose parents smoke around them get more ear infections. They also have fluid in their ears more often and have more operations to put in ear tubes for drainage.
- Secondhand smoke can trigger an asthma attack in a child. Children with asthma who are around secondhand smoke have more severe and frequent asthma attacks. A severe asthma attack can put a child's life in danger.[2]

[2] "Health Problems Caused by Secondhand Smoke," Centers for Disease Control and Prevention (CDC), November 1, 2022. Available online. URL: www.cdc.gov/tobacco/secondhand-smoke/health.html. Accessed September 28, 2023.

PART 4 | COMMON CANCERS LINKED TO TOBACCO USE

CHAPTER 27
SMOKING AND CANCER

What Is Cancer?

Cancer refers to diseases in which abnormal cells divide out of control and are able to invade other tissues. Cancer cells can spread to other parts of the body through the blood and lymph systems, which help the body get rid of toxins.

There are more than 100 different types of cancer. Most cancers are named after the organ or type of cell in which they start—for example, lung cancer begins in the lung, and laryngeal cancer begins in the larynx (voice box).

Symptoms can include the following:

- a thickening or lump in any part of the body
- weight loss or gain with no known reason
- a sore that does not heal
- hoarseness or a cough that does not go away
- a hard time swallowing
- discomfort after eating
- changes in bowel or bladder habits
- unusual bleeding or discharge
- feeling weak or very tired

How Is Smoking Related to Cancer?

Smoking can cause cancer and then block your body from fighting it.

- Poisons in cigarette smoke can weaken the body's immune system, making it harder to kill cancer cells. When this happens, cancer cells keep growing without being stopped.
- Poisons in tobacco smoke can damage or change a cell's deoxyribonucleic acid (DNA). DNA is the cell's "instruction manual" that controls a cell's normal growth and function. When DNA is damaged, a cell can begin growing out of control and create a cancer tumor.

Doctors have known for years that smoking causes most lung cancers. It is still true when nearly 9 out of 10 lung cancer deaths are caused by smoking cigarettes or secondhand smoke exposure. In fact, people who smoke have a greater risk for lung cancer today than they did in 1964, even though they smoke fewer cigarettes. One reason may be changes in how cigarettes are made and what chemicals they contain.

Treatments are getting better, but lung cancer still kills more men and women than any other type of cancer. In the United States, more than 7,300 nonsmokers die each year from lung cancer caused by secondhand smoke. Secondhand smoke is the combination of smoke from the burning end of a cigarette and the smoke breathed out by someone smoking.

Smoking can cause cancer almost anywhere in your body (see Figure 27.1), including the following:

- blood (acute myeloid leukemia (AML))
- bladder
- cervix
- colon and rectum
- esophagus
- kidney and renal pelvis
- larynx
- liver
- lungs, trachea, and bronchus
- mouth and throat
- pancreas
- stomach

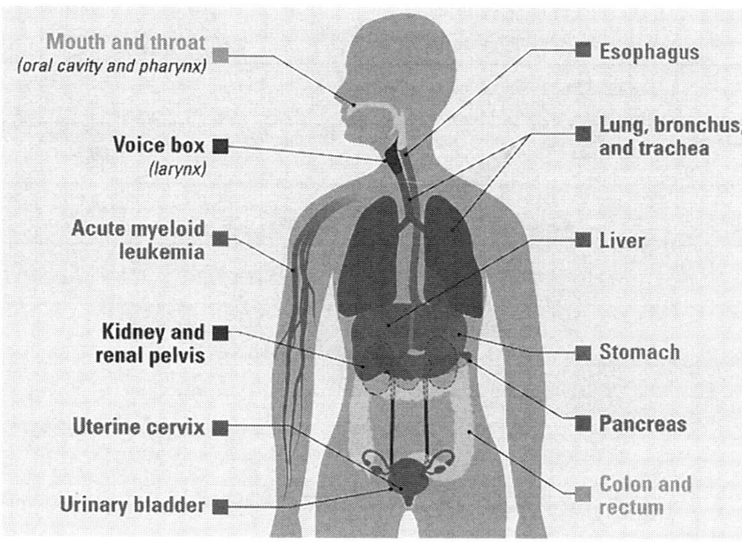

Figure 27.1. Cancers Caused by Tobacco Use
Centers for Disease Control and Prevention (CDC)

Men with prostate cancer who smoke may be more likely to die from prostate cancer than nonsmokers.

Smokeless tobacco, such as chewing tobacco, also causes cancer, including cancers of the:

- esophagus
- mouth and throat
- pancreas

How Can Smoking-Related Cancers Be Prevented?

The most important thing you can do to prevent smoking-related cancer is not to smoke cigarettes or to quit if you do. It is also important to avoid secondhand smoke.

Quitting smoking lowers the risk for 12 types of cancer: cancers of the lung, larynx, oral cavity and pharynx, esophagus, pancreas, bladder, stomach, colon and rectum, liver, cervix, kidney, and AML.

- Within 5–10 years of quitting, your chance of getting cancer of the mouth, throat, or voice box drops by half.
- Within 10 years of quitting, your chance of getting cancer of the bladder, esophagus, or kidney decreases.
- Within 10–15 years after you quit smoking, your risk of lung cancer drops by half.
- Within 20 years after you quit smoking, your risk of getting cancer of the mouth, throat, voice box, or pancreas drops to close to that of someone who does not smoke. Also, the risk of cervical cancer drops by about half.[1]

[1] "Smoking and Cancer," Centers for Disease Control and Prevention (CDC), May 5, 2022. Available online. URL: www.cdc.gov/tobacco/campaign/tips/diseases/cancer.html. Accessed September 28, 2023.

CHAPTER 28
LUNG CANCER

What Is Lung Cancer?

Cancer is a disease in which cells in the body grow out of control. When cancer starts in the lungs, it is called "lung cancer."

Lung cancer begins in the lungs and may spread to lymph nodes or other organs in the body, such as the brain. Cancer from other organs also may spread to the lungs. When cancer cells spread from one organ to another, they are called "metastases."

Lung cancers usually are grouped into two main types called "small cell" and "non-small cell" (non-small cell includes adenocarcinoma and squamous cell carcinoma (SCC)). These types of lung cancer grow differently and are treated differently. Non-small cell lung cancer is more common than small cell lung cancer.

What Are the Risk Factors for Lung Cancer?

Research has found several risk factors that may increase your chances of getting lung cancer.

Smoking

Cigarette smoking is the number one risk factor for lung cancer. In the United States, cigarette smoking is linked to about 80–90 percent of lung cancer deaths. Using other tobacco products, such as cigars or pipes also increases the risk for lung cancer. Tobacco smoke is a toxic mix of more than 7,000 chemicals. Many are poisons. At least 70 are known to cause cancer in people or animals.

People who smoke cigarettes are 15–30 times more likely to get lung cancer or die from lung cancer than people who do not smoke. Even smoking a few cigarettes a day or smoking occasionally increases the risk of lung cancer. The more years a person smokes and the more cigarettes smoked each day, the more risk goes up.

People who quit smoking have a lower risk of lung cancer than if they had continued to smoke, but their risk is higher than the risk for people who never smoked. Quitting smoking at any age can lower the risk of lung cancer.

Cigarette smoking can cause cancer almost anywhere in the body. Cigarette smoking causes cancer of the mouth and throat, esophagus, stomach, colon, rectum, liver, pancreas, voicebox (larynx), lung, trachea, bronchus, kidney, and renal pelvis, urinary bladder, and cervix, and causes acute myeloid leukemia (AML).

Secondhand Smoke

Smoke from other people's cigarettes, pipes, or cigars (secondhand smoke) also causes lung cancer. In the United States, one out of four people who do not smoke, including 14 million children, were exposed to secondhand smoke during 2013–2014.

Radon

After smoking, radon is the second leading cause of lung cancer in the United States. Radon is a naturally occurring gas that forms in rocks, soil, and water. It cannot be seen, tasted, or smelled. When radon gets into homes or buildings through cracks or holes, it can get trapped and build up in the air inside. People who live or work in these homes and buildings breathe in high radon levels. Over long periods of time, radon can cause lung cancer.

The U.S. Environmental Protection Agency (EPA) estimates that radon causes about 21,000 lung cancer deaths each year. The risk of lung cancer from radon exposure is higher for people who smoke than for people who do not smoke. However, the EPA estimates that more than 10 percent of radon-related lung cancer deaths occur among people who have never smoked cigarettes. Nearly 1 out of every 15 homes in the United States has high radon levels.

Other Substances

Examples of substances found at some workplaces that increase risk include asbestos, arsenic, diesel exhaust, and some forms of silica and chromium. For many of these substances, the risk of getting lung cancer is even higher for those who smoke. Living in areas with higher levels of air pollution may increase the risk of getting lung cancer.

Personal or Family History of Lung Cancer

If you are a lung cancer survivor, there is a risk that you may develop another lung cancer, especially if you smoke. Your risk of lung cancer may be higher if your parents, brothers or sisters, or children have had lung cancer. This could be true because they also smoke, they live or work in the same place where they are exposed to radon and other substances that can cause lung cancer, or because of an inherited genetic mutation.

Radiation Therapy to the Chest

Cancer survivors who had radiation therapy to the chest are at higher risk of lung cancer.

Diet

Scientists are studying many different foods and dietary supplements to see whether they change the risk of getting lung cancer. There is much we still need to know. We do know that people who smoke and take beta-carotene supplements have increased risk of lung cancer.

What Are the Symptoms of Lung Cancer?

Different people have different symptoms for lung cancer. Some people have symptoms related to the lungs. Some people whose lung cancer has spread to other parts of the body (metastasized) have symptoms specific to that part of the body. Some people just have general symptoms of not feeling well. Most people with lung cancer do not have symptoms until the cancer is advanced. Lung cancer symptoms may include the following:

- coughing that gets worse or does not go away
- chest pain
- shortness of breath
- wheezing
- coughing up blood
- feeling very tired all the time
- weight loss with no known cause

Other changes that can sometimes occur with lung cancer may include repeated bouts of pneumonia and swollen or enlarged lymph nodes (glands) inside the chest in the area between the lungs.

These signs and symptoms can happen with other illnesses, too. If you have some of these signs and symptoms, talk to your doctor, who can help find the cause.

What Can You Do to Reduce Your Risk of Lung Cancer?

You can help lower your risk of lung cancer in the following ways:

- **Do not smoke**. Cigarette smoking causes about 80–90 percent of lung cancer deaths in the United States. The most important thing you can do to prevent lung cancer is to not start smoking or to quit if you smoke.
- **Avoid secondhand smoke**. Smoke from other people's cigarettes, cigars, or pipes is called "secondhand smoke." Make your home and car smoke-free.
- **Get your home tested for radon**. The EPA recommends that all homes be tested for radon.
- **Be careful at work**. Follow health and safety guidelines to avoid carcinogens (things that can cause cancer).

Screening for Lung Cancer

Screening means testing for a disease when there are no symptoms or history of that disease. Doctors recommend a screening test to find a disease early, when treatment may work better.

The only recommended screening test for lung cancer is low-dose computed tomography (also called a "low-dose CT scan," or "LDCT"). During an LDCT scan, you lie on a table and an x-ray machine uses a low dose (amount) of radiation to make detailed images of your lungs. The scan only takes a few minutes and is not painful.

Who Should Be Screened?

The U.S. Preventive Services Task Force (USPSTF) recommends yearly lung cancer screening with LDCT for people who:

- have a 20-pack-year or more smoking history
- smoke now or have quit within the past 15 years
- are between 50 and 80 years old

A pack-year is smoking an average of one pack of cigarettes per day for one year. For example, a person could have a 20-pack-year history by smoking one pack a day for 20 years or two packs a day for 10 years.

Risks of Screening

Lung cancer screening has at least three risks:

- A lung cancer screening test can suggest that a person has lung cancer when no cancer is present. This is called a "false-positive result." False-positive results can lead to follow-up tests and surgeries that are not needed and may have risks.
- A lung cancer screening test can find cases of cancer that may never have caused a problem for the patient. This is called "overdiagnosis." Overdiagnosis can lead to treatment that is not needed.
- Radiation from repeated LDCT tests can cause cancer in otherwise healthy people.

That is why lung cancer screening is recommended only for adults who are at high risk for developing the disease because of their smoking history and age, and who do not have a health problem that substantially limits their life expectancy or their ability or willingness to have lung surgery, if needed.

If you are thinking about getting screened, talk to your doctor. If lung cancer screening is right for you, your doctor can refer you to a high-quality screening facility.

Some people with a smoking history may blame themselves or feel that others blame them for being at risk for getting cancer. Lung cancer can be caused by many different things. If you do get lung cancer, lung cancer screening can help find it early, when treatment may work better.

When you get lung cancer screening, your doctor may ask you if you smoke, ask if you are ready to quit smoking, and tell you about proven steps that can help you quit. No matter how long you have used tobacco, quitting can reduce your risk for lung cancer and other chronic diseases. Many people who use tobacco become addicted to nicotine, a drug found naturally in tobacco. This can make it hard to quit using tobacco. Most people who use tobacco try to quit several times before they succeed.

When Should Screening Stop?

The USPSTF recommends that yearly lung cancer screening stop when the person being screened:

- turns 81 years old
- has not smoked in 15 or more years
- develops a health problem that makes him or her unwilling or unable to have surgery if lung cancer is found

How Is Lung Cancer Diagnosed and Treated?

Types of Lung Cancer

The two main types of lung cancer are small cell lung cancer and non-small cell lung cancer. These categories refer to what the cancer cells look like under a microscope. Non-small cell lung cancer is more common than small cell lung cancer.

If you have lung cancer (especially non-small cell lung cancer), your doctor may run tests to find out if you have a change in your genes (genetic mutation). The results of these tests help your doctor know which treatments will work best for you.

Staging

If lung cancer is diagnosed, other tests are done to find out how far it has spread through the lungs, lymph nodes, and the rest of the body. This process is called "staging." The type and stage of lung cancer tells doctors what kind of treatment you need.

Screening can help find lung cancer at an early stage, when treatment may work better.

Types of Treatment

Lung cancer is treated in several ways, depending on the type of lung cancer and how far it has spread. People with non-small cell lung cancer can be treated with surgery, chemotherapy, radiation therapy (RT), targeted therapy, or a combination of these treatments. People with small cell lung cancer are usually treated with radiation therapy and chemotherapy.

- **Surgery**. An operation where doctors cut out cancer tissue.
- **Chemotherapy**. Using special medicines to shrink or kill the cancer. The drugs can be pills you take or medicines given in your veins, or sometimes both.
- **Radiation therapy**. Using high-energy rays (similar to x-rays) to kill the cancer.

- **Targeted therapy**. Using drugs to block the growth and spread of cancer cells. The drugs can be pills you take or medicines given in your veins. You will get tests to see if targeted therapy is right for your cancer type before this treatment is used.

Doctors from different specialties often work together to treat lung cancer. Pulmonologists are doctors who are experts in diseases of the lungs. Surgeons are doctors who perform operations. Thoracic surgeons specialize in chest, heart, and lung surgery. Medical oncologists are doctors who treat cancer with medicines. Radiation oncologists are doctors who treat cancers with radiation.

Complementary and Alternative Medicine

Complementary and alternative medicine (CAM) are medicines and health practices that are not standard treatments doctors usually use to treat cancer.

Complementary medicine is used in addition to standard treatments. Examples include acupuncture and meditation.

Alternative medicine is used instead of standard treatments. Examples include special diets, megadose vitamins, herbal preparations, special teas, and magnet therapy.

Many kinds of CAM have not been tested scientifically and may not be safe. Some CAMs may make your cancer medicine not work as well. Talk to your doctor about the risks and benefits before you start any kind of CAM.

Living with Lung Cancer

When you have been diagnosed with cancer, you are considered a cancer survivor from that moment throughout the rest of your life.

Finding lung cancer earlier and making new treatments available are helping more lung cancer survivors live longer. We offer some tips to help you live with lung cancer as long and well as possible.

It is important to get the treatment you need at the best time. You deserve timely and appropriate care for your lung cancer and its symptoms (including pain), as well as any side effects of treatment. Molecular testing (also called "tumor" or "biomarker testing") may help you make decisions about treatment. You may also consider genetic testing to identify inherited characteristics.

Talk with your health-care provider about how a survivorship care plan can help you coordinate your follow-up care to support your physical and emotional health.

Take steps to stay healthy. This can lower your risk of getting cancer again or having the cancer come back.

Some cancer survivors may blame themselves or feel that others blame them for having cancer. Lung cancer survivors may have feelings of blame or stigma. You may find it helpful to talk about your experiences and feelings with a social worker or other mental health professional.

Source: "Living with Lung Cancer," Centers for Disease Control and Prevention (CDC), July 31, 2023. Available online. URL: www.cdc.gov/cancer/lung/living/index.htm. Accessed September 28, 2023.

Which Treatment Is Right for You?

Choosing the treatment that is right for you may be hard. Talk to your cancer doctor about the treatment options available for your type and stage of cancer. Your doctor can explain the risks and benefits of each treatment and their side effects. Side effects are how your body reacts to drugs or other treatments.

Sometimes, people get an opinion from more than one cancer doctor. This is called a "second opinion." Getting a second opinion may help you choose the treatment that is right for you.[1]

[1] "What Is Lung Cancer?" Centers for Disease Control and Prevention (CDC), July 31, 2023. Available online. URL: www.cdc.gov/cancer/lung/basic_info/what-is-lung-cancer.htm. Accessed September 28, 2023.

CHAPTER 29
COLORECTAL CANCER

What Is Colorectal Cancer?

Colorectal cancer is cancer that develops in the tissues of the colon or rectum. Your colon and rectum are part of your digestive system (see Figure 29.1).

Your colon is the first and longest part of your large intestine. It absorbs water and some nutrients from foods. It also changes the leftover waste products into stool (poop).

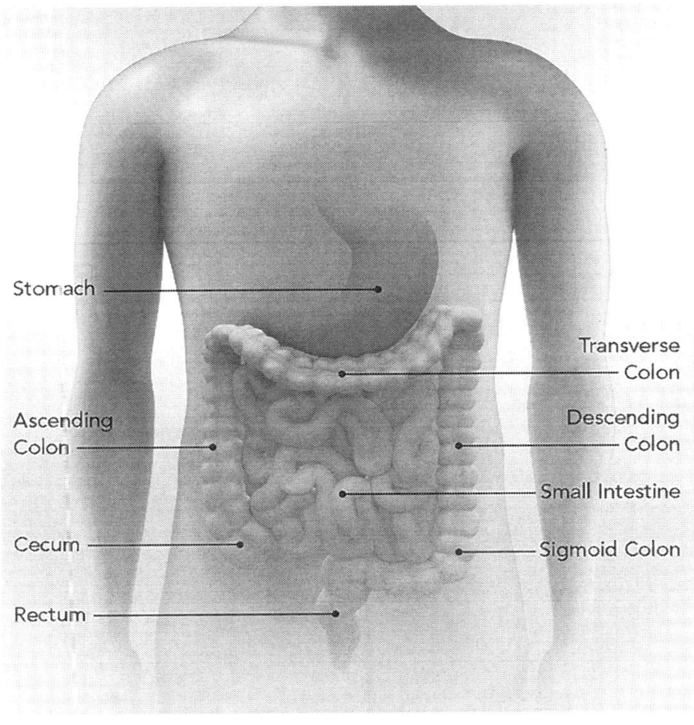

Figure 29.1. Illustration of Colon and Rectum
Centers for Disease Control and Prevention (CDC)

Your rectum is the lower part of your large intestine. It is where your body stores stool.

Cancer that begins in the colon is called "colon cancer," and cancer that begins in the rectum is called "rectal cancer." Cancer that affects either of these parts may also be called "colorectal cancer."

What Causes Colorectal Cancer?

Colorectal cancer happens when there are changes in your genetic material (DNA). These changes are also called "mutations" or "variants." Often, the genetic changes that lead to colorectal cancer happen during your lifetime, and the exact cause is unknown. But certain genetic changes that raise your risk for colorectal cancer are inherited, meaning that you are born with them.

Besides genetics, other factors, including your lifestyle and the environment, can affect your risk of colorectal cancer.

What Are the Symptoms of Colorectal Cancer?

Colorectal cancer may not always cause symptoms, especially at first. If you do have symptoms, they could include the following:

- a change in bowel habits that lasts more than a few days, such as:
  - diarrhea
  - constipation
  - feeling that the bowel does not empty completely
  - your stool being narrower or having been a different shape than usual
- blood (either bright red or very dark) in the stool
- frequent gas pains, bloating, fullness, or cramps
- weight loss for no known reason
- fatigue

What Is Screening for Colorectal Cancer, and Who Needs It?

Because colorectal cancer may not cause symptoms at first, it is important to have screening tests for colorectal cancer. Screening tests look for signs of a disease before you have any symptoms. They can help find cancer early when it may be easier to treat.

Most experts recommend that start screenings at 45 and continue until at least age 75. People over 75 and those who are at high risk should talk to their providers about how often they need screening and what type of test they should get.

The types of tests include different stool tests and procedures, such as colonoscopies and flexible sigmoidoscopy. Talk with your provider about how often you need screening and what type of test you should get.

How Is Colorectal Cancer Diagnosed?

If you have symptoms that could be caused by colorectal cancer or if your screening test results are abnormal, you may need to have more tests to find out if you have cancer. Possible tests include the following:

- a physical exam
- a digital rectal exam (For this exam, your provider inserts a lubricated, gloved finger into your rectum to feel for lumps or anything unusual.)
- the tests that are also used for screening (colonoscopy, stool tests, etc.) and biopsy if you have not already had them
- other blood and tissue tests

What Are the Treatments for Colorectal Cancer?

Your treatment options usually depend on your age, your general health, how serious the cancer is, and which type of cancer you have.

For colon cancer, your treatment may include one or more of the following options:

- surgery
- radiofrequency ablation (a procedure that uses radio waves to heat and destroy abnormal cells. The radio waves travel through electrodes (small devices that carry electricity).)
- cryosurgery (a procedure in which an extremely cold liquid or an instrument called a "cryoprobe" is used to freeze and destroy abnormal tissue)
- chemotherapy
- radiation therapy
- targeted therapy (which uses drugs or other substances that mainly attack specific cancer cells and cause less harm to normal cells)
- immunotherapy

For rectal cancer, your treatment may include one or more of the following options:

- surgery
- radiation therapy
- chemotherapy
- active surveillance (which means having regular tests to see if your rectal cancer has changed. If the tests show the cancer is starting to grow, then you will have treatment to try to cure the cancer.)
- targeted therapy (which uses drugs or other substances that mainly attack specific cancer cells and cause less harm to normal cells)
- immunotherapy[1]

[1] MedlinePlus, "Colorectal Cancer," National Institutes of Health (NIH), December 21, 2022. Available online. URL: https://medlineplus.gov/colorectalcancer.html. Accessed September 28, 2023.

Colorectal Cancer Prevention

Avoiding cancer risk factors may help prevent certain cancers. Risk factors include smoking, being overweight, and not getting enough exercise. Increasing protective factors such as quitting smoking and exercising may also help prevent some cancers. Talk to your doctor or other health-care professional about how you might lower your risk of cancer.

The following risk factors increase the risk of colorectal cancer:

- **Age**. The risk of colorectal cancer increases after age 50. Most cases of colorectal cancer are diagnosed after age 50.
- **Family history of colorectal cancer**. Having a parent, brother, sister, or child with colorectal cancer doubles a person's risk of colorectal cancer.
- **Personal history**. Having a personal history of the following conditions increases the risk of colorectal cancer:
  - previous colorectal cancer
  - high-risk adenomas (colorectal polyps that are 1 cm or larger in size or that have cells that look abnormal under a microscope)
  - ovarian cancer
  - inflammatory bowel disease (IBD, such as ulcerative colitis or Crohn's disease)
- **Inherited risk**. The risk of colorectal cancer is increased when certain gene changes linked to FAP or hereditary nonpolyposis colon cancer (HNPCC or Lynch syndrome) are inherited.
- **Alcohol**. Drinking three or more alcoholic beverages per day increases the risk of colorectal cancer. Drinking alcohol is also linked to the risk of forming large colorectal adenomas (benign tumors).
- **Cigarette smoking**. It is linked to an increased risk of colorectal cancer and death from colorectal cancer. Smoking cigarettes is also linked to an increased risk of forming colorectal adenomas. Cigarette smokers who have had surgery to remove colorectal adenomas are at an increased risk for the adenomas to recur (come back).
- **Race**. Black individuals have an increased risk of colorectal cancer and death from colorectal cancer compared to other races.
- **Obesity**. Obesity is linked to an increased risk of colorectal cancer and death from colorectal cancer.

The following protective factors decrease the risk of colorectal cancer:

- **Physical activity**. A lifestyle that includes regular physical activity is linked to a decreased risk of colorectal cancer.
- **Aspirin**. Studies have shown that taking aspirin lowers the risk of colorectal cancer and the risk of death from colorectal cancer. The decrease in risk begins 10–20 years after patients start taking aspirin.

The possible harms of aspirin use daily or every other day include an increased risk of stroke and bleeding in the stomach and intestines. These risks may be greater among the elderly, men, and those with conditions linked to a higher-than-normal risk of bleeding.

- **Combination hormone replacement therapy (HRT)**. Studies have shown that combination HRT that includes both estrogen and progestin lowers the risk of invasive colorectal cancer in postmenopausal women. However, in women who take combination HRT and do develop colorectal cancer, the cancer is more likely to be advanced when it is diagnosed and the risk of dying from colorectal cancer is not decreased. The possible harms of combination HRT include an increased risk of having:
  - breast cancer
  - heart disease
  - blood clots
- **Polyp removal**. Most colorectal polyps are adenomas, which may develop into cancer. Removing colorectal polyps that are larger than 1 cm (pea-sized) may lower the risk of colorectal cancer. It is not known if removing smaller polyps lowers the risk of colorectal cancer. The possible harms of polyp removal during colonoscopy or sigmoidoscopy include a tear in the wall of the colon and bleeding.[2]

[2] "Colorectal Cancer Prevention (PDQ®)—Patient Version," National Cancer Institute (NCI), June 26, 2023. Available online. URL: www.cancer.gov/types/colorectal/patient/colorectal-prevention-pdq. Accessed September 28, 2023.

CHAPTER 30
BLADDER CANCER

What Is Bladder Cancer?

Bladder cancer occurs when cells in the bladder start to grow without control. The bladder is a hollow, balloon-shaped organ in the lower part of the abdomen that stores urine.

The bladder has a muscular wall that allows it to get larger to store urine made by the kidneys and to shrink to squeeze urine out of the body. There are two kidneys, one on each side of the backbone, above the waist. The bladder and kidneys work together to remove toxins and wastes from your body through urine:

- Tiny tubules in the kidneys filter and clean the blood.
- These tubules take out waste products and make urine.
- The urine passes from each kidney through a long tube called a "ureter" into the bladder.
- The bladder holds the urine until it passes through a tube called the "urethra" and leaves the body.

Types of Bladder Cancer

Urothelial carcinoma (also called "transitional cell carcinoma" (TCC)) is cancer that begins in the urothelial cells, which line the urethra, bladder, ureters, renal pelvis, and some other organs. Almost all bladder cancers are urothelial carcinomas.

Urothelial cells are also called "transitional cells" because they change shape. These cells are able to stretch when the bladder is full of urine and shrink when it is emptied.

Other types of bladder cancer are rare:

- **Squamous cell carcinoma (SCC)**. It is a cancer that begins in squamous cells (thin, flat cells lining the inside of the bladder). This type of cancer may form after long-term irritation or infection with a tropical parasite called "schistosomiasis," which is common in Africa and the Middle East but rare in the United States. When chronic irritation occurs, transitional cells that line the bladder can gradually change to squamous cells.

- **Adenocarcinoma**. It is a cancer that begins in glandular cells that are found in the lining of the bladder. Glandular cells in the bladder make mucus and other substances.
- **Small cell carcinoma of the bladder**. It is a cancer that begins in neuroendocrine cells (nerve-like cells that release hormones into the blood in response to a signal from the nervous system).

There are other ways to describe bladder cancer:

- **Nonmuscle-invasive bladder cancer**. It is a cancer that has not reached the muscle wall of the bladder. Most bladder cancers are nonmuscle-invasive.
- **Muscle-invasive bladder cancer**. It is a cancer that has spread through the lining of the bladder and into the muscle wall of the bladder or beyond it.

Causes of Bladder Cancer

Bladder cancer is caused by certain changes in how bladder cells function, especially how they grow and divide into new cells. There are many risk factors for bladder cancer, but many do not directly cause cancer. Instead, they increase the chance of deoxyribonucleic acid (DNA) damage in cells that may lead to bladder cancer.

A risk factor is anything that increases the chance of getting a disease. Some risk factors for bladder cancer, such as using tobacco, can be changed. Risk factors also include things people cannot change, such as their age and family history. It is important to learn about risk factors for bladder cancer because it can help you make choices that might lower your risk of getting it.

Risk Factors for Bladder Cancer

In the United States, bladder cancer occurs more often in men than in women, and more often in White individuals than in Black individuals. Bladder cancer can be diagnosed at any age, but the risk increases as a person gets older.

Using tobacco, especially smoking cigarettes, is a major risk factor for bladder cancer. Tobacco contains harmful chemicals called "carcinogens." When you use tobacco, these chemicals get absorbed into the bloodstream, are filtered by the kidneys, and then collect in the urine. This exposes your bladder to high levels of these chemicals, which can damage the DNA in the cells lining your bladder.

Other risk factors for bladder cancer include the following:

- having a family history of bladder cancer
- having certain changes in the genes that are linked to bladder cancer, such as *HRAS*, *RB1*, *PTEN/MMAC1*, *NAT2*, and *GSTM1*
- being exposed to paints, dyes, metals, or petroleum products in the workplace
- past treatment with radiation therapy to the pelvis or with certain anticancer drugs, such as cyclophosphamide or ifosfamide

- taking the Chinese herb *Aristolochia fangchi*
- drinking water from a well that has high levels of arsenic
- drinking water that has been treated with chlorine
- having a bladder infection caused by a parasite called "*Schistosoma haematobium*," which is common in Africa and the Middle East but rare in the United States
- using urinary catheters for a long time

Having one or more of these risk factors does not necessarily mean you will get bladder cancer. Many people with risk factors never develop bladder cancer, while others with no known risk factors do. Talk with your doctor if you think you might be at risk of bladder cancer. Bladder cancer screening options may be available to you.

Symptoms of Bladder Cancer

The symptoms of bladder cancer can vary from person to person. The most common symptom is blood in the urine, called "hematuria." It is often slightly rusty to bright red in color. You may see blood in your urine at one point, then not see it again for a while. Sometimes there are very small amounts of blood in the urine that can only be found by having a test done.

Other common symptoms of bladder cancer include the following:

- frequent urination
- pain or burning during urination
- feeling as if you need to urinate even if your bladder is not full
- urinating often during the night

When the cancer has grown large or spread beyond the bladder to other parts of the body, symptoms may include the following:

- being unable to urinate
- lower back pain on one side of the body
- pain in the abdomen
- bone pain or tenderness
- unintended weight loss and loss of appetite
- swelling in the feet
- feeling tired

It is important to check with your doctor if you have any of these symptoms. Keep in mind that urinary tract infections (UTIs), kidney or bladder stones, or other problems related to the kidney could be the cause, not cancer. Your doctor will ask you when your symptoms started and how often you are having them. They will most likely ask you to give a urine sample as a first step in diagnosing what is causing your symptoms.

Screening of Bladder Cancer

Tests to Screen for Bladder Cancer

There is no standard screening test for bladder cancer in people at average risk. When enough evidence has been collected to show that a screening test is safe, accurate, and useful for people at average risk of bladder cancer, it will become a standard test. However, certain tests may be used to screen for bladder cancer in people who have had bladder cancer in the past or who are at an increased risk of developing it.

Hematuria Test

Hematuria is red blood cells (RBCs) in the urine. It may be caused by cancer or by other conditions. A hematuria test is used to check for blood in a sample of urine by viewing it under a microscope or using a special test strip. The test may be repeated over time.

Urine Cytology

Urine cytology is a lab test in which a sample of urine is checked under a microscope for abnormal cells.

Urine Tumor Marker Tests

Urinary tumor markers are substances found in the urine that are either made by bladder cancer cells or that the body makes in response to bladder cancer. For this test, a sample of urine is checked in the lab to detect the presence of these substances. Urine tumor marker tests may also be used to help diagnose some types of bladder cancer.

Cystoscopy

Cystoscopy is a procedure to look inside the bladder and urethra to check for abnormal areas. A cystoscope (a thin, lighted tube) is inserted through the urethra into the bladder. Tissue samples may be taken for biopsy.

Risks of Bladder Cancer Screening

Screening tests have benefits and risks. Talk with your doctor about whether bladder cancer screening is right for you.

Potential risks of harm from bladder cancer screening include false-positive and false-negative test results:

- **False-positive test results**. Screening test results may appear to be abnormal even though no cancer is present. A false-positive test result (one that shows there is cancer when there is not) can cause anxiety and is usually followed by more tests (such as cystoscopy or other invasive procedures), which also have risks. False-positive results often occur with hematuria testing; blood in the urine is usually caused by conditions other than cancer.

- **False-negative test results**. Screening test results may appear to be normal even though bladder cancer is present. A person who receives a false-negative test result (one that shows there is no cancer when there is) may delay seeking medical care even if there are symptoms.

Diagnosis of Bladder Cancer

If you have symptoms or lab test results that suggest bladder cancer, your doctor will need to find out if they are due to cancer or another condition. Your doctor may:

- ask about your personal and family medical history to learn more about your symptoms and possible risk factors for bladder cancer
- ask for a sample of your urine so it can be checked in the lab for blood, abnormal cells, or infection
- do a physical exam, which for women, may include a pelvic exam, to check for signs of cancer

Depending on your symptoms, medical history, and results of your urine lab tests and physical exam, your doctor may recommend more tests to find out if you have bladder cancer, and if so, its extent (stage).

Tests to Diagnose Bladder Cancer

The following tests and procedures are used to diagnose bladder cancer. The results will also help you and your doctor plan treatment.

Cystoscopy

Cystoscopy is a procedure in which the doctor looks inside the bladder and urethra (the tube that carries urine out of your body) to check for abnormal areas. A cystoscope is slowly inserted through the urethra into the bladder to allow the doctor to see inside. A cystoscope is a thin, tube-like instrument with a light and a lens for viewing. It may also have a tool to remove very small bladder tumors or tissue samples for biopsy. Cystoscopy helps to diagnose, and sometimes treat, bladder cancer and other conditions.

Biopsy

A biopsy is usually done during a cystoscopy procedure. It is a procedure in which a sample of cells or tissue is removed from the bladder so that a pathologist can view it under a microscope to check for signs of cancer. It may be possible to remove the entire tumor at the time of the biopsy.

Talk with your doctor to learn what to expect during and after your cystoscopy and biopsy. Some people have blood in the urine or discomfort and a burning sensation while urinating for a day or two.

Computed Tomography Urogram or Intravenous Pyelogram

Computed tomography (CT) urogram is a test that takes a CT scan of the urinary tract using a contrast dye injected into a vein. To begin the procedure, a CT machine takes a series of detailed pictures of the kidneys. The contrast dye is then injected, and another CT scan of the kidneys, bladder, and ureters is done. About 10 minutes later, a final scan is taken as the contrast dye drains from the kidneys into the bladder. CT urogram also captures detailed pictures of nearby bones, soft tissues, and blood vessels. This allows the doctor to see how well your urinary tract is working and to check for signs of disease.

Intravenous pyelogram (IVP) is an x-ray imaging test of your urinary tract. After a contrast dye is injected into a vein, a series of x-ray pictures of the kidneys, ureters, and bladder are taken to find out if cancer is present in these organs. As the contrast dye moves through the kidneys, ureters, and bladder, more x-ray pictures are taken at specific times. This allows your doctor to see how well your urinary tract is working and to check for signs of disease.

Urine Tumor Marker Test

Urinary tumor markers are substances found in the urine that are either made by bladder cancer cells or that the body makes in response to bladder cancer. For this test, a sample of urine is checked in the lab to detect the presence of these substances. Urine tumor marker tests may be used to help diagnose some types of bladder cancer.

Tests to Stage Bladder Cancer

If you are diagnosed with bladder cancer, you will be referred to an urologic oncologist. This is a doctor who specializes in diagnosing and treating cancers of the male and female urinary tract and the male reproductive organs. They will recommend tests to determine the extent of cancer. Sometimes the cancer is only in the bladder. Or, it may have spread from the bladder to other parts of the body. The process of learning the extent of cancer in the body is called "staging." It is important to know the stage of the bladder cancer to plan treatment.

The following imaging tests may be used to determine the bladder cancer stage:

- **Computed tomography scan**. It uses a computer linked to an x-ray machine to make a series of detailed x-ray pictures of areas inside the body from different angles. A dye may be injected into a vein or swallowed to help the organs or tissues show up more clearly.
- **Magnetic resonance imaging (MRI)**. It uses a magnet, radio waves, and a computer to make a series of detailed pictures of areas inside the body, such as the bladder. This procedure is also called "nuclear magnetic resonance imaging" (NMRI). Images may be taken at three different times after the dye is injected, to get the best picture of abnormal areas in the bladder. This is called "triple-phase MRI."

- **Chest x-ray**. It is an x-ray of the organs and bones inside the chest. An x-ray is a type of high-energy radiation that can go through the body and onto film, making a picture of areas inside the chest.
- **Bone scan**. It is a procedure that checks to see if there are rapidly dividing cells, such as cancer cells, in the bone. A very small amount of radioactive material is injected into a vein and travels through the bloodstream. The radioactive material collects in the bones with cancer and is detected by a scanner.

Getting a Second Opinion

Some people may want to get a second opinion to confirm their bladder cancer diagnosis and treatment plan. If you choose to seek a second opinion, you will need to get important medical test results and reports from the first doctor to share with the second doctor. The second doctor will review the pathology report, slides, and scans before giving a recommendation. The doctor who gives the second opinion may agree with your first doctor, suggest changes or another approach, or provide more information about your cancer.

Prognosis of Bladder Cancer

If you have been diagnosed with bladder cancer, you may have questions about how serious the cancer is and your chances of survival. The likely outcome or course of a disease is called "prognosis."

The prognosis for bladder cancer depends on many factors:

- the stage of the cancer, including whether the cancer:
    - has not reached the muscle wall of the bladder (called "nonmuscle-invasive" or "superficial bladder cancer") or
    - has spread through the inner lining of the bladder and into the muscle wall of the bladder or beyond it (called "muscle-invasive bladder cancer" or "invasive bladder cancer")
- the type of bladder cancer
- whether the cancer is low- or high-grade
- the patient's age and general health

For nonmuscle-invasive bladder cancer, prognosis also depends on whether:

- there are many tumors or large tumors
- the cancer has grown into the connective tissue next to the lining of the bladder
- the cancer has come back after treatment

Nonmuscle-invasive bladder cancer can often be cured.

For muscle-invasive bladder cancer, prognosis also depends on whether carcinoma in situ is also present.

Treatment for Bladder Cancer

Different types of treatment are available for bladder cancer. You and your cancer care team will work together to decide your treatment plan, which may include more than one type of treatment. Many factors will be considered, such as the stage and grade of the cancer, your overall health, and your preferences. Your plan will include information about your cancer, the goals of treatment, your treatment options and the possible side effects, and the expected length of treatment.

It will be helpful to talk with your cancer care team before treatment begins about what to expect. Some things you will want to learn about include what you need to do before treatment begins, how you will feel while going through it, and what kind of help you will need.

Survival Rates for Bladder Cancer

Doctors estimate bladder cancer prognosis by using statistics collected over many years from people with bladder cancer. One statistic that is commonly used in making a prognosis is the five-year relative survival rate. The five-year relative survival rate tells you what percent of people with the same type and stage of bladder cancer are alive five years after their cancer was diagnosed, compared with people in the overall population. For example, the five-year relative survival rate for localized bladder cancer is 71 percent. This means that people diagnosed with localized bladder cancer are 71 percent as likely as someone who does not have bladder cancer to be alive five years after diagnosis.

The five-year relative survival rates for bladder cancer are as follows:

- 97 percent for carcinoma in situ of the bladder alone (abnormal cells found in the tissue lining the inside of the bladder)
- 71 percent for localized bladder cancer (cancer is in the bladder only)
- 39 percent for regional bladder cancer (cancer has spread beyond the bladder to nearby lymph nodes or organs)
- 8 percent for metastatic bladder cancer (cancer has spread beyond the bladder to a distant part of the body)

Source: "Bladder Cancer Prognosis and Survival Rates," National Cancer Institute (NCI), April 27, 2023. Available online. URL: www.cancer.gov/types/bladder/survival. Accessed September 28, 2023.

Surgery

Surgery is the main treatment for bladder cancer. The type of surgery depends on where the cancer is located. Other treatments may be given in addition to surgery:

- Treatment given before surgery is called "preoperative therapy" or "neoadjuvant therapy." Chemotherapy may be given before surgery to shrink the tumor and reduce the amount of tissue that needs to be removed during surgery.
- Treatment given after surgery, to lower the risk that the cancer will come back, is called "adjuvant therapy." After the doctor removes all the cancer that

can be seen, some patients may be given chemotherapy, radiation therapy, immunotherapy, and/or targeted therapy to kill any cancer cells that are left.

The types of surgery done to treat bladder cancer are as follows:

- **Transurethral resection (TUR) with fulguration**. During TUR with fulguration, the doctor inserts a cystoscope (a thin lighted tube) into the bladder through the urethra. A tool with a small wire loop on the end is then used to remove the cancer or to burn the tumor away with high-energy electricity. This is known as "fulguration."
- **Partial cystectomy**. It is a surgery to remove part of the bladder. This may be done for patients who have a low-grade tumor that has invaded the wall of the bladder but is limited to one area of the bladder. Because only a part of the bladder is removed, patients are able to urinate normally after recovering from this surgery. This is also called "segmental cystectomy."
- **Radical cystectomy with urinary diversion**. It is a surgery to remove the bladder and any lymph nodes and nearby organs that contain cancer. This surgery may be done when the bladder cancer invades the muscle layers or when nonmuscle-invasive bladder cancer involves a large part of the bladder:
    - In men, the nearby organs that are removed are the prostate and the seminal vesicles.
    - In women, the uterus, the ovaries, and part of the vagina are removed.

Sometimes, when the cancer has spread outside the bladder and cannot be completely removed, surgery to remove only the bladder may be done to reduce urinary symptoms caused by the cancer.

When the bladder must be removed, the surgeon performs a procedure called "urinary diversion" to create another way for the body to store and pass urine. It may involve redirecting urine into the colon, using catheters to drain the bladder, or making an opening in the abdomen that connects to a bag outside the body for collecting urine.

Radiation Therapy

Radiation therapy uses high-energy x-rays or other types of radiation to kill cancer cells or keep them from growing. Bladder cancer is sometimes treated with external beam radiation therapy. This type of radiation therapy uses a machine outside the body to send radiation toward the area of the body with cancer. Radiation therapy may be given alone or with other types of treatment, such as chemotherapy.

Chemotherapy

Chemotherapy (also called "chemo") uses drugs to stop the growth of cancer cells, either by killing the cells or by stopping them from dividing. Chemotherapy may be given alone or with other types of treatment. The way the chemotherapy is given depends on the type and stage of the cancer being treated.

Systemic Chemotherapy

Systemic chemotherapy for bladder cancer is when chemotherapy drugs are injected into a vein. When given this way, the drugs enter the bloodstream to reach cancer cells throughout the body. Systemic chemotherapy drugs that may be used to treat bladder cancer are:

- carboplatin
- cisplatin
- doxorubicin
- fluorouracil (5-FU)
- gemcitabine
- methotrexate
- mitomycin
- paclitaxel
- vinblastine

Combinations of these drugs may be used. Other chemotherapy drugs not listed here may also be used.

Intravesical Chemotherapy

For bladder cancer, chemotherapy may be intravesical, meaning it is put into the bladder through a tube inserted into the urethra. Intravesical treatments flush the bladder with drugs that kill cancer cells that remain after surgery. This lowers the chance of the cancer coming back.

Mitomycin and gemcitabine are two chemotherapy drugs given as intravesical chemotherapy to treat bladder cancer. These drugs can also be given systemically.

Immunotherapy

Immunotherapy helps a person's immune system fight cancer. Your doctor may suggest biomarker tests to help predict your response to certain immunotherapy drugs.

Systemic Immunotherapy

Systemic immunotherapy drugs used to treat urothelial cancer (a type of bladder cancer) include the following:

- avelumab
- nivolumab
- pembrolizumab

These drugs work in more than one way to kill cancer cells. They are also considered targeted therapy because they target specific changes or substances in cancer cells.

Intravesical Immunotherapy

The bacillus Calmette-Guérin (BCG) is an intravesical immunotherapy drug used to treat bladder cancer. BCG is given in a solution that is placed directly into the bladder using a catheter (thin tube). Intravesical treatments flush the bladder with drugs that kill cancer cells that remain after surgery. This lowers the chance of the cancer coming back.

Targeted Therapy

Targeted therapy uses drugs or other substances to block the action of specific enzymes, proteins, or other molecules involved in the growth and spread of cancer cells. Your doctor may suggest biomarker tests to help predict your response to certain targeted therapy drugs. Targeted therapies used to treat bladder cancer include the following:

- enfortumab vedotin
- erdafitinib
- ramucirumab
- sacituzumab govitecan-hziy[1]

[1] "What Is Bladder Cancer?" National Cancer Institute (NCI), February 16, 2023. Available online. URL: www.cancer.gov/types/bladder. Accessed September 28, 2023.

CHAPTER 31
ORAL CANCER

Oral cancer includes cancers of the mouth and the back of the throat. Oral cancers develop on the tongue, on the tissue lining the mouth and gums, under the tongue, at the base of the tongue, and the area of the throat at the back of the mouth.

Oral cancer accounts for roughly 3 percent of all cancers diagnosed annually in the United States, or about 54,000 new cases in 2022.

Oral cancer most often occurs in people over the age of 40 and affects more than twice as many men as women. Most cancers in the mouth are related to tobacco use, drinking alcohol, or both, and most throat cancers are caused by the human papillomavirus (HPV). The incidence of HPV-positive oral cancer has risen in recent years.

Causes of Oral Cancer

- **Tobacco and alcohol use**. Tobacco use of any kind, including cigarette, pipe, cigar, and electronic cigarette smoking, as well as chewing tobacco and snuff, puts you at risk for developing oral cancers. Heavy alcohol use also increases the risk. Using both tobacco and alcohol increases the risk even further.
- **HPV**. Infection with the sexually transmitted HPV (specifically the HPV 16 type) has been linked to oral cancers.
- **Age**. Risk increases with age. Oral cancers most often occur in people over the age of 40.
- **Sun exposure**. Cancer of the lip can be caused by sun exposure.
- **Poor nutrition**. A diet low in fruits and vegetables has been linked with an increased risk of oral cancer.
- **Genetics**. People with inherited defects in certain genes have a high risk of mouth and middle throat cancer.

Symptoms of Oral Cancer

If you have any of the following symptoms for more than two weeks, see a dentist or a doctor:

- a sore, irritation, lump, or thick patch in your mouth, lip, or throat
- a white or red patch in your mouth
- persistent sore throat, a feeling that something is caught in your throat, or hoarseness or loss of your voice
- a lump in the neck
- difficulty chewing, swallowing, or speaking
- difficulty moving your jaw or tongue
- swelling of your jaw that causes dentures to fit poorly or become uncomfortable
- pain or bleeding in the mouth
- numbness in your tongue or other areas of your mouth
- ear pain

Diagnosis of Oral Cancer

- Because oral cancer can spread quickly, early detection is important. An oral cancer examination can detect early signs of cancer. The exam is painless and takes only a few minutes. Your regular dental checkup is an excellent opportunity to have the examination.
- During the examination, your dentist or dental hygienist will check your face, neck, lips, entire mouth, and the back of the throat for possible signs of cancer.
- If the dentist finds anything unusual, he or she will recommend additional tests and/or refer you to a specialist.

Helpful Tips

Oral cancer and its treatment can cause dental problems. It is important that your mouth is in good health before cancer treatment begins.

- See a dentist for a thorough examination one month, if possible, before starting cancer treatment to give your mouth time to heal after any dental work you might need.
- Before, during, and after cancer treatment, ask your health-care provider for ways to control pain and other symptoms and to relieve the side effects of therapy.
- Talk to your health-care team about financial aid, transportation, home care, and emotional and social support for yourself and your family.

Source: "Oral Cancer," National Institute of Dental and Craniofacial Research (NIDCR), June 2023. Available online. URL: www.nidcr.nih.gov/health-info/oral-cancer. Accessed September 28, 2023.

Treatment of Oral Cancer

Oral cancer is treated with surgery and possibly radiation therapy or chemotherapy. Oral cancer that is further along when it is diagnosed may need a combination of treatments.

Another treatment option is targeted therapy, which is a newer type of cancer treatment that uses drugs to precisely identify and attack cancer cells. Immunotherapy may also be a potential treatment; it can work with the body's natural defenses to improve immune function. The choice of treatment depends on your general health, where in your mouth or throat the cancer began, the size and type of the tumor, and whether the cancer has spread.

Your doctor may refer you to a specialist. Specialists who treat oral cancer include the following:

- head and neck surgeons
- dentists who specialize in surgery of the mouth, face, and jaw (oral and maxillofacial surgeons)
- ear, nose, and throat doctors (otolaryngologists)
- doctors who specifically treat cancer (medical and radiation oncologists)

Other health-care professionals who may be part of a treatment team include dentists, plastic surgeons, reconstructive surgeons, speech pathologists, oncology nurses, registered dietitians, genetic counselors, and mental health counselors.[1]

[1] "Oral Cancer," National Institute of Dental and Craniofacial Research (NIDCR), June 2023. Available online. URL: www.nidcr.nih.gov/health-info/oral-cancer. Accessed September 28, 2023.

CHAPTER 32
ESOPHAGEAL CANCER

Esophageal cancer is a disease in which malignant (cancer) cells form in the tissues of the esophagus. The esophagus is the hollow, muscular tube that moves food and liquid from the throat to the stomach. The wall of the esophagus is made up of several layers of tissue, including mucous membrane, muscle, and connective tissue. Esophageal cancer starts on the inside lining of the esophagus and spreads outward through the other layers as it grows.

The two most common forms of esophageal cancer are named for the type of cells that become malignant (cancerous):

- **Squamous cell carcinoma (SCC)**. Cancer that forms in the thin, flat cells lining the inside of the esophagus. This cancer is most often found in the upper and middle part of the esophagus but can occur anywhere along the esophagus. This is also called "epidermoid carcinoma."
- **Adenocarcinoma**. Cancer that begins in glandular cells. Glandular cells in the lining of the esophagus produce and release fluids such as mucus. Adenocarcinomas usually form in the lower part of the esophagus, near the stomach.

Risk Factors of Esophageal Cancer

Smoking, heavy alcohol use, and Barrett esophagus can increase the risk of esophageal cancer. Anything that increases your risk of getting a disease is called a "risk factor." Having a risk factor does not mean that you will get cancer; not having risk factors does not mean that you will not get cancer. Talk with your doctor if you think you may be at risk. Risk factors include the following:

- tobacco use
- heavy alcohol use
- Barrett esophagus (This is a condition in which the cells lining the lower part of the esophagus have changed or been replaced with abnormal cells that could lead to cancer of the esophagus. Gastric reflux (heartburn) is the most common cause of Barrett esophagus.)
- older age

Signs and Symptoms of Esophageal Cancer

The signs and symptoms of esophageal cancer are weight loss and painful or difficult swallowing. These and other signs and symptoms may be caused by esophageal cancer or by other conditions. Check with your doctor if you have any of the following:

- painful or difficult swallowing
- weight loss
- pain behind the breastbone
- hoarseness and cough
- indigestion and heartburn
- a lump under the skin

Tests That Examine Esophageal Cancer

The following tests and procedures may be used:

- **Physical exam and health history**. An exam of the body to check general signs of health, including checking for signs of disease, such as lumps or anything else that seems unusual. A history of the patient's health habits and past illnesses and treatments will also be taken.
- **Chest x-ray**. An x-ray of the organs and bones inside the chest. An x-ray is a type of energy beam that can go through the body and onto film, making a picture of areas inside the body.
- **Esophagoscopy**. A procedure to look inside the esophagus to check for abnormal areas. An esophagoscope is inserted through the mouth or nose and down the throat into the esophagus. An esophagoscope is a thin, tube-like instrument with a light and a lens for viewing. It may also have a tool to remove tissue samples, which are checked under a microscope for signs of cancer. When the esophagus and stomach are looked at, it is called an "upper endoscopy."
- **Biopsy**. The removal of cells or tissues so they can be viewed under a microscope by a pathologist to check for signs of cancer. The biopsy is usually done during an esophagoscopy. Sometimes a biopsy shows changes in the esophagus that are not cancer but may lead to cancer.

Prognosis of Esophageal Cancer

Certain factors affect prognosis (chance of recovery) and treatment options. The prognosis and treatment options depend on the following:

- the stage of the cancer (Whether it affects part of the esophagus, involves the whole esophagus, or has spread to other places in the body.)
- whether the tumor can be completely removed by surgery
- the patient's general health

When esophageal cancer is found very early, there is a better chance of recovery. Esophageal cancer is often in an advanced stage when it is diagnosed. At later stages, esophageal cancer can be treated but rarely can be cured. Taking part in one of the clinical trials being done to improve treatment should be considered.

Treatment of Esophageal Cancer

Different types of treatment are available for patients with esophageal cancer. Some treatments are standard (the currently used treatment), and some are being tested in clinical trials. A treatment clinical trial is a research study meant to help improve current treatments or obtain information on new treatments for patients with cancer. When clinical trials show that a new treatment is better than the standard treatment, the new treatment may become the standard treatment. Patients may want to think about taking part in a clinical trial. Some clinical trials are open only to patients who have not started treatment.

Risks of Esophageal Cancer Screening

Screening tests have risks. Decisions about screening tests can be difficult. Not all screening tests are helpful and most have risks. Before having any screening test, you may want to discuss the test with your doctor. It is important to know the risks of the test and whether it has been proven to reduce the risk of dying from cancer.

The risks of esophageal cancer screening tests include the following:

- **Finding esophageal cancer may not improve health or help a person live longer**. Screening may not improve your health or help you live longer if you have advanced esophageal cancer or if it has already spread to other places in your body.
  Some cancers never cause symptoms or become life-threatening, but if found by a screening test, the cancer may be treated. It is not known if treatment of these cancers will help you live longer than if no treatment were given, and treatments for cancer may have serious side effects.
- **False-negative test results can occur**. Screening test results may appear to be normal even though esophageal cancer is present. A person who receives a false-negative test result (one that shows there is no cancer when there really is) may delay seeking medical care even if there are symptoms.
- **False-positive test results can occur**. Screening test results may appear to be abnormal even though no cancer is present. A false-positive test result (one that shows there is cancer when there really is not) can cause anxiety and is usually followed by more tests (such as biopsy), which also have risks.
- **Side effects may be caused by the test itself**. There are rare but serious side effects that may occur with esophagoscopy and biopsy. These include the following:
  - a small hole (puncture) in the esophagus
  - problems with breathing
  - heart attack
  - passage of food, water, stomach acid, or vomit into the airway
  - severe bleeding that may need to be treated in a hospital

Source: "Esophageal Cancer Screening (PDQ®)—Patient Version," National Cancer Institute (NCI), June 26, 2023. Available online. URL: www.cancer.gov/types/esophageal/patient/esophageal-screening-pdq. Accessed September 28, 2023.

Patients have special nutritional needs during treatment for esophageal cancer. Many people with esophageal cancer find it hard to eat because they have trouble swallowing. The esophagus may be narrowed by the tumor or as a side effect of treatment. Some patients may receive nutrients directly into a vein. Others may need a feeding tube (a flexible plastic tube that is passed through the nose or mouth into the stomach) until they are able to eat on their own.

Types of Treatment Used in Esophageal Cancer

Surgery

Surgery is the most common treatment for cancer of the esophagus. Part of the esophagus may be removed in an operation called an "esophagectomy."

The doctor will connect the remaining healthy part of the esophagus to the stomach so the patient can still swallow. A plastic tube or part of the intestine may be used to make the connection. Lymph nodes near the esophagus may also be removed and viewed under a microscope to see if they contain cancer. If the esophagus is partly blocked by the tumor, an expandable metal stent (tube) may be placed inside the esophagus to help keep it open.

Small, early-stage cancer and high-grade dysplasia of the esophagus may be removed by endoscopic resection. An endoscope (a thin, tube-like instrument with a light and a lens for viewing) is inserted through a small incision (cut) in the skin or through an opening in the body, such as the mouth. A tool attached to the endoscope is used to remove tissue.

Radiation Therapy

Radiation therapy is a cancer treatment that uses high-energy x-rays or other types of radiation to kill cancer cells or keep them from growing. There are two types of radiation therapy:

- External radiation therapy uses a machine outside the body to send radiation toward the area of the body with cancer.
- Internal radiation therapy uses a radioactive substance sealed in needles, seeds, wires, or catheters that are placed directly into or near the cancer.

The way the radiation therapy is given depends on the type and stage of the cancer being treated. External and internal radiation therapy are used to treat esophageal cancer.

A plastic tube may be inserted into the esophagus to keep it open during radiation therapy. This is called "intraluminal intubation" and "dilation."

Chemotherapy

Chemotherapy is a cancer treatment that uses drugs to stop the growth of cancer cells, either by killing the cells or by stopping them from dividing. When chemotherapy is taken by mouth or injected into a vein or muscle, the drugs enter the bloodstream and can reach cancer cells throughout the body (systemic chemotherapy). When chemotherapy is placed directly into the cerebrospinal fluid (CF), an organ, or a body cavity such as the abdomen, the drugs mainly affect cancer cells in those areas (regional chemotherapy). The way the chemotherapy is given depends on the type and stage of the cancer being treated.

Chemoradiation Therapy

Chemoradiation therapy combines chemotherapy and radiation therapy to increase the effects of both.

Laser Therapy

Laser therapy is a cancer treatment that uses a laser beam (a narrow beam of intense light) to kill cancer cells.

Electrocoagulation

Electrocoagulation is the use of an electric current to kill cancer cells.

Immunotherapy

Immunotherapy is a treatment that uses the patient's immune system to fight cancer. Substances made by the body or made in a laboratory are used to boost, direct, or restore the body's natural defenses against cancer.

Immune checkpoint inhibitor therapy is a type of immunotherapy being studied to treat patients with advanced esophageal cancer that cannot be removed by surgery and recurrent esophageal cancer. Some types of immune cells, such as T cells, and some cancer cells have certain proteins, called "checkpoint proteins," on their surface that keep immune responses in check. When cancer cells have large amounts of these proteins, they will not be attacked and killed by T cells. Immune checkpoint inhibitors block these proteins and the ability of T cells to kill cancer cells is increased.

There are two types of immune checkpoint inhibitor therapy:

- **CTLA-4 inhibitor therapy**. CTLA-4 is a protein on the surface of T cells that helps keep the body's immune responses in check. When CTLA-4 attaches to another protein called "B7" on a cancer cell, it stops the T cell from killing the cancer cell. CTLA-4 inhibitors attach to CTLA-4 and allow the T cells to kill cancer cells. Ipilimumab is a type of CTLA-4 inhibitor.
- **PD-1 and PD-L1 inhibitor therapy**. PD-1 is a protein on the surface of T cells that helps keep the body's immune responses in check. PD-L1 is a protein found on some types of cancer cells. When PD-1 attaches to PD-L1, it stops the T cell from killing the cancer cell. PD-1 and PD-L1 inhibitors keep PD-1 and PD-L1 proteins from attaching to each other. This allows the T cells to kill cancer cells. Nivolumab is a type of PD-1 inhibitor.

Targeted Therapy

Targeted therapy is a type of treatment that uses drugs or other substances to identify and attack specific cancer cells. Monoclonal antibody therapy is a type of targeted therapy used in the treatment of esophageal cancer.

Monoclonal antibodies are immune system proteins made in the laboratory to treat many diseases, including cancer. As a cancer treatment, these antibodies can attach to a specific target on cancer cells or other cells that may help cancer cells grow. The antibodies are able to kill the cancer cells, block their growth, or keep them from spreading. Monoclonal antibodies are given by infusion. They may be used alone or to carry drugs, toxins, or radioactive material directly to cancer cells. Treatment for esophageal cancer may cause side effects.

Follow-Up Tests

Some of the tests that were done to diagnose the cancer or to find out the stage of the cancer may be repeated. Some tests will be repeated in order to see how well the treatment is working. Decisions about whether to continue, change, or stop treatment may be based on the results of these tests.

Some of the tests will continue to be done from time to time after treatment has ended. The results of these tests can show if your condition has changed or if the cancer has recurred (come back). These tests are sometimes called "follow-up tests" or "checkups."[1]

[1] "Esophageal Cancer Treatment (PDQ®)—Patient Version," National Cancer Institute (NCI), September 21, 2023. Available online. URL: www.cancer.gov/types/esophageal/patient/esophageal-treatment-pdq. Accessed September 28, 2023.

CHAPTER 33
PANCREATIC CANCER

The pancreas is a gland about six inches long that is shaped like a thin pear lying on its side. The wider end of the pancreas is called the "head," the middle section is called the "body," and the narrow end is called the "tail." The pancreas lies between the stomach and the spine.

The pancreas has two main jobs in the body:

- to make juices that help digest (break down) food
- to make hormones, such as insulin and glucagon, that help control blood sugar levels. Both of these hormones help the body use and store the energy it gets from food

The digestive juices are made by exocrine pancreas cells and the hormones are made by endocrine pancreas cells. About 95 percent of pancreatic cancers begin in exocrine cells.

Anything that increases your risk of getting a disease is called a "risk factor." Having a risk factor does not mean that you will get cancer; not having risk factors does not mean that you will not get cancer. Talk with your doctor if you think you may be at risk.

Risk factors for pancreatic cancer include the following:

- smoking
- being very overweight
- having a personal history of diabetes or chronic pancreatitis
- having a family history of pancreatic cancer or pancreatitis
- having certain hereditary conditions, such as:
    - multiple endocrine neoplasia type 1 (MEN1) syndrome
    - hereditary nonpolyposis colon cancer (HNPCC; Lynch syndrome)
    - von Hippel-Lindau syndrome
    - Peutz-Jeghers syndrome
    - hereditary breast and ovarian cancer syndrome
    - familial atypical multiple mole melanoma (FAMMM) syndrome
    - ataxia telangiectasia

Signs and Symptoms of Pancreatic Cancer

Pancreatic cancer may not cause early signs or symptoms. Signs and symptoms may be caused by pancreatic cancer or by other conditions. Check with your doctor if you have any of the following:

- jaundice (yellowing of the skin and whites of the eyes)
- light-colored stools
- dark urine
- pain in the upper or middle abdomen and back
- weight loss for no known reason
- loss of appetite
- feeling very tired

Early Diagnosis of Pancreatic Cancer Is Difficult

Pancreatic cancer is difficult to detect and diagnose for the following reasons:

- There are not any noticeable signs or symptoms in the early stages of pancreatic cancer.
- The signs and symptoms of pancreatic cancer, when present, are like the signs and symptoms of many other illnesses.
- The pancreas is hidden behind other organs, such as the stomach, small intestine, liver, gallbladder, spleen, and bile ducts.

Source: "Pancreatic Cancer Treatment (PDQ®)—Patient Version," National Cancer Institute (NCI), May 5, 2023. Available online. URL: www.cancer.gov/types/pancreatic/patient/pancreatic-treatment-pdq. Accessed September 29, 2023.

Tests Used to Diagnose and Stage Pancreatic Cancer

Pancreatic cancer is usually diagnosed with tests and procedures that make pictures of the pancreas and the area around it. The process used to find out if cancer cells have spread within and around the pancreas is called "staging." Tests and procedures to detect, diagnose, and stage pancreatic cancer are usually done at the same time. In order to plan treatment, it is important to know the stage of the disease and whether or not the pancreatic cancer can be removed by surgery.

The following tests and procedures may be used:

- **Physical exam and health history**. An exam of the body to check general signs of health, including checking for signs of disease, such as lumps or anything else that seems unusual. A history of the patient's health habits and past illnesses and treatments will also be taken.
- **Blood chemistry studies**. A procedure in which a blood sample is checked to measure the amounts of certain substances, such as bilirubin, released into the blood by organs and tissues in the body. An unusual (higher or lower than normal) amount of a substance can be a sign of disease.

- **Tumor marker test**. A procedure in which a sample of blood, urine, or tissue is checked to measure the amounts of certain substances, such as CA 19-9, and carcinoembryonic antigen (CEA), made by organs, tissues, or tumor cells in the body. Certain substances are linked to specific types of cancer when found in increased levels in the body. These are called "tumor markers."
- **Magnetic resonance imaging (MRI)**. A procedure that uses a magnet, radio waves, and a computer to make a series of detailed pictures of areas inside the body. This procedure is also called "nuclear magnetic resonance imaging" (NMRI).
- **Computed tomography (CT) scan**. A procedure that makes a series of detailed pictures of areas inside the body, taken from different angles. The pictures are made by a computer linked to an x-ray machine. A dye may be injected into a vein or swallowed to help the organs or tissues show up more clearly. This procedure is also called "computed tomography," "computerized tomography," or "computerized axial tomography." A spiral or helical CT scan makes a series of very detailed pictures of areas inside the body using an x-ray machine that scans the body in a spiral path.
- **Positron emission tomography (PET) scan.** A procedure to find malignant tumor cells in the body. A small amount of radioactive glucose (sugar) is injected into a vein. The PET scanner rotates around the body and makes a picture of where glucose is being used in the body. Malignant tumor cells show up brighter in the picture because they are more active and take up more glucose than normal cells do. A PET scan and CT scan may be done at the same time. This is called a "positron emission tomography-computed tomography" (PET-CT).
- **Abdominal ultrasound**. An ultrasound exam used to make pictures of the inside of the abdomen. The ultrasound transducer is pressed against the skin of the abdomen and directs high-energy sound waves (ultrasound) into the abdomen. The sound waves bounce off the internal tissues and organs and make echoes. The transducer receives the echoes and sends them to a computer, which uses the echoes to make pictures called "sonograms." The picture can be printed to be looked at later.
- **Endoscopic ultrasound (EUS).** A procedure in which an endoscope is inserted into the body, usually through the mouth or rectum. An endoscope is a thin, tube-like instrument with a light and a lens for viewing. A probe at the end of the endoscope is used to bounce high-energy sound waves (ultrasound) off internal tissues or organs and make echoes. The echoes form a picture of body tissues called a "sonogram." This procedure is also called "endosonography."
- **Endoscopic retrograde cholangiopancreatography (ERCP).** A procedure used to x-ray the ducts (tubes) that carry bile from the liver to the

gallbladder and from the gallbladder to the small intestine. Sometimes pancreatic cancer causes these ducts to narrow and block or slow the flow of bile, causing jaundice. An endoscope (a thin, lighted tube) is passed through the mouth, esophagus, and stomach into the first part of the small intestine. A catheter (a smaller tube) is then inserted through the endoscope into the pancreatic ducts. A dye is injected through the catheter into the ducts and an x-ray is taken. If the ducts are blocked by a tumor, a fine tube may be inserted into the duct to unblock it. This tube (or stent) may be left in place to keep the duct open. Tissue samples may also be taken.

- **Percutaneous transhepatic cholangiography (PTC)**. A procedure used to x-ray the liver and bile ducts. A thin needle is inserted through the skin below the ribs and into the liver. Dye is injected into the liver or bile ducts and an x-ray is taken. If a blockage is found, a thin, flexible tube called a "stent" is sometimes left in the liver to drain bile into the small intestine or a collection bag outside the body. This test is done only if ERCP cannot be done.
- **Laparoscopy**. A surgical procedure to look at the organs inside the abdomen to check for signs of disease. Small incisions (cuts) are made in the wall of the abdomen and a laparoscope (a thin, lighted tube) is inserted into one of the incisions. The laparoscope may have an ultrasound probe at the end in order to bounce high-energy sound waves off internal organs, such as the pancreas. This is called "laparoscopic ultrasound." Other instruments may be inserted through the same or other incisions to perform procedures such as taking tissue samples from the pancreas or a sample of fluid from the abdomen to check for cancer.
- **Biopsy**. The removal of cells or tissues so they can be viewed under a microscope by a pathologist to check for signs of cancer. There are several ways to do a biopsy for pancreatic cancer. A fine needle or a core needle may be inserted into the pancreas during an x-ray or ultrasound to remove cells. Tissue may also be removed during a laparoscopy or surgery to remove the tumor.

Prognosis for Pancreatic Cancer

The prognosis and treatment options depend on the following:

- whether or not the tumor can be removed by surgery
- the stage of the cancer (the size of the tumor and whether the cancer has spread outside the pancreas to nearby tissues or lymph nodes or to other places in the body)
- the patient's general health
- whether the cancer has just been diagnosed or has recurred (come back)

Pancreatic cancer can be controlled only if it is found before it has spread when it can be completely removed by surgery. If the cancer has spread, palliative treatment can improve the patient's quality of life (QOL) by controlling the symptoms and complications of this disease.

Treatment for Pancreatic Cancer

Different types of treatment are available for patients with pancreatic cancer. Some treatments are standard (the currently used treatment), and some are being tested in clinical trials. A treatment clinical trial is a research study meant to help improve current treatments or obtain information on new treatments for patients with cancer. When clinical trials show that a new treatment is better than the standard treatment, the new treatment may become the standard treatment. Patients may want to think about taking part in a clinical trial. Some clinical trials are open only to patients who have not started treatment.

Types of Treatment Used for Pancreatic Cancer

Surgery

One of the following types of surgery may be used to take out the tumor:

- **Whipple procedure**. A surgical procedure in which the head of the pancreas, the gallbladder, part of the stomach, part of the small intestine, and the bile duct are removed. Enough of the pancreas is left to produce digestive juices and insulin.
- **Total pancreatectomy**. This operation removes the whole pancreas, part of the stomach, part of the small intestine, the common bile duct, the gallbladder, the spleen, and nearby lymph nodes.
- **Distal pancreatectomy**. Surgery to remove the body and the tail of the pancreas. The spleen may also be removed if cancer has spread to the spleen.

If the cancer has spread and cannot be removed, the following types of palliative surgery may be done to relieve symptoms and improve QOL:

- **Biliary bypass**. If cancer is blocking the bile duct and bile is building up in the gallbladder, a biliary bypass may be done. During this operation, the doctor will cut the gallbladder or bile duct in the area before the blockage and sew it to the small intestine to create a new pathway around the blocked area.
- **Endoscopic stent placement**. If the tumor is blocking the bile duct, surgery may be done to put in a stent (a thin tube) to drain bile that has built up in the area. The doctor may place the stent through a catheter that drains the bile into a bag on the outside of the body or the stent may go around the blocked area and drain the bile into the small intestine.

- **Gastric bypass**. If the tumor is blocking the flow of food from the stomach, the stomach may be sewn directly to the small intestine so the patient can continue to eat normally.

Radiation Therapy

Radiation therapy is a cancer treatment that uses high-energy x-rays or other types of radiation to kill cancer cells or keep them from growing. External radiation therapy uses a machine outside the body to send radiation toward the area of the body with cancer.

Chemotherapy

Chemotherapy is a cancer treatment that uses drugs to stop the growth of cancer cells, either by killing the cells or by stopping them from dividing. When chemotherapy is taken by mouth or injected into a vein or muscle, the drugs enter the bloodstream and can reach cancer cells throughout the body (systemic chemotherapy). Combination chemotherapy is treatment using more than one anticancer drug.

Chemoradiation Therapy

Chemoradiation therapy combines chemotherapy and radiation therapy to increase the effects of both.

Targeted Therapy

Targeted therapy is a type of treatment that uses drugs or other substances to identify and attack specific cancer cells. Tyrosine kinase inhibitors (TKIs) are targeted therapy drugs that block signals needed for tumors to grow. Erlotinib is a type of TKI used to treat pancreatic cancer.

Treatments for Pain Caused by Pancreatic Cancer

Pain can occur when the tumor presses on nerves or other organs near the pancreas. When pain medicine is not enough, there are treatments that act on nerves in the abdomen to relieve the pain. The doctor may inject medicine into the area around the affected nerves or may cut the nerves to block the feeling of pain. Radiation therapy with or without chemotherapy can also help relieve pain by shrinking the tumor.

Nutritional Needs for Patients with Pancreatic Cancer

Surgery to remove the pancreas may affect its ability to make pancreatic enzymes that help to digest food. As a result, patients may have problems digesting food and absorbing nutrients into the body. To prevent malnutrition, the doctor may prescribe medicines that replace these enzymes.

Follow-Up Tests

Some of the tests that were done to diagnose the cancer or to find out the stage of the cancer may be repeated. Some tests will be repeated in order to see how well the treatment is working. Decisions about whether to continue, change, or stop treatment may be based on the results of these tests.

Some of the tests will continue to be done from time to time after treatment has ended. The results of these tests can show if your condition has changed or if the cancer has recurred (come back). These tests are sometimes called "follow-up tests" or "checkups."[1]

[1] "Pancreatic Cancer Treatment (PDQ®)—Patient Version," National Cancer Institute (NCI), May 5, 2023. Available online. URL: www.cancer.gov/types/pancreatic/patient/pancreatic-treatment-pdq. Accessed September 29, 2023.

CHAPTER 34
LARYNGEAL CANCER

Laryngeal cancer is a disease in which malignant (cancer) cells form in the tissues of the larynx. The larynx is a part of the throat, between the base of the tongue and the trachea. The larynx contains the vocal cords, which vibrate and make sound when air is directed against them. The sound echoes through the pharynx, mouth, and nose to make a person's voice.

The following are the three main parts of the larynx:

- **Supraglottis**. The upper part of the larynx above the vocal cords, including the epiglottis.
- **Glottis**. The middle part of the larynx where the vocal cords are located.
- **Subglottis**. The lower part of the larynx between the vocal cords and the trachea (windpipe).

Most laryngeal cancers form in squamous cells, the thin, flat cells lining the inside of the larynx.

Laryngeal cancer is a type of head and neck cancer.

Risk of Laryngeal Cancer

The use of tobacco products and drinking too much alcohol can affect the risk of laryngeal cancer. Anything that increases a person's chance of getting a disease is called a "risk factor." Not every person with one or more of these risk factors will develop laryngeal cancer, and it will develop in people who do not have any known risk factors. Talk with your doctor if you think you may be at risk.

Signs and Symptoms of Laryngeal Cancer

These and other signs and symptoms may be caused by laryngeal cancer or by other conditions. Check with your doctor if you have any of the following:

- a sore throat or cough that does not go away
- trouble or pain when swallowing
- ear pain

- a lump in the neck or throat
- a change or hoarseness in the voice

Tests Used to Diagnose Laryngeal Cancer

In addition to asking about your personal and family health history, your doctor may perform the following tests and procedures:

- **Physical exam of the throat and neck**. An exam to check the throat and neck for abnormal areas. The doctor will feel the inside of the mouth with a gloved finger and examine the mouth and throat with a small long-handled mirror and light. This will include checking the insides of the cheeks and lips; the gums; the back, roof, and floor of the mouth; the top, bottom, and sides of the tongue; and the throat. The neck will be felt for swollen lymph nodes. A history of the patient's health habits and past illnesses and medical treatments will also be taken.
- **Biopsy**. The removal of cells or tissues, so they can be viewed under a microscope by a pathologist to check for signs of cancer. The sample of tissue may be removed during one of the following procedures:
  - **Laryngoscopy**. A procedure in which the doctor checks the larynx (voice box) with a mirror or a laryngoscope to check for abnormal areas. A laryngoscope is a thin, tube-like instrument with a light and a lens for viewing the inside of the throat and voice box. It may also have a tool to remove tissue samples, which are checked under a microscope for signs of cancer.
  - **Endoscopy**. A procedure to look at organs and tissues inside the body, such as the throat, esophagus, and trachea to check for abnormal areas. An endoscope (a thin, lighted tube with a light and a lens for viewing) is inserted through an opening in the body, such as the mouth. A special tool on the endoscope may be used to remove samples of tissue.
- **Computerized tomography (CT) scan**. A procedure that makes a series of detailed pictures of areas inside the body, taken from different angles. The pictures are made by a computer linked to an x-ray machine. A dye may be injected into a vein or swallowed to help the organs or tissues show up more clearly.
- **Magnetic resonance imaging (MRI)**. A procedure that uses a magnet, radio waves, and a computer to make a series of detailed pictures of areas inside the body. This procedure is also called "nuclear magnetic resonance imaging" (NMRI).
- **Positron emission tomography (PET) scan**. A procedure to find malignant tumor cells in the body. A small amount of radioactive glucose (sugar) is injected into a vein. The PET scanner rotates around the body and makes a picture of where glucose is being used in the body. Malignant tumor cells

show up brighter in the picture because they are more active and take up more glucose than normal cells do.

- **PET-CT scan**. A procedure that combines the pictures from a positron emission tomography (PET) scan and a computed tomography scan. The PET and CT scans are done at the same time with the same machine. The combined scans give more detailed pictures of areas inside the body than either scan gives by itself. A PET-CT scan may be used to help diagnose diseases, such as cancer; plan treatment; or find out how well treatment is working.
- **Bone scan**. A procedure to check if there are rapidly dividing cells, such as cancer cells, in the bone. A very small amount of radioactive material is injected into a vein and travels through the bloodstream. The radioactive material collects in the bones with cancer and is detected by a scanner.
- **Barium swallow**. A series of x-rays of the esophagus and stomach. The patient drinks a liquid that contains barium (a silver-white metallic compound). The liquid coats the esophagus and stomach, and x-rays are taken. This procedure is also called an "upper GI series."

Factors Affecting Prognosis and Treatment Options

The prognosis depends on the following:

- the stage of the disease
- the location and size of the tumor
- the grade of the tumor
- the patient's age, gender, and general health, including whether the patient is anemic

Treatment options depend on the following:

- the stage of the disease
- the location and size of the tumor
- keeping the patient's ability to talk, eat, and breathe as normal as possible
- whether the cancer has come back (recurred)

Smoking tobacco and drinking alcohol decrease the effectiveness of treatment for laryngeal cancer. Patients with laryngeal cancer who continue to smoke and drink are less likely to be cured and more likely to develop a second tumor. After treatment for laryngeal cancer, frequent and careful follow-up is important.

Treatment for Laryngeal Cancer

Different types of treatment are available for patients with laryngeal cancer. Some treatments are standard (the currently used treatment), and some are being tested in clinical trials. A treatment clinical trial is a research study meant to help improve current treatments or obtain information on new treatments for patients with cancer. When clinical trials show that a new treatment is better than the standard treatment, the new treatment may become the standard treatment. Patients may want to think about taking part in a clinical trial. Some clinical trials are open only to patients who have not started treatment.

Types of Treatment Used in Laryngeal Cancer

Radiation Therapy

Radiation therapy is a cancer treatment that uses high-energy x-rays or other types of radiation to kill cancer cells or keep them from growing. External radiation therapy uses a machine outside the body to send radiation toward the area of the body with cancer.

Radiation therapy may work better in patients who have stopped smoking before beginning treatment. External radiation therapy to the thyroid or the pituitary gland may change the way the thyroid gland works. A blood test to check the thyroid hormone level in the body may be done before and after therapy to make sure the thyroid gland is working properly.

Hyperfractionated radiation therapy may be used to treat laryngeal cancer. Hyperfractionated radiation therapy is radiation treatment in which a smaller-than-usual total daily dose of radiation is divided into two doses and the treatments are given twice a day. Hyperfractionated radiation therapy is given over the same period of time (days or weeks) as standard radiation therapy. New types of radiation therapy are being studied in the treatment of laryngeal cancer.

Surgery

Surgery (removing the cancer in an operation) is a common treatment for all stages of laryngeal cancer. The following surgical procedures may be used:

- **Cordectomy**. Surgery to remove the vocal cords only.
- **Supraglottic laryngectomy**. Surgery to remove the supraglottis only.
- **Hemilaryngectomy**. Surgery to remove half of the larynx (voice box). A hemilaryngectomy saves the voice.
- **Partial laryngectomy**. Surgery to remove part of the larynx (voice box). A partial laryngectomy helps keep the patient's ability to talk.
- **Total laryngectomy**. Surgery to remove the whole larynx. During this operation, a hole is made in the front of the neck to allow the patient to breathe. This is called a "tracheostomy."
- **Thyroidectomy**. The removal of all or part of the thyroid gland.
- **Laser surgery**. A surgical procedure that uses a laser beam (a narrow beam of intense light) as a knife to make bloodless cuts in tissue or to remove a surface lesion such as a tumor in the larynx.

After the doctor removes all the cancer that can be seen at the time of the surgery, some patients may be given chemotherapy or radiation therapy after surgery to kill any cancer cells that are left. Treatment given after the surgery, to lower the risk that the cancer will come back, is called "adjuvant therapy."

Chemotherapy

Chemotherapy is a cancer treatment that uses drugs to stop the growth of cancer cells, either by killing the cells or by stopping the cells from dividing. When chemotherapy is taken by mouth or injected into a vein or muscle, the drugs enter the bloodstream and can reach cancer cells throughout the body (systemic chemotherapy).

Immunotherapy

Immunotherapy is a treatment that uses the patient's immune system to fight cancer. Substances made by the body or made in a laboratory are used to boost, direct, or restore the body's natural defenses against cancer. This cancer treatment is a type of biologic therapy.

- **Programmed cell death protein 1 (PD-1) and programmed cell death ligand 1 (PD-L1) inhibitor therapy**. PD-1 is a protein on the surface of T cells that helps keep the body's immune responses in check. PD-L1 is a protein found in some types of cancer cells. When PD-1 attaches to PD-L1, it stops the T cell from killing the cancer cell. PD-1 and PD-L1 inhibitors keep PD-1 and PD-L1 proteins from attaching to each other. This allows the T cells to kill cancer cells. Nivolumab and pembrolizumab are types of PD-1 inhibitors used to treat metastatic or recurrent laryngeal cancer.

Treatments That Are Tested in Clinical Trials

Targeted Therapy

Targeted therapy is a type of treatment that uses drugs or other substances to identify and attack specific cancer cells.

- **Monoclonal antibodies**. Monoclonal antibodies are immune system proteins made in the laboratory to treat many diseases, including cancer. As a cancer treatment, these antibodies can attach to a specific target on cancer cells or other cells that may help cancer cells grow. The antibodies are able to then kill the cancer cells, block their growth, or keep them from spreading. Monoclonal antibodies are given by infusion. They may be used alone or to carry drugs, toxins, or radioactive material directly to cancer cells. Cetuximab is being studied in the treatment of laryngeal cancer.

Radiosensitizers

Radiosensitizers are drugs that make tumor cells more sensitive to radiation therapy. Combining radiation therapy with radiosensitizers may kill more tumor cells.

Follow-Up Tests

Some of the tests that were done to diagnose the cancer or to find out the stage of the cancer may be repeated. Some tests will be repeated in order to see how well the treatment is working. Decisions about whether to continue, change, or stop treatment may be based on the results of these tests.

Some of the tests will continue to be done from time to time after treatment has ended. The results of these tests can show if your condition has changed or if the cancer has recurred (come back). These tests are sometimes called "follow-up tests" or "check-ups."[1]

[1] "Laryngeal Cancer Treatment (PDQ®)–Patient Version," National Cancer Institute (NCI), March 31, 2023. Available online. URL: www.cancer.gov/types/head-and-neck/patient/adult/laryngeal-treatment-pdq. Accessed September 29, 2023.

CHAPTER 35
KIDNEY CANCER

What Are the Kidneys?

The body has two kidneys, one on each side of the body, located behind the liver and stomach. The kidneys make urine, which is how the body washes liquid waste out of the body. The kidneys also play a role in controlling blood pressure and stimulating the bone marrow to make red blood cells (RBCs).

What Is the Renal Pelvis?

The renal pelvis is in the center of the kidney and is responsible for collecting the urine and feeding it into the ureters, two tubes that connect the kidneys with the bladder. The bladder holds urine until it is peed out.

What Are the Symptoms of Kidney and Renal Pelvis Cancers?

A person with kidney or renal pelvis cancer may or may not have one or more of the following symptoms. The same symptoms can also come from other causes. If you have any of the following symptoms, talk to your doctor.

- blood in the urine
- a lump or swelling in the kidney area or abdomen
- lower back pain or pain in the side that does not go away
- feeling tired often
- fever that keeps coming back
- not feeling like eating
- losing weight for no reason
- something blocking your bowels
- a general feeling of poor health

What Causes Kidney and Renal Pelvis Cancers?

Risk factors for kidney and renal pelvis cancers include the following:

- being overweight or obesity
- smoking

- having high blood pressure (HBP, which is not known whether the increased risk is due to HBP itself or the medicines used to treat it)
- taking certain pain medicines for a long time
- having certain genetic conditions
- having a long-lasting infection with hepatitis C
- having kidney stones
- having sickle cell trait, which is associated with a very rare form of kidney cancer (renal medullary carcinoma (RMC))
- being exposed to a chemical called "trichloroethylene," which is used to remove grease from metal

Treatment and Diagnosis of Kidney Cancer

Tests to diagnose kidney cancer include blood, urine, and imaging tests. You may also have a biopsy.

Treatment depends on your age, your overall health, and how advanced the cancer is. It might include surgery, chemotherapy, or radiation, biologic, or targeted therapies. Biologic therapy boosts your body's own ability to fight cancer. Targeted therapy uses drugs or other substances that attack specific cancer cells with less harm to normal cells.

Source: MedlinePlus, "Kidney Cancer," National Institutes of Health (NIH), August 11, 2020. Available online. URL: https://medlineplus.gov/kidneycancer.html. Accessed September 29, 2023.

How Can You Reduce Your Risk for Kidney and Renal Pelvis Cancers?

To lower your risk of kidney and renal pelvis cancers, do the following:

- Do not smoke or quit if you do.
- Keep a healthy weight.
- Eat a healthy diet.
- Be physically active.
- Be very careful if you use certain kinds of chemicals, especially trichloroethylene. This chemical is used by workers in some jobs, such as those who work with metals.[1]

[1] "Kidney Cancer," Centers for Disease Control and Prevention (CDC), June 28, 2023. Available online. URL: www.cdc.gov/cancer/kidney/index.htm. Accessed September 29, 2023.

CHAPTER 36
LIVER CANCER

What Is Liver Cancer?

Primary liver cancer is a disease in which malignant (cancer) cells form in the tissues of the liver. Cancer that forms in other parts of the body and spreads to the liver is not primary liver cancer. The liver is one of the largest organs in the body. It has two lobes and fills the upper right side of the abdomen inside the rib cage. The main functions of the liver include the following:

- to make bile to help digest fat that comes from food
- to store glycogen (sugar), which the body uses for energy
- to filter harmful substances from the blood so they can be passed from the body in stools and urine

Types of Liver Cancer

Hepatocellular carcinoma and bile duct cancer (cholangiocarcinoma) are the main types of adult primary liver cancer.

Most adult primary liver cancers are hepatocellular carcinomas. This type of liver cancer is the third leading cause of cancer-related deaths worldwide.

Primary liver cancer can occur in both adults and children. However, treatment for children is different than treatment for adults.

Signs and Symptoms of Liver Cancer

These and other signs and symptoms may be caused by adult primary liver cancer or by other conditions. Check with your doctor if you have any of the following:

- a hard lump on the right side just below the rib cage
- discomfort in the upper abdomen on the right side
- a swollen abdomen
- pain near the right shoulder blade or in the back
- jaundice (yellowing of the skin and whites of the eyes)
- easy bruising or bleeding

- unusual tiredness or weakness
- nausea and vomiting
- loss of appetite or feelings of fullness after eating a small meal
- weight loss for no known reason
- pale, chalky bowel movements and dark urine
- fever

Liver Cancer Causes, Risk Factors, and Prevention

Worldwide, liver cancer is the sixth most common cancer and the third leading cause of cancer death. In the United States, rates are highest in American Indian or Alaska Native individuals. Liver cancer is the sixth leading cause of cancer deaths in the United States.

Liver Cancer Causes and Risk Factors

The most common type of liver cancer in adults, hepatocellular carcinoma (HCC), typically develops in people with chronic (long-lasting) liver disease caused by hepatitis virus infection or cirrhosis. Men are more likely to develop HCC than women. People with multiple risk factors have an even higher risk.

Many risk factors have been associated with liver cancer. Not everyone with one or more of these risk factors will develop the disease, and the disease will develop in some people who do not have any known risk factors. Risk factors include the following:

- **Hepatitis B virus (HBV) infection**. HBV can be transmitted in blood, semen, or other body fluids. The infection can be passed from mother to child during childbirth, through sexual contact, or by sharing needles that are used to inject drugs. It can cause inflammation (swelling) of the liver that leads to cancer. Routine HBV vaccination in infancy is reducing the incidence of HBV infection. Chronic HBV infection is the leading cause of liver cancer in Asia and Africa.
- **Hepatitis C virus (HCV) infection**. HCV can be transmitted in the blood. The infection can be spread by sharing needles that are used to inject drugs or, less often, through sexual contact. In the past, it was also spread during blood transfusions or organ transplants. Nowadays, blood banks test all donated blood for HCV, which greatly lowers the risk of getting the virus from blood transfusions. It can cause cirrhosis that may lead to liver cancer. Chronic HCV infection is the leading cause of liver cancer in North America, Europe, and Japan.
- **Cirrhosis**. The risk of developing liver cancer is increased for people who have cirrhosis, a disease in which healthy liver tissue is replaced by scar tissue. The scar tissue blocks the flow of blood through the liver and keeps it from working as it should. Chronic alcoholism and chronic hepatitis infections are common causes of cirrhosis. People with HCV-related

cirrhosis have a higher risk of developing liver cancer than people with cirrhosis related to HBV or alcohol use.

- **Heavy alcohol use**. Heavy alcohol use can cause cirrhosis, which is a risk factor for liver cancer. Liver cancer can also occur in heavy alcohol users who do not have cirrhosis. Heavy alcohol users who have cirrhosis are 10 times more likely to develop liver cancer, compared with heavy alcohol users who do not have cirrhosis.
  Studies have shown there is also an increased risk of liver cancer in people with HBV or HCV infection who use alcohol heavily.
- **Aflatoxin B1**. The risk of developing liver cancer may be increased by eating foods that contain aflatoxin B1 (poison from a fungus that can grow on foods, such as corn and nuts, that have been stored in hot, humid places). It is most common in sub-Saharan Africa, Southeast Asia, and China.
- **Nonalcoholic steatohepatitis (NASH)**. NASH is a condition that can cause cirrhosis that may lead to liver cancer. It is the most severe form of nonalcoholic fatty liver disease, where there is an abnormal amount of fat in the liver. In some people, this can cause inflammation and injury to the cells of the liver. Having NASH-related cirrhosis increases the risk of developing liver cancer. Liver cancer has also been found in people with NASH who do not have cirrhosis.
- **Cigarette smoking**. Cigarette smoking has been linked to a higher risk of liver cancer. The risk increases with the number of cigarettes smoked per day and the number of years the person has smoked.
- **Other conditions**. Certain rare medical and genetic conditions may increase the risk of liver cancer. These conditions include the following:
  - untreated hereditary hemochromatosis
  - alpha-1 antitrypsin deficiency
  - glycogen storage disease
  - porphyria cutanea tarda
  - Wilson disease

Liver Cancer Prevention

Cancer prevention is action taken to lower the chance of getting cancer. By preventing cancer, the number of new cases of cancer in a group or population is lowered. Hopefully, this will lower the number of deaths caused by cancer.

Anything that increases your chance of getting cancer is called a "risk factor." Anything that lowers your chance of getting cancer is called a "cancer protective factor." Prevention includes avoiding risk factors and increasing protective factors.

The following are protective factors for liver cancer:

- **Getting the hepatitis B vaccine**. Preventing HBV infection (by being vaccinated for HBV as a newborn) has been shown to lower the risk of liver cancer in children. It is not yet known if being vaccinated lowers the risk of liver cancer in adults.

- **Getting treatment for chronic hepatitis B infection**. Treatment options for people with chronic HBV infection include interferon and nucleos(t)ide analog therapy. These treatments may reduce the risk of developing liver cancer.
- **Reducing exposure to aflatoxin B1**. Replacing foods that contain high amounts of aflatoxin B1 with foods that contain a much lower level of the poison can reduce the risk of liver cancer.

Liver Cancer Screening

Screening is looking for cancer before a person has any symptoms. This can help find cancer at an early stage. When abnormal tissue or cancer is found early, it may be easier to treat.

It is important to remember that your doctor does not necessarily think you have cancer if he or she suggests a screening test. Screening tests are given when you have no cancer symptoms. If a screening test result is abnormal, you may need to have more tests done to find out if you have cancer. These are called "diagnostic tests."

Risks of Liver Cancer Screening

Decisions about screening tests can be difficult. Not all screening tests are helpful and most have risk of harms associated with them. Before having any screening test, you may want to discuss the test with your doctor. It is important to be aware of any possible harms of the test and whether the test has been proven to reduce the risk of dying from cancer.

The risks of liver cancer screening include the following:

- **False-negative test results can occur**. Screening test results may appear to be normal even though liver cancer is present. A person who receives a false-negative test result (one that shows there is no cancer when there really is) may delay seeking medical care even if there are symptoms.
- **False-positive test results can occur**. Screening test results may appear to be abnormal even though no cancer is present. A false-positive test result (one that shows there is cancer when there really is not) can cause anxiety and is usually followed by diagnostic tests and procedures, such as a liver biopsy, which also have risks.
- **Procedures to diagnose liver cancer can cause complications**. Abnormal screening results may be followed up with a liver biopsy to diagnose liver cancer. Liver biopsy may cause the following rare, but serious, complications:
    - hemorrhage
    - trouble breathing

- leakage of bile, which can cause an infection of the lining of the abdomen
- a small puncture (hole) in an organ in the abdomen
- spread of cancer cells along the needle path where the biopsy needle is inserted and withdrawn (taken out)

Liver Cancer Diagnosis

How Is Liver Cancer Diagnosed?

Tests that examine the liver and the blood are used to detect and diagnose liver cancer. Not every person will receive all the following tests.

The following tests and procedures may be used:

- **Physical exam and health history**. A physical exam of the body will be done to check a person's health, including checking for signs of disease, such as lumps or anything else that seems unusual. A history of the patient's health habits and past illnesses and treatments will also be taken.
- **Alpha-fetoprotein (AFP) tumor marker test**. Tumor markers are released into the blood by organs, tissues, or tumor cells in the body. An increased level of AFP in the blood may be a sign of liver cancer. Other cancers and certain noncancerous conditions, including cirrhosis and hepatitis, may also increase AFP levels. Sometimes the AFP level is normal even when there is liver cancer.
- **Liver function tests**. These blood tests measure the amounts of certain substances released into the blood by the liver. A higher-than-normal amount of a substance can be a sign of liver cancer.
- **Computed tomography (CT or CAT) scan**. This procedure uses a computer linked to an x-ray machine to make a series of detailed pictures of areas inside the body, such as the abdomen, taken from different angles. A dye may be injected into a vein or swallowed to help the organs or tissues show up more clearly. This procedure is also called "computed tomography," "computerized tomography," or "computerized axial tomography." Images may be taken at three different times after the dye is injected, to get the best picture of abnormal areas in the liver. This is called "triple-phase CT." A spiral or helical CT scan makes a series of very detailed pictures of areas inside the body using an x-ray machine that scans the body in a spiral path.
- **Magnetic resonance imaging (MRI)**. This procedure uses a magnet, radio waves, and a computer to make a series of detailed pictures of areas inside the body, such as the liver. To create detailed pictures of blood vessels in and near the liver, dye is injected into a vein. This procedure is called "magnetic resonance angiography." Images may be taken at three different times after the dye is injected, to get the best picture of abnormal areas in the liver. This is called "triple-phase MRI."

- **Ultrasound exam**. This procedure uses high-energy sound waves (ultrasound) that are bounced off the liver and make echoes. The echoes form a picture of the liver called a "sonogram."
- **Biopsy**. During a biopsy, cells or tissues are removed so they can be viewed under a microscope by a pathologist to check for signs of cancer. Procedures used to collect the sample of cells or tissues include the following:
  - **Fine-needle aspiration biopsy**. A sample of fluid, tissue, or cells is removed using a thin needle.
  - **Core needle biopsy**. A sample of cells or tissue is removed using a slightly wider needle.
- **Laparoscopy**. This surgical procedure is done to look at the organs inside the abdomen to check for signs of disease. Small incisions (cuts) are made in the wall of the abdomen and a laparoscope (a thin, lighted tube) is inserted into one of the incisions. Another instrument is inserted through the same or another incision to remove the tissue samples.

  A biopsy is not always needed to diagnose liver cancer. Sometimes the doctors can diagnose liver cancer based on the results of imaging tests, such as CT scans and MRI.

After primary liver cancer has been diagnosed, tests are done to find out if cancer cells have spread within the liver or to other parts of the body. The process of determining the size and location of the cancer and whether it has spread is called "staging."

Some of the tests and procedures used to diagnose liver cancer, such as CT scan and MRI, may be used in the staging process. A positron emission tomography (PET) scan may also be used:

- **PET scan**. This procedure is used to find malignant tumor cells in the body. A small amount of radioactive glucose (sugar) is injected into a vein. The PET scanner rotates around the body and makes a picture of where glucose is being used in the body. Malignant tumor cells show up brighter in the picture because they are more active and take up more glucose than normal cells do.

What Affects Liver Cancer Prognosis?

Once liver cancer has been diagnosed, the prognosis (chance of recovery) and treatment options depend on the following:

- the stage of the cancer (the size of the tumor, whether it affects part or all of the liver, or has spread to other places in the body)
- how well the liver is working
- the patient's general health, including whether there is cirrhosis of the liver

Finding and treating liver cancer early may prevent death from liver cancer.

Liver Cancer Treatment

There are different types of treatment for patients with liver cancer. Some treatments are standard (the currently used treatment), and some are being tested in clinical trials.

Types of Liver Cancer Treatment

Surveillance

Surveillance is used for lesions smaller than one centimeter found during screening. Follow-up every three months is common. Surveillance is closely watching a patient's condition but not giving any treatment unless there are changes in test results that show the condition is getting worse. During active surveillance, certain exams and tests are done on a regular schedule.

Surgery

A partial hepatectomy (surgery to remove the part of the liver where cancer is found) may be done. A wedge of tissue, an entire lobe, or a larger part of the liver, along with some of the healthy tissue around it is removed. The remaining liver tissue takes over the functions of the liver and may regrow.

Liver Transplant

In a liver transplant, the entire liver is removed and replaced with a healthy donated liver. A liver transplant may be done when the disease is in the liver only and a donated liver can be found. If the patient has to wait for a donated liver, other treatment is given as needed.

Ablation Therapy

Ablation therapy removes or destroys tissue. Different types of ablation therapy are used for liver cancer:

- **Radiofrequency ablation**. Special needles are inserted directly through the skin or through an incision in the abdomen to reach the tumor. High-energy radio waves heat the needles and tumor, which kills cancer cells.
- **Microwave therapy**. The tumor is exposed to high temperatures created by microwaves. This can damage and kill cancer cells or make them more sensitive to the effects of radiation and certain anticancer drugs.
- **Percutaneous ethanol injection**. A small needle is used to inject ethanol (pure alcohol) directly into a tumor to kill cancer cells. Several treatments may be needed. Usually, local anesthesia is used, but if the patient has many tumors in the liver, general anesthesia may be used.
- **Cryoablation**. An instrument is used to freeze and destroy cancer cells. This type of treatment is also called "cryotherapy" and "cryosurgery." The doctor may use ultrasound to guide the instrument.

- **Electroporation therapy**. Electrical pulses are sent through an electrode placed in a tumor to kill cancer cells. Electroporation therapy is being studied in clinical trials.

Embolization Therapy

Embolization therapy is used for patients who cannot have surgery to remove the tumor or ablation therapy and whose tumor has not spread outside the liver. Embolization therapy is the use of substances to block or decrease the flow of blood through the hepatic artery to the tumor. When the tumor does not get the oxygen and nutrients it needs, it will not continue to grow.

The liver receives blood from the hepatic portal vein and the hepatic artery. Blood that comes into the liver from the hepatic portal vein usually goes to the healthy liver tissue. Blood that comes from the hepatic artery usually goes to the tumor. When the hepatic artery is blocked during embolization therapy, the healthy liver tissue continues to receive blood from the hepatic portal vein.

There are two main types of embolization therapy:

- **Transarterial embolization (TAE)**. A small incision (cut) is made in the inner thigh and a catheter (thin, flexible tube) is inserted and threaded up into the hepatic artery. Once the catheter is in place, a substance that blocks the hepatic artery and stops blood flow to the tumor is injected.
- **Transarterial chemoembolization (TACE)**. This procedure is like TAE except an anticancer drug is also given. The procedure can be done by attaching the anticancer drug to small beads that are injected into the hepatic artery or by injecting the anticancer drug through the catheter into the hepatic artery and then injecting the substance to block the hepatic artery. Most of the anticancer drug is trapped near the tumor and only a small amount of the drug reaches other parts of the body. This type of treatment is also called "chemoembolization."

Targeted Therapy

Targeted therapy is a type of treatment that uses drugs or other substances to identify and attack specific cancer cells. Targeted therapies usually cause less harm to normal cells than chemotherapy or radiation therapy do. Targeted therapies used to treat advanced liver cancer include the following:

- bevacizumab
- cabozantinib
- lenvatinib
- ramucirumab
- regorafenib
- sorafenib

Immunotherapy

Immunotherapy is a treatment that uses the patient's immune system to fight cancer. Substances made by the body or made in a laboratory are used to boost, direct, or restore the body's natural defenses against cancer.

Immune checkpoint inhibitors are a type of immunotherapy. Immune checkpoint inhibitors that may be used to treat liver cancer include the following:

- atezolizumab with the targeted therapy bevacizumab
- nivolumab with ipilimumab
- pembrolizumab

Radiation Therapy

External radiation therapy uses a machine outside the body to send high-energy x-rays or other types of radiation toward the area of the body with cancer. This kills cancer cells or keeps them from growing. Certain ways of giving external radiation therapy can help keep radiation from damaging nearby healthy tissue:

- **Conformal radiation therapy**. Conformal radiation therapy uses a computer to make a three-dimensional (3-D) picture of the tumor and shapes the radiation beams to fit the tumor. This allows a high dose of radiation to reach the tumor and causes less damage to nearby healthy tissue.
- **Stereotactic body radiation therapy**. Stereotactic body radiation therapy uses special equipment to place the patient in the same position for each radiation treatment. Once a day for several days, a radiation machine aims a larger-than-usual dose of radiation directly at the tumor. By having the patient in the same position for each treatment, there is less damage to nearby healthy tissue. This procedure is also called "stereotactic external-beam radiation therapy" and "stereotaxic radiation therapy."
- **Proton beam radiation therapy**. Proton beam radiation therapy is a type of high-energy, external radiation therapy that uses streams of protons (tiny particles with a positive charge) to kill tumor cells. This type of treatment can lower the amount of radiation damage to healthy tissue near a tumor.[1]

[1] "What Is Liver Cancer?" National Cancer Institute (NCI), May 18, 2022. Available online. URL: www.cancer.gov/types/liver/what-is-liver-cancer. Accessed September 29, 2023.

CHAPTER 37
CERVICAL CANCER

What Is Cervical Cancer?

Cervical cancer is cancer that starts in the cells of the cervix. The cervix is the lower, narrow end of the uterus (womb). The cervix connects the uterus to the vagina (birth canal). Cervical cancer usually develops slowly over time. Before cancer appears in the cervix, the cells of the cervix go through changes known as "dysplasia," in which abnormal cells begin to appear in the cervical tissue. Over time, if not destroyed or removed, the abnormal cells may become cancer cells and start to grow and spread more deeply into the cervix and to surrounding areas.

The cervix has two main parts:

- The ectocervix (also called "exocervix") is the outer part of the cervix that can be seen during a gynecologic exam. The ectocervix is covered with thin, flat cells called "squamous cells."
- The endocervix is the inner part of the cervix that forms a canal that connects the vagina to the uterus. The endocervix is covered with column-shaped glandular cells that make mucus.

The squamocolumnar junction (also called the "transformation zone") is the border where the endocervix and ectocervix meet. Most cervical cancers begin in this area.

Types of Cervical Cancer

Cervical cancers are named after the type of cell where the cancer started. The two main types are as follows:

- **Squamous cell carcinoma (SCC)**. Most cervical cancers (up to 90%) are SCC. These cancers develop from cells in the ectocervix.
- **Adenocarcinoma**. Cervical adenocarcinomas develop in the glandular cells of the endocervix. Clear cell adenocarcinoma, also called "clear cell carcinoma" or "mesonephroma," is a rare type of cervical adenocarcinoma.

Sometimes, cervical cancer has features of both SCC and adenocarcinoma. This is called "mixed carcinoma" or "adenosquamous carcinoma." Very rarely, cancer develops in other cells in the cervix.

Causes of Cervical Cancer

Long-lasting (persistent) infection with high-risk types of human papillomavirus (HPV) causes virtually all cervical cancers. Two high-risk types, HPV 16 and HPV 18, cause 70 percent of cervical cancers worldwide.

Nearly all people who are sexually active will become infected with HPV at some point in their lives. Most HPV infections go away on their own within a year or two as the immune system controls the infection. These short-term infections do not cause cancer. When a high-risk HPV infection lasts for years, it can lead to changes in the cervical cells, resulting in a precancerous lesion. If the precancerous lesion is not found and removed, it may eventually develop into cervical cancer.

People who become sexually active at a young age, especially before age 18, or have multiple sexual partners are more likely to become infected with a high-risk type of HPV.

Rare Cause of Cervical Cancer

Being exposed to a drug called "diethylstilbestrol" (DES) in the womb is an independent risk factor for a type of cervical cancer called "clear cell adenocarcinoma." Between 1940 and 1971, DES was given to some pregnant women in the United States to prevent miscarriage (premature birth of a fetus that cannot survive) and early labor. Women whose mothers took DES while pregnant have an increased risk of cervical cell abnormalities and of clear cell adenocarcinoma of the vagina and cervix.

Risk Factors in Cervical Cancer

Some risk factors make it more likely for a person who has a high-risk HPV infection of the cervix to develop cervical cancer. These risk factors include the following:

- **Having a weakened immune system**. This can lower the body's ability to fight an HPV infection. HPV infections are more likely to be persistent and progress to cancer in people who are immunocompromised than in people who are not immunocompromised. You may be immunocompromised if you:
  - have a human immunodeficiency virus (HIV) infection or another disease that weakens your immune system
  - take medicine to suppress your immune response, such as to prevent organ rejection after a transplant, to treat an autoimmune disease, or to treat cancer
- **Smoking or breathing in secondhand smoke**. People who smoke or breathe in secondhand smoke have an increased risk of developing cervical cancer.

The risk increases the more a person smokes or is exposed to secondhand smoke.

- **Reproductive factors**. Both the use of oral contraceptives (birth control pills) and giving birth to many children are associated with an increased risk of cervical cancer. The reasons for these associations are not well understood.
- **Obesity**. Cervical cancer screening may be more difficult in those with obesity, leading to lower detection of precancers and a higher risk of cancer.

Symptoms of Cervical Cancer

Early on, cervical cancer usually does not have symptoms, making it hard to detect. Symptoms usually begin after the cancer has spread.

When symptoms of early-stage cervical cancer do occur, they may include the following:

- vaginal bleeding after sex
- vaginal bleeding after menopause
- vaginal bleeding between periods or periods that are heavier or longer than normal
- vaginal discharge that is watery and has a strong odor or that contains blood
- pelvic pain or pain during sex

Symptoms of advanced cervical cancer (cancer has spread beyond the cervix to other parts of the body) may include the symptoms of early-stage cervical cancer and:

- difficult or painful bowel movements or bleeding from the rectum when having a bowel movement
- difficult or painful urination or blood in the urine
- dull backache
- swelling of the legs
- pain in the abdomen
- feeling tired

These symptoms may be caused by many conditions other than cervical cancer. The only way to know is to see a health professional. If it is cervical cancer, ignoring symptoms can delay treatment and make it less effective.

Screening of Cervical Cancer

The goal of screening for cervical cancer is to find precancerous cervical cell changes, when treatment can prevent cervical cancer from developing. Sometimes, cancer is found during cervical screening. Cervical cancer found at an early stage is usually easier to treat. By the time symptoms appear, cervical cancer may have begun to spread, making treatment more difficult.

There are three main ways to screen for cervical cancer:

- The HPV test checks cells for infection with high-risk HPV types that can cause cervical cancer.
- The Pap test (also called a "Pap smear" or "cervical cytology") collects cervical cells so they can be checked for changes caused by HPV that may—if left untreated—turn into cervical cancer. It can find precancerous cells and cervical cancer cells. A Pap test also sometimes finds conditions that are not cancer, such as infection or inflammation.
- The HPV/Pap cotest uses an HPV test and Pap test together to check for both high-risk HPV and cervical cell changes.

When to Get Screened for Cervical Cancer

Cervical screening recommendations are developed by several organizations, including the United States Preventive Services Task Force (USPSTF) and the American Cancer Society (ACS). How often you should be screened for cervical cancer and which tests you should get will depend on your age and health history. Because HPV vaccination does not prevent infection with all high-risk HPV types, vaccinated people who have a cervix should follow cervical cancer screening recommendations:

- **Age 21–29 years**. If you are in this age group, the USPSTF recommends getting your first Pap test at age 21, followed by Pap testing every three years. Even if you are sexually active, you do not need a Pap test before age 21.
- **Age 30–65 years**. If you are in this age group, the USPSTF recommends getting screened for cervical cancer using one of the following methods:
  - HPV test every five years
  - HPV/Pap cotest every five years
  - Pap test every three years

  Updated cervical cancer screening guidelines from the ACS recommend starting screening at age 25 with an HPV test and having HPV testing every five years through age 65. However, testing with an HPV/Pap cotest every five years or with a Pap test every three years is still acceptable.
- **Older than 65 years**. If you are in this age group, talk with your health-care provider to learn if screening is still needed. If you have been screened regularly and had normal test results, your health-care provider will probably advise you that you no longer need screening. However, if your recent test results were abnormal or you have not been screened regularly, you may need to continue screening beyond age 65.

Exceptions to the Cervical Cancer Screening Guidelines

Your health-care provider may recommend more frequent screening if you:

- are HIV positive
- have a weakened immune system
- were exposed before birth to a medicine called "diethylstilbestrol" (DES), which was prescribed to some pregnant women through the mid-1970s
- had a recent abnormal cervical screening test or biopsy result
- have had cervical cancer

If you have had an operation to remove both the uterus and cervix (called a "total hysterectomy") for reasons not related to cancer or abnormal cervical cells, you do not need to be screened for cervical cancer. However, if your hysterectomy was related to cervical cancer or precancer, talk with your health-care provider to learn what follow-up care you need. If you have had an operation to remove the uterus but not the cervix (sometimes called a "partial" or "supracervical hysterectomy") you should continue routine cervical cancer screening.

Where to Get Screened for Cervical Cancer

Doctors' offices, clinics, and community health centers offer HPV and Pap tests. Many people receive these tests from their obstetrics/gynecology (OB/GYN) or primary care provider.

If you do not have a primary care provider or doctor you see regularly, you can find a clinic near you that offers cervical cancer screening by contacting:

- your state or local health department
- the National Breast and Cervical Cancer Early Detection Program (NBCCEDP) or calling 800-232-4636 (The NBCCEDP provides low-income, uninsured, and underserved people access to timely cervical cancer screening and diagnostic services.)
- a Planned Parenthood clinic or calling 800-230-7526
- National Cancer Institute (NCI) Cancer Information Service or calling 800-422-6237

Cervical screening test results usually come back from the lab in about one to three weeks. If you do not hear from your health-care provider, call and ask for your test results. Make sure you understand any follow-up visits or tests you may need.

What to Expect during a Cervical Cancer Screening Test

Cervical cancer screening tests are usually done during a pelvic exam, which takes only a few minutes. During the exam, you lie on your back on an exam table, bend your knees, and put your feet into supports at the end of the table. The health-care provider uses a speculum to gently open your vagina to see the cervix. A soft, narrow brush or tiny spatula is used to collect a small sample of cells from your cervix.

The sample is then sent to a lab, where the cells can be checked to see if they are infected with the types of HPV that cause cancer (an HPV test). The same sample can be checked for abnormal cells (a Pap test). When both an HPV test and a Pap test are done on the same sample, this is called an "HPV/Pap cotest."

A pelvic exam may include more than taking samples for an HPV and/or Pap test. Your health-care provider may also check the size, shape, and position of the uterus and ovaries and feel for any lumps or cysts. The rectum may also be checked for lumps or abnormal areas. You may talk with your health-care provider about being tested for sexually transmitted infections (STIs).

Most health-care providers will tell you what to expect at each step of the exam, so you will be at ease.

Researchers have found that cervical cancer screening may be less effective for people with obesity, possibly because of challenges in visualizing the cervix and obtaining a cell sample. Approaches to improve cervical visualization, including the use of a larger speculum, may be helpful.

Does Cervical Cancer Screening Have Any Risks?

Cervical cancer screening saves lives. Very few people screened for cervical cancer at routine intervals develop cervical cancer. Screening can detect cervical changes early, lowering a person's chance of dying from cervical cancer. Despite these benefits, cervical screening is not perfect, and there are several possible harms to be aware of. Before having any screening test, you may want to discuss the test with your doctor.

Potential risks of harm from cervical cancer screening include the following:

- **Unnecessary follow-up tests and treatment**. Finding a condition through screening that would not have caused problems may lead to unnecessary follow-up tests and possibly treatment. The current recommended screening intervals and tests reduce the chance of finding and treating cervical cell abnormalities that would have gone away on their own.
- **False-positive test results**. Screening test results may sometimes appear abnormal even though no precancer or cancer is present. When a Pap test shows a false-positive result (one that shows there is precancer or cancer when there is not), it can cause anxiety and is usually followed by more tests and procedures (such as colposcopy, cryotherapy, or loop electrosurgical excision procedure), which also have harms.
- **False-negative test results**. Screening test results may appear normal even though cervical precancer or cancer is present. A person who receives a false-negative test result (one that shows there is no cancer when there is) may delay seeking medical care even if there are symptoms.

Tests for Cervical Cancer

People who have cervical cancer screening at regular intervals are rarely found to have cancer. Most people who receive abnormal cervical cancer screening results either have HPV infections or have early cell changes that can be monitored (since they often go away on their own) or treated early (to prevent the development of cervical cancer).

Human papillomavirus Test

HPV test results show whether high-risk HPV types were found in cervical cells. An HPV test will come back as a negative test result or a positive test result.

- **Negative HPV test result**. High-risk HPV was not found. You should have the next test in five years. You may need to come back sooner if you had abnormal results in the past.
- **Positive HPV test result**. High-risk HPV was found. Your health-care provider will recommend follow-up steps you need to take, based on your specific test result.

What Does It Mean If You Have a Positive Human papillomavirus Test after Years of Negative Tests?

Sometimes, after several negative HPV tests, a woman may have a positive HPV test result. This is not necessarily a sign of a new HPV infection. Sometimes an HPV infection can become active again after many years. Some other viruses behave this way. For example, the virus that causes chickenpox can reactivate later in life to cause shingles.

Researchers do not know whether a reactivated HPV infection has the same risk of causing cervical cell changes or cervical cancer as a new HPV infection.

Pap Test

Pap test results show whether cervical cells are normal or abnormal. A Pap test may also come back as unsatisfactory.

- **Normal Pap test results**. No abnormal cervical cells were found. A normal test result may also be called a "negative test result" or "negative for intraepithelial lesion" (area of abnormal growth) or "malignancy."
- **Unsatisfactory Pap test results**. The lab sample may not have had enough cells, or the cells may have been clumped together or hidden by blood or mucus. Your health-care provider will ask you to come in for another Pap test in two to four months.
- **Abnormal Pap test results**. An abnormal test result may also be called a "positive test result." Some of the cells of the cervix look different from the normal cells. An abnormal test result does not mean you have cancer. Your health-care provider will recommend monitoring, more testing, or treatment.

Diagnosis of Cervical Cancer

If you have symptoms or screening test results that suggest the possibility of cervical cancer, your doctor will do follow-up tests to find out if it is due to cancer or some other cause. They will usually start by asking about your personal and family medical history and by doing a physical exam, which will include a pelvic exam and rectovaginal exam. They may recommend diagnostic tests to find out if you have cervical cancer, and if so, whether it has spread to another part of the body. The results of these tests will also help you and your doctor plan treatment.

The following procedures are used to diagnose cervical cancer.

Colposcopy

Colposcopy is a procedure in which the health-care provider inserts a speculum to gently open the vagina and view the cervix. A vinegar solution will be applied to the cervix to help show abnormal areas. The health-care provider then places an instrument called a "colposcope" close to the vagina. It has a bright light and a magnifying lens and allows the health-care provider to look closely at the cervix. A colposcopy usually includes a biopsy.

Biopsy

A biopsy is a procedure in which a sample of tissue is removed from the cervix so that a pathologist can view it under a microscope to check for signs of cancer. The following types of biopsies are used to check for cervical cancer:

- **Punch biopsy**. It is a procedure in which a small, round piece of tissue is removed using a sharp, hollow circular instrument. Sometimes several different areas of the cervix will be checked with a punch biopsy. This procedure is usually done in the doctor's office.
- **Endocervical curettage**. It is a procedure to collect cells or tissue from the cervical canal using a curette (spoon-shaped instrument). This procedure removes only a small amount of tissue and is usually done in the doctor's office.
- **Loop electrosurgical excision procedure (LEEP)**. It uses a thin wire loop, through which an electrical current is passed, to remove tissue from the cervix. LEEP may be used to diagnose cervical cancer. It may also be used to remove precancer or early-stage cancer. This procedure is typically done in a doctor's office. It usually takes only a few minutes, and local anesthesia is used to numb the area.
- **Cone biopsy**. It is surgery to remove a larger, cone-shaped piece of tissue from the cervix and cervical canal. A cone biopsy may be used to diagnose cervical cancer. It may also be used to remove precancer or early-stage cancer. This procedure is also called "conization." A cone biopsy is done at the hospital under general anesthesia.

Talk with your health-care provider to learn what to expect during and after your biopsy procedure. Some people have bleeding and/or discharge after a biopsy. Others have pain that feels like cramps during menstruation.

Getting a Second Opinion

Some people want to get a second opinion to confirm their cervical cancer diagnosis and treatment plan. If you choose to seek a second opinion, you will need to get important medical test results and reports from the first doctor to share with the second doctor. The second doctor will review the pathology report, slides, and scans before giving a recommendation. The doctor who gives the second opinion may agree with your first doctor, suggest changes or another approach, or provide more information about your cancer.

Prognosis of Cervical Cancer

If you have been diagnosed with cervical cancer, you may have questions about how serious the cancer is and your chances of survival. The likely outcome or course of a disease is called "prognosis."

The prognosis for cervical cancer depends on many factors:

- the stage of the cancer (the size of the tumor and whether the cancer has spread beyond the cervix)
- the type of cervical cancer (adenocarcinoma or squamous cell carcinoma (SCC))
- your age and general health
- whether you have other health problems or diseases, including if you are immunocompromised or have HIV
- whether the cancer is newly diagnosed or has recurred (come back)

Treatment for Cervical Cancer

Different types of treatment are available for cervical cancer. You and your cancer care team will work together to decide your treatment plan, which may include more than one type of treatment. Many factors will be considered, such as the stage of the cancer, your overall health, and your preferences. Your treatment plan will include information about your cancer, the goals of treatment, the treatment options and possible side effects, and the expected length of treatment.

If you are concerned about whether treatment will affect your fertility, talk with your cancer care team before treatment begins about what to expect.

Surgery

Surgery (also called an "operation") is sometimes used to treat cervical cancer. The type of surgery depends on where the cancer is located. The following surgical procedures may be used.

Cold Knife Conization

Cold knife conization uses a scalpel to remove a cone-shaped piece of tissue from the cervix and cervical canal. Sometimes all the cancer can be removed during this procedure. Cold knife conization is done in the hospital under general anesthesia.

Survival Rates for Cervical Cancer

Doctors estimate cervical cancer prognosis by using statistics collected over many years from people with cervical cancer. One statistic that is commonly used in making a prognosis is the five-year relative survival rate. The five-year relative survival rate tells you what percent of people with the same type and stage of cervical cancer are alive five years after their cancer was diagnosed, compared with people in the overall population. For example, the five-year relative survival rate for cervical cancer diagnosed at an early stage is 91 percent. This means that people diagnosed with early-stage cervical cancer are 91 percent as likely as people who do not have cervical cancer to be alive five years after diagnosis. The five-year relative survival rates for cervical cancer are as follows:

- When cervical cancer is diagnosed at an early stage, the five-year relative survival rate is 91 percent.
- When cervical cancer is diagnosed after it has spread to nearby tissues, organs, or regional lymph nodes, the five-year relative survival rate is 60 percent.
- When cervical cancer is diagnosed after it has spread to a distant part of the body, the five-year relative survival rate is 19 percent.
- The five-year relative survival rate for all people with cervical cancer is 67 percent.

Source: "What Is Cervical Cancer?" National Cancer Institute (NCI), June 15, 2023. Available online. URL: www.cancer.gov/types/cervical/survival. Accessed September 29, 2023.

Sentinel Lymph Node Biopsy

Sentinel lymph node biopsy removes the sentinel lymph node during surgery. The sentinel lymph node is the first lymph node in a group of lymph nodes to receive lymphatic drainage from the primary tumor. It is therefore the first lymph node the cancer is likely to spread to from the primary tumor. To identify the sentinel lymph node, a radioactive substance and/or blue dye is injected near the tumor. The substance or dye flows through the lymph ducts to the lymph nodes. The first lymph node to receive the substance or dye is removed. A pathologist views the tissue under a microscope to look for cancer cells. If cancer cells are found, more lymph nodes will be removed through a separate incision (cut). This is called a "lymph node dissection." After the sentinel lymph node biopsy, the surgeon removes the cancer.

Hysterectomy

A hysterectomy is surgery to remove the uterus. As a treatment for cervical cancer, the cervix, and sometimes the surrounding structures, are removed. Several types of hysterectomy may be used to treat cervical cancer:

- **Total hysterectomy**. This removes the uterus and the cervix. When the surgery is done entirely through the vagina (with no incisions on the abdomen) and the uterus and cervix are removed through the vagina, the operation is called a "total vaginal hysterectomy." If the surgery is done through a large incision on the abdomen (either vertical or horizontal) and the uterus and cervix are removed through this incision, the operation is called a "total abdominal hysterectomy." If the surgery is done through small incisions on the abdomen, the operation is called a "total laparoscopic hysterectomy." The uterus and cervix are usually taken out through the vagina, although sometimes an abdominal incision is made to remove the uterus and cervix.

- **Radical hysterectomy**. This removes the uterus, cervix, part of the vagina, and a wide area of ligaments and tissues around these organs. The ovaries, fallopian tubes, or nearby lymph nodes may also be removed.
- **Modified radical hysterectomy**. This removes the uterus, cervix, upper part of the vagina, and ligaments and tissues that closely surround these organs. This type of surgery removes fewer tissues and/or organs than radical hysterectomy. The ovaries, fallopian tubes, or nearby lymph nodes may also be removed.

Radical Trachelectomy

Radical trachelectomy (also called "radical cervicectomy") removes the cervix, nearby tissue, and the upper part of the vagina. Lymph nodes may also be removed. After the surgeon removes the cervix, they attach the uterus to the remaining part of the vagina. A special stitch or band is placed on the uterus (in a procedure called a "cerclage") to help keep the uterus closed during pregnancy. If you have this surgery, you may still be able to become pregnant.

Bilateral Salpingo-Oophorectomy

Bilateral salpingo-oophorectomy removes both ovaries and both fallopian tubes. This is done when the cancer has spread to these organs.

Total Pelvic Exenteration

A total pelvic exenteration removes the lower colon, rectum, and bladder. The cervix, vagina, ovaries, and nearby lymph nodes are also removed. Artificial openings (stoma) are made for urine and stool to flow from the body to a collection bag. Plastic surgery may be needed to make an artificial vagina after this operation.

Radiation Therapy

Radiation therapy uses high-energy x-rays or other types of radiation to kill cancer cells or keep them from growing by damaging their deoxyribonucleic acid (DNA). The two main types of radiation therapy are external radiation therapy and internal radiation therapy (also called "brachytherapy").

Both external and internal radiation therapy are used to treat cervical cancer and may also be used as palliative therapy to relieve symptoms and improve quality of life (QOL) in people with advanced cervical cancer.

External Radiation Therapy

External-beam radiation therapy uses a machine outside the body to send radiation toward the area of the body with cancer. Intensity-modulated radiation therapy (IMRT) is a way of giving external radiation therapy that can help keep radiation from damaging nearby healthy tissue.

IMRT is a type of three-dimensional (3D) radiation therapy that uses a computer to make pictures of the size and shape of the tumor. Thin beams of radiation of different intensities (strengths) are aimed directly at the tumor from many angles. IMRT is being studied for the treatment of cervical cancer.

Internal Radiation Therapy

Internal radiation therapy uses a radioactive substance sealed in needles, seeds, wires, or catheters that are placed directly into or near the cancer. Internal radiation therapy is also called "brachytherapy."

Chemotherapy

Chemotherapy (also called "chemo") uses drugs to stop the growth of cancer cells, either by killing the cells or by stopping them from dividing. Chemotherapy may be given alone or with other types of treatment.

Chemotherapy drugs used to treat cervical cancer include the following:

- cisplatin
- carboplatin
- gemcitabine
- ifosfamide
- irinotecan
- paclitaxel
- topotecan
- vinorelbine

Combinations of these drugs may be used. Other chemotherapy drugs not listed here may also be used.

Targeted therapy

Targeted therapy uses drugs or other substances to block the action of specific enzymes, proteins, or other molecules involved in the growth and spread of cancer cells.

Targeted therapies used to treat cervical cancer include the following:

- bevacizumab
- tisotumab vedotin

Immunotherapy

Immunotherapy helps a person's immune system fight cancer. Biomarker tests can be used to help predict your response to certain immunotherapy drugs.

Pembrolizumab is an immunotherapy drug used to treat certain patients whose cervical cancer has the biomarker PD-L1.

Follow-Up Testing during and after Treatment

Some of the tests that were done to diagnose cervical cancer or to find out the stage of the cancer may be repeated during treatment to see how well the treatment is working. Decisions about whether to continue, change, or stop treatment may be based on the results of these tests.

Some of the tests will continue to be done from time to time after treatment has ended. The results of these tests can show if your condition has changed or if the cancer has recurred (come back). These tests are sometimes called "follow-up tests" or "checkups."

Tell your doctor if you have any of the following signs or symptoms, which may mean the cancer has come back:

- vaginal bleeding or discharge
- pain in the abdomen, back, or leg
- swelling in the leg
- trouble urinating
- change in your bowel movements
- cough
- feeling tired

For cervical cancer, follow-up tests are usually done every three to four months for the first two years, followed by check-ups every six months. The check-up includes a current health history and exam of the body to check for signs and symptoms of recurrent cervical cancer and for late effects of treatment. A Pap test may or may not be done during your visits.

Prevention of Cervical Cancer

Cervical cancer is highly preventable and highly curable if caught early. Nearly all cervical cancers could be prevented by HPV vaccination, routine cervical cancer screening, and appropriate follow-up treatment when needed.

Human Papillomavirus Vaccination

HPV vaccination is a safe and effective way to help prevent cervical cancer. Gardasil 9 is the vaccine approved by the U.S. Food and Drug Administration (FDA) for females and males aged 9–45 in the United States. Gardasil 9 is approved to prevent precancers and cancers caused by seven cancer-causing HPV types (16, 18, 31, 33, 45, 52, and 58) and to prevent genital warts caused by HPV types 6 and 11. The HPV vaccine does not treat an existing HPV infection.

Cervical Cancer Screening

Because HPV vaccination does not protect against all HPV types that can cause cervical cancer, getting screened at regular intervals is still important.

Condoms

Condoms, which prevent some sexually transmitted diseases (STDs), can decrease the risk of HPV transmission. However, they do not completely prevent it. Therefore, exposure to HPV is still possible in areas that are not covered by the condom.[1]

[1] "What Is Cervical Cancer?" National Cancer Institute (NCI), June 15, 2023. Available online. URL: www.cancer.gov/types/cervical. Accessed September 29, 2023.

CHAPTER 38
OVARIAN CANCER

Ovarian, fallopian tube, and primary peritoneal cancers are diseases in which malignant (cancer) cells form in the ovaries, fallopian tubes, or peritoneum.

The ovaries are a pair of organs in the female reproductive system. They are in the pelvis, one on each side of the uterus (the hollow, pear-shaped organ where a fetus grows). Each ovary is about the size and shape of an almond. The ovaries make eggs and female hormones (chemicals that control the way certain cells or organs work in the body).

The fallopian tubes are a pair of long, slender tubes, one on each side of the uterus. Eggs pass from the ovaries, through the fallopian tubes, to the uterus. Cancer sometimes begins at the end of the fallopian tube near the ovary and spreads to the ovary.

The peritoneum is the tissue that lines the abdominal wall and covers organs in the abdomen. Primary peritoneal cancer forms in the peritoneum and has not spread there from another part of the body. Cancer sometimes begins in the peritoneum and spreads to the ovary.

Ovarian cancer is the leading cause of death from cancer of the female reproductive system. Ovarian cancer is most common in postmenopausal women. Over the past 10 years, the number of new cases of ovarian cancer decreased slightly each year. There was also a slight decrease in the number of deaths from ovarian cancer each year from 2009 to 2018.

Women who have a family history of ovarian cancer and/or certain inherited gene changes, such as *BRCA1* or *BRCA2* gene changes, have a higher risk than women who do not have a family history or who have not inherited these gene changes. For women with inherited risk, genetic counseling and genetic testing can be used to find out more about how likely they are to develop ovarian cancer.

It is hard to find ovarian cancer early. Early ovarian cancer may not cause any symptoms. When symptoms do appear, ovarian cancer is often advanced.

Risk and Protective Factors of Ovarian Cancer

Avoiding risk factors and increasing protective factors may help prevent cancer. Avoiding these risk factors may help prevent certain cancers. Risk factors include smoking, being overweight, and not getting enough exercise. Increasing protective factors, such as quitting smoking and exercising, may also help prevent some cancers. Talk to your doctor or other health-care professional about how you might lower your risk of cancer.

The following are risk factors for ovarian, fallopian tube, and primary peritoneal cancers:

- **Family history of ovarian, fallopian tube, and primary peritoneal cancers**. A woman whose mother or sister had ovarian cancer has an increased risk of ovarian cancer. A woman with two or more relatives with ovarian cancer also has an increased risk of ovarian cancer.
- **Inherited risk**. The risk of ovarian cancer is increased in women who have inherited certain changes in the *BRCA1*, *BRCA2*, or other genes.
  The risk of ovarian cancer is also increased in women who have certain inherited syndromes that include the following:
  - familial site-specific ovarian cancer syndrome
  - familial breast/ovarian cancer syndrome
  - hereditary nonpolyposis colorectal cancer (HNPCC; Lynch syndrome)
- **Hormone replacement therapy**. There is a slightly increased risk of ovarian cancer in women who are taking hormone replacement therapy (HRT) after menopause. There is also an increased risk of ovarian cancer in women who have recently used HRT, even if they used it for less than five years. The risk of ovarian cancer is the same for HRT with estrogen only or with combined estrogen and progestin. HRT taken through the skin may have a lower risk than HRT taken by mouth. When HRT is stopped, the risk of ovarian cancer decreases over time. The risk of ovarian cancer is not affected by the age of the woman when taking HRT.
- **Weight and height**. Being overweight or having obesity is linked to an increased risk of ovarian cancer. Obesity is also linked to an increased risk of death from ovarian cancer. Being tall may also be linked to a slight increase in the risk of ovarian cancer.
- **Endometriosis**. Women who have endometriosis have an increased risk of ovarian cancer.

The following are protective factors for ovarian, fallopian tube, and primary peritoneal cancers:

- **Oral contraceptives**. Taking oral contraceptives ("the pill") lowers the risk of ovarian cancer. The longer oral contraceptives are used, the lower the risk may be. The decrease in risk may last up to 30 years after a woman has stopped taking oral contraceptives. Taking oral contraceptives increases the risk of blood clots. This risk is higher in women who also smoke.
- **Tubal ligation**. The risk of ovarian cancer is decreased in women who have tubal ligation (surgery to close both fallopian tubes).

- **Giving birth**. Women who have given birth have a decreased risk of ovarian cancer compared to women who have not given birth. Giving birth to more than one child further decreases the risk of ovarian cancer.
- **Salpingectomy**. Some studies have shown that salpingectomy (surgery to remove one or both fallopian tubes) is linked with a decreased risk of ovarian cancer. When both fallopian tubes are removed, the risk of ovarian cancer is lowered more than when one fallopian tube is removed.
- **Breastfeeding**. Breastfeeding is linked to a decreased risk of ovarian cancer. The longer a woman breastfeeds, the lower her risk of ovarian cancer. Women who breastfeed for at least 8–10 months have the greatest decrease in risk of ovarian cancer.
- **Risk-reducing salpingo-oophorectomy**. Some women who have a high risk of ovarian cancer may choose to have a risk-reducing salpingo-oophorectomy (surgery to remove the fallopian tubes and ovaries when there are no signs of cancer). This includes women who have inherited certain changes in the *BRCA1* and *BRCA2* genes or have an inherited syndrome.

  It is very important to have a cancer risk assessment and counseling before making this decision. These and other factors may be discussed:
  - infertility
  - early menopause (The drop in estrogen levels caused by removing the ovaries can cause early menopause. Symptoms of menopause can worsen and include: hot flashes, night sweats, trouble sleeping, mood changes, decreased sex drive, heart disease, vaginal dryness, frequent urination, and osteoporosis (decreased bone density).)

  These symptoms may not be the same in all women. HRT may be used to lessen these symptoms.

  Women who have had a risk-reducing salpingo-oophorectomy continue to have a small risk of ovarian cancer in the peritoneum (a thin layer of tissue that lines the inside of the abdomen). This is rare but may occur if ovarian cancer cells had already spread to the peritoneum before the surgery or if some ovarian tissue remains after surgery.

It is not clear whether the following affect the risk of ovarian, fallopian tube, and primary peritoneal cancers:

- **Diet**. Studies of dietary factors have not found a strong link to ovarian cancer.
- **Alcohol**. Studies have not shown a link between drinking alcohol and the risk of ovarian cancer.
- **Aspirin and nonsteroidal antiinflammatory drugs (NSAIDs)**. Some studies of aspirin and NSAIDs have found a decreased risk of ovarian cancer, and others have not.

- **Talc**. Studies of women who used talcum powder (talc) dusted on the perineum (the area between the vagina and the anus) have not found clear evidence of an increased risk of ovarian cancer.
- **Infertility treatment**. Overall, studies in women using fertility drugs have not found clear evidence of an increased risk of ovarian cancer. The risk of invasive ovarian cancer may be higher in women who do not get pregnant after taking fertility drugs.

Cancer Prevention Clinical Trials Are Used to Study Ways to Prevent Cancer

Cancer prevention clinical trials are used to study ways to lower the risk of developing certain types of cancer. Some cancer prevention trials are conducted with healthy people who have not had cancer but who have an increased risk for cancer. Other prevention trials are conducted with people who have had cancer and are trying to prevent another cancer of the same type or to lower their chance of developing a new type of cancer. Other trials are done with healthy volunteers who are not known to have any risk factors for cancer.

The purpose of some cancer prevention clinical trials is to find out whether actions people take can prevent cancer. These may include eating fruits and vegetables, exercising, quitting smoking, or taking certain medicines, vitamins, minerals, or food supplements.[1]

[1] "Ovarian, Fallopian Tube, and Primary Peritoneal Cancers Prevention (PDQ®)—Patient Version" National Cancer Institute (NCI), February 17, 2023. Available online. URL: www.cancer.gov/types/ovarian/patient/ovarian-prevention-pdq. Accessed September 29, 2023.

CHAPTER 39
STOMACH CANCER

What Is Stomach Cancer?

Stomach (gastric) cancer is cancer that starts in the cells lining the stomach. The stomach is an organ on the left side of the upper abdomen that digests food. The stomach is part of the digestive tract, a series of hollow, muscular organs joined in a long, twisting tube from the mouth to the anus. The digestive tract processes nutrients in foods that are eaten and helps pass waste material out of the body:

- Food moves from the throat to the stomach through a tube called the "esophagus."
- After food enters the stomach, it is broken down by stomach muscles that mix the food and liquid with digestive juices.
- After leaving the stomach, partly digested food passes into the small intestine and then into the large intestine.
- The end of the large intestine, called the "rectum," stores the waste from the digested food until it is pushed out of the anus during a bowel movement.

Types of Stomach Cancer

- **Adenocarcinoma of the stomach**. It begins in the mucus-producing cells in the innermost lining of the stomach. Nearly all stomach cancers are adenocarcinomas.

  Adenocarcinoma of the stomach is divided into two main classes, depending on where it forms in the stomach:

  - Gastric cardia cancer begins in the top inch of the stomach, just below where it meets the esophagus. Most adenocarcinomas are found in the gastric cardia.
  - Noncardia gastric cancer is cancer that begins in all other sections of the stomach.

  Adenocarcinoma of the stomach may also be described as intestinal or diffuse, depending on how the cells look under a microscope:

  - **Intestinal adenocarcinomas**. These are well differentiated, meaning the cancer cells look similar to normal cells under a microscope.

- **Diffuse adenocarcinomas**. These are undifferentiated or poorly differentiated, meaning the cancer cells look different from normal cells under a microscope. Diffuse adenocarcinomas tend to grow and spread more quickly than the intestinal type and be harder to treat.
- **Gastroesophageal junction adenocarcinoma (GEJ)**. It is a type of cancer that forms in the area where the esophagus meets the gastric cardia. GEJ may be treated similarly to stomach cancer or esophageal cancer.
- **Gastrointestinal neuroendocrine tumors**. These cancers begin in neuroendocrine cells (a type of cell that is like a nerve cell and a hormone-making cell) that line the gastrointestinal tract. Neuroendocrine cells make hormones that help control digestive juices and the muscles used in moving food through the stomach and intestines.
- **Gastrointestinal stromal tumors (GIST)**. These cancers begin in nerve cells that are found in the wall of the stomach and other digestive organs. GIST is a type of soft tissue sarcoma.
- **Primary gastric lymphoma**. This is a type of non-Hodgkin lymphoma (NHL) that forms in the stomach. Most primary gastric lymphomas are either mucosa-associated lymphoid tissue (MALT) gastric lymphoma or diffuse large B-cell lymphoma of the stomach.

Rarely, other types of cancer, such as squamous cell carcinoma (SCC), small cell carcinoma, and leiomyosarcoma (LMS), can also begin in the stomach.

Causes of Stomach Cancer

Stomach cancer is caused by certain changes to the way stomach cells function, especially how they grow and divide into new cells. There are many risk factors for stomach cancer, but many do not directly cause cancer. Instead, they increase the chance of deoxyribonucleic acid (DNA) damage in cells that may lead to stomach cancer.

A risk factor is anything that increases the chance of getting a disease. Some risk factors for stomach cancer, such as tobacco use, can be changed. However, risk factors also include things people cannot change, such as their age and family history.

Risk Factors for Stomach Cancer

There are several risk factors for stomach cancer. Different risk factors may increase the risk of cancer in different parts of the stomach. For example, *Helicobacter pylori* (*H. pylori*) infection increases the risk of cancer in the lower and middle part of the stomach, while obesity and gastroesophageal reflux disease (GERD) increase the risk of cancer in the upper stomach.

Helicobacter pylori infection

Chronic infection of the mucosal layer of the stomach with *H. pylori* is a major risk factor for stomach cancer. This bacterium spreads from person to person through direct contact with saliva, vomit, or stool. Although many people with chronic *H. pylori* infections do not have symptoms, some develop stomach ulcers or an inflammation of the stomach called "atrophic gastritis." In some people, atrophic gastritis leads to increasingly severe changes in the stomach lining and eventually to stomach cancer or gastric mucosa-associated lymphoid tissue (MALT) lymphoma.

Other Medical Conditions

The risk of stomach cancer is increased in people who have:

- chronic atrophic gastritis (thinning of the stomach lining caused by long-term inflammation of the stomach)
- atrophic gastritis with intestinal metaplasia (a condition in which the cells that line the stomach are replaced by cells that normally line the intestines)
- Epstein-Barr virus (EBV) infection
- pernicious anemia (an autoimmune condition in which the intestines cannot properly absorb vitamin B_{12}, resulting in a low RBC count)
- obesity (excess body weight)
- GERD (a condition in which stomach acid repeatedly flows back into the esophagus)

Genetics and Family History

The risk of stomach cancer is increased, sometimes to very high levels, in people who have:

- a first-degree relative (parent, sibling, or child) who has had stomach cancer
- a family cancer syndrome, such as:
  - familial adenomatous polyposis
  - familial intestinal gastric cancer (FIGC) (a type of stomach cancer that runs in families but does not have a known genetic cause)
  - gastric adenocarcinoma and proximal polyposis of the stomach (GAPPS)
  - hereditary diffuse gastric cancer (HDGC)
  - juvenile polyposis syndrome
  - Li-Fraumeni syndrome
  - Lynch syndrome (also called "hereditary nonpolyposis colon cancer" (HNPCC))
  - Peutz-Jeghers syndrome
- Type A blood

Diet
Eating a diet that is low in fruits and vegetables or that is high in salted, smoked, or poorly preserved foods may increase the risk of stomach cancer.

Tobacco Use
People who smoke have a higher risk of stomach cancer than nonsmokers. Smoking also makes treatment for *H. pylori* infection less effective. Smokers who stop smoking lower their risk of having stomach cancer over time.

Environmental and Occupational Exposures
The risk of stomach cancer is increased in people who:

- work in the rubber or coal industry
- have been exposed to very high levels of radiation

Having one or more of these risk factors does not necessarily mean you will get stomach cancer. Many people with risk factors never develop stomach cancer, whereas others with no known risk factors do. Talk with your doctor if you think you might be at increased risk.

Stomach cancer screening or preventive surgery may be available to people at very high risk of stomach cancer, such as those with certain genetic conditions or family histories.

Symptoms of Stomach Cancer
Early on, stomach cancer usually does not have symptoms, making it hard to detect. Symptoms usually begin after the cancer has spread.

When symptoms of early-stage stomach cancer do occur, they may include the following:

- indigestion and stomach discomfort
- a bloated feeling after eating
- mild nausea
- loss of appetite
- heartburn

Symptoms of advanced stomach cancer (cancer has spread beyond the stomach to other parts of the body) may include the symptoms of early-stage stomach cancer and:

- blood in the stool
- vomiting
- weight loss for no known reason
- stomach pain
- jaundice (yellowing of eyes and skin)
- ascites (build-up of fluid in the abdomen)
- trouble swallowing

These symptoms may be caused by many conditions other than stomach cancer. It is important to check with your doctor if you have any of these symptoms. Your doctor will ask when your symptoms started and how often you have been having them. If it is stomach cancer, ignoring symptoms can delay treatment and make it less effective.

Screening of Stomach Cancer

Screening is looking for cancer before a person has any symptoms. This can help detect cancer at an early stage. When abnormal tissue or cancer is found early, it may be easier to treat.

In the United States, there are no standard or routine screening tests to detect stomach cancer in people at average risk. Researchers are working to develop such tests. If a test reduces the number of deaths from stomach cancer, it may become a standard screening test.

Tests to Screen for Stomach Cancer

Some people who have a higher risk of stomach cancer may benefit from screening with upper endoscopy, including the following:

- older people with chronic gastric atrophy or pernicious anemia
- people who have had
  - partial gastrectomy
  - a family history of stomach cancer
- people who have certain genetic syndromes
- people from countries where stomach cancer is more common

Upper Endoscopy

Upper endoscopy is a procedure to look inside the esophagus, stomach, and duodenum (first part of the small intestine) to check for abnormal areas. An endoscope is passed through the mouth and down the throat into the esophagus. An endoscope is a thin, tube-like instrument with a light and a lens for viewing. It may also have a tool to remove tissue, which is checked under a microscope for signs of disease.

Screening Risks of Stomach Cancer

Talk with your doctor about whether stomach cancer screening is right for you.

Potential risks of stomach cancer screening include the following:

- **False-negative test results**. Screening test results may appear to be normal even though stomach cancer is present. A person who receives a false-negative test result (one that shows there is no cancer when there really is) may delay seeking medical care even if there are symptoms.
- **False-positive test results**. Screening test results may appear to be abnormal even though no cancer is present. A false-positive test result (one that shows there is cancer when there really is not) can cause anxiety and is usually followed by more tests and procedures which also have risks.

- **Risks of the screening test itself**. Upper endoscopy may cause the following rare, but serious, complications:
  - a small hole (puncture) in the esophagus or stomach
  - heart problems
  - breathing problems
  - lung infection from inhaling food, fluid, or stomach acid into the lung
  - severe bleeding that needs to be treated at a hospital
  - reactions to medicine used during the procedure

Diagnosis of Stomach Cancer

If you have symptoms that suggest stomach cancer, your doctor will need to find out if they are due to cancer or another condition. They may:

- ask about your personal and family medical history to learn about your possible risk factors for stomach cancer
- do a physical exam, which will include feeling your abdomen for anything abnormal
- run blood tests to check for anemia (a low red blood cell (RBC) count), which could be a sign of bleeding in the stomach
- check your stool for hidden (occult) blood, which could be a sign of bleeding in the stomach

Depending on these results, your doctor may recommend tests to find out if you have stomach cancer.

Tests to Diagnose Stomach Cancer

The following tests and procedures are used to diagnose stomach cancer. The results will also help you and your doctor plan treatment.

Upper Endoscopy with Biopsy

An endoscope (a thin, lighted tube) is passed through the mouth and down the throat into the esophagus. It may also have a tool to remove a sample of cells or tissue (biopsy) so a pathologist can view it under a microscope to check for signs of cancer.

The sample of tissue may be checked for *Helicobacter pylori* (*H. pylori*) infection and used for biomarker testing.

Talk with your doctor to learn what to expect during and after your biopsy.

Barium Swallow

Barium swallow is a series of x-rays of the esophagus and stomach. The patient drinks a liquid that contains barium (a silver-white metallic compound). The liquid coats the esophagus and stomach, and x-rays are taken. This procedure is also called an "upper GI series."

Computerized Tomography Scan

A computed tomography (CT) scan uses a computer linked to an x-ray machine to make a series of detailed pictures of areas inside the body from different angles. A dye may be injected into a vein or swallowed to help the organs or tissues show up more clearly. This procedure is also called "computed tomography," "computerized tomography," or "computerized axial tomography."

Biomarker Testing

Biomarker testing is a way to look for genes, proteins, and other substances (called "biomarkers" or "tumor markers") that can provide information about cancer. Some biomarkers affect how certain cancer treatments work. Biomarker testing may help you and your doctor choose a cancer treatment for you.

To check for these biomarkers, samples of tissue containing stomach cancer cells are removed during a biopsy or surgery. The samples are tested in a laboratory to see whether the stomach cancer cells have these biomarkers.

For stomach cancer, biomarker testing includes the following:

- **Human epidermal growth factor receptor 2 (HER2)**. The cancer cells may have larger than normal amounts of a protein called "HER2."
- **Programmed death-ligand 1 (PD-L1)**. The cells may have larger than normal amounts of an immune checkpoint protein called "PD-L1."
- **Microsatellite instability**. The cells may have microsatellite instability. This may be caused by mistakes that do not get corrected when DNA is copied in a cell.
- **Mismatch repair deficiency**. The cells may have a defect in a mismatch repair gene.
- **Tumor mutational burden**. If the cells have a high tumor mutational burden, it means they have many gene mutations.
- **Neurotrophic tyrosine receptor kinase (NTRK)**. The cells may have changes in one of the *NTRK* genes.

Tests to Stage Stomach Cancer

If you are diagnosed with stomach cancer, you will be referred to a gastrointestinal oncologist. This is a doctor who specializes in diagnosing and treating cancers of the stomach and intestines. Your doctor will recommend tests to find out if the cancer has spread and if so, how far. Sometimes the cancer is only in the stomach. Or, it may have spread from the stomach to other parts of the body. The process of learning the extent of cancer in the body is called "staging." It is important to know the stage of stomach cancer to plan treatment.

The following imaging tests and procedures may be used to find out your stage:

- **Endoscopic ultrasound**. This is a procedure in which an endoscope is inserted into the body, usually through the mouth or rectum. An endoscope is a thin, tube-like instrument with a light and a lens for viewing. A probe at the end of the endoscope is used to bounce high-energy sound waves (ultrasound) off internal tissues or organs and make echoes. The echoes form a picture of body tissues called a "sonogram." This procedure is also called "endosonography."

- **PET-CT scan**. The scan combines the pictures from a positron emission tomography (PET) scan and a CT scan. The PET and CT scans are done at the same time on the same machine. The pictures from both scans are combined to make a more detailed picture than either test would make by itself.
    - For the PET scan, a small amount of radioactive glucose is injected into a vein. The scanner rotates around the body and makes a picture of where glucose is being used in the body. Cancer cells show up brighter in the picture because they are more active and take up more glucose than normal cells.
    - For the CT scan, a series of detailed x-ray pictures of areas inside the body is taken from different angles. A dye may be injected into a vein or swallowed to help the organs or tissues show up more clearly.
- **Magnetic resonance imaging (MRI) with gadolinium**. This is a procedure that uses a magnet, radio waves, and a computer to make a series of detailed pictures of areas inside the body. A substance called "gadolinium" is injected into a vein. The gadolinium collects around the cancer cells so they show up brighter in the picture. This procedure is also called "nuclear magnetic resonance imaging" (NMRI).
- **Laparoscopy**. This is a surgical procedure to look at the organs inside the abdomen to check for signs of disease. Small incisions (cuts) are made in the wall of the abdomen and a laparoscope (a thin, lighted tube) is inserted into one of the incisions. Other instruments may be inserted through the same or other incisions to perform procedures such as removing organs or taking tissue samples to be checked under a microscope for signs of cancer. A solution may be washed over the surface of the organs in the abdomen and then removed to collect cells. These cells are also looked at under a microscope to check for signs of cancer.

Getting a Second Opinion

You may want to get a second opinion to confirm your stomach cancer diagnosis and treatment plan. If you seek a second opinion, you will need to get important medical test results and reports from the first doctor to share with the second doctor. The second doctor will review the pathology report, slides, and scans before giving a recommendation. The doctor who gives the second opinion may agree with your first doctor, suggest changes or another approach, or provide more information about your cancer.

Prognosis of Stomach Cancer

If you have been diagnosed with stomach cancer, you may have questions about how serious the cancer is and your chances of survival. The likely outcome or course of a disease is called "prognosis."

The prognosis for stomach cancer depends on:

- the stage of the cancer, including whether the cancer is only in the stomach or has spread to lymph nodes or other places in the body
- your overall health

When stomach cancer is found early, there is a better chance of recovery. Stomach cancer is often advanced when it is diagnosed. At advanced stages, stomach cancer can be treated but is rarely cured.

Survival Rates for Stomach Cancer

Doctors estimate stomach cancer prognosis by using statistics collected over many years from people with stomach cancer. One statistic that is commonly used in making a prognosis is the five-year relative survival rate. The five-year relative survival rate tells you what percent of people with the same type and stage of stomach cancer are alive five years after their cancer was diagnosed, compared with people in the overall population. For example, the five-year relative survival rate for stomach cancer is 36 percent. This means that, overall, people diagnosed with stomach cancer are 36 percent as likely as similar people who do not have stomach cancer to be alive five years after diagnosis.

The five-year relative survival rates for different stages of stomach cancer are:

- 75 percent for localized stomach cancer (cancer is in the stomach only)
- 35 percent for regional stomach cancer (cancer has spread beyond the stomach to nearby lymph nodes or organs)
- 7 percent for metastatic stomach cancer (cancer has spread beyond the stomach to a distant part of the body)

Source: "What Is Stomach Cancer?" National Cancer Institute (NCI), May 31, 2023. Available online. URL: www.cancer.gov/types/stomach/survival. Accessed October 3, 2023.

Treatment for Stomach Cancer

Different types of treatments are available for stomach cancer. You and your cancer care team will work together to decide your treatment plan, which may include more than one type of treatment. Many factors will be considered, such as the stage of the cancer, your overall health, and your preferences. Your plan will include information about your cancer, the goals of treatment, your treatment options and the possible side effects, and the expected length of treatment.

Talking with your cancer care team before treatment begins about what to expect will be helpful. You will want to learn what you need to do before treatment begins, how you will feel while going through it, and what kind of help you will need.

Endoscopic Mucosal Resection

Endoscopic mucosal resection is a procedure that uses an endoscope to remove carcinoma in situ and early-stage cancer from the lining of the digestive tract. An endoscope is a thin, tube-like instrument with a light and a lens and tools to remove tissue.

Surgery

Surgery is a common treatment for stomach cancer. The type of surgery depends on where the cancer is located.

Other treatments may be given in addition to surgery:

- Treatment given before surgery is called "preoperative therapy" or "neoadjuvant therapy." Chemotherapy may be given before surgery to shrink the tumor and reduce the amount of tissue that needs to be removed during surgery.
- Treatment given after surgery, to lower the risk that the cancer will come back, is called "adjuvant therapy." After the doctor removes all the cancer that can be seen, some patients may be given chemotherapy, radiation therapy, or both to kill any cancer cells that are left.

Gastrectomy

Gastrectomy, the removal of part or all of the stomach, is the main surgery for stomach cancer:

- **Subtotal gastrectomy**. This is the removal of the part of the stomach that contains cancer, nearby lymph nodes, and parts of other tissues and organs near the tumor. The spleen may also be removed.
- **Total gastrectomy**. This is the removal of the entire stomach, nearby lymph nodes, and parts of the esophagus, small intestine, and other tissues near the tumor. The spleen may also be removed. Then the surgeon attaches the esophagus to the small intestine so the patient can continue to eat and swallow.

Endoluminal Stent Placement

Endoluminal stent placement may be done when the tumor blocks the passage into or out of the stomach. In this procedure, the surgeon places a stent (a thin, expandable tube) from the esophagus to the stomach or from the stomach to the small intestine to allow the patient to eat normally.

Endoluminal Laser Therapy

Endoluminal laser therapy is a procedure in which an endoscope (a thin, lighted tube) with a laser attached is used as a knife to open a gastrointestinal blockage.

Gastrojejunostomy

Gastrojejunostomy is the removal of the part of the stomach with cancer that is blocking the opening into the small intestine. Then the surgeon connects the stomach to the jejunum (a part of the small intestine) to allow food and medicine to pass from the stomach into the small intestine.

Radiation Therapy

Radiation therapy uses high-energy x-rays or other types of radiation to kill cancer cells or keep them from growing. Stomach cancer is sometimes treated with external radiation therapy. This type of radiation therapy uses a machine outside the body to send radiation toward the area of the body with cancer.

Chemotherapy

Chemotherapy (also called "chemo") uses drugs to stop the growth of cancer cells, either by killing the cells or by stopping them from dividing.

Chemotherapy for stomach cancer is usually systemic, meaning it is injected into a vein or given by mouth. When given this way, the drugs enter the bloodstream to reach cancer cells throughout the body.

Chemotherapy drugs used to treat stomach cancer include the following:

- capecitabine
- cisplatin
- docetaxel
- doxorubicin
- epirubicin
- fluorouracil (5-FU)
- irinotecan
- leucovorin
- oxaliplatin
- paclitaxel
- trifluridine/tipiracil

Targeted Therapy

Targeted therapy uses drugs or other substances to identify and attack specific cancer cells. Your doctor may suggest biomarker tests to help predict your response to certain targeted therapy drugs.

Targeted therapies used to treat stomach cancer include the following:

- ramucirumab
- regorafenib
- trastuzumab
- trastuzumab deruxtecan

Immunotherapy

Immunotherapy helps a person's immune system fight cancer. Your doctor may suggest biomarker tests to help predict your response to certain immunotherapy drugs.

Immunotherapy drugs used to treat stomach cancer include the following:

- nivolumab
- pembrolizumab

These drugs work in more than one way to kill cancer cells. They are also considered targeted therapy because they target specific changes or substances in cancer cells.

Hyperthermic Intraperitoneal Chemotherapy

Regional chemotherapy is a method of placing chemotherapy directly into an organ or a body cavity, such as the abdomen, to mainly affect cancer cells in those areas.

A type of regional chemotherapy called "hyperthermic intraperitoneal chemotherapy," or "hot chemotherapy," is being studied to treat stomach cancer and may be offered at certain treatment centers. After the surgeon has removed as much of the cancer as possible during surgery, a chemotherapy drug, such as mitomycin or cisplatin, is warmed and pumped directly into the peritoneal cavity through a thin tube for about two hours. The surgeon then drains the chemotherapy from the abdomen and rinses the abdomen before closing the incision.

Follow-Up Testing

Some tests that were done to diagnose or stage the cancer may be repeated to see how well the treatment is working. Decisions about whether to continue, change, or stop treatment may be based on the results of these tests. These tests are sometimes called "follow-up tests" or "check-ups."

You may also have blood tests for tumor markers such as carcinoembryonic antigen (CEA) and cancer antigen 19-9 (CA 19-9). Increased levels of these markers may mean your stomach cancer has come back.[1]

[1] "What Is Stomach Cancer?" National Cancer Institute (NCI), March 15, 2006. Available online. URL: www.cancer.gov/types/stomach. Accessed October 3, 2023.

CHAPTER 40
ACUTE MYELOID LEUKEMIA

Acute myeloid leukemia (AML) is a type of cancer in which the bone marrow makes a large number of abnormal blood cells. AML is a cancer of the blood and bone marrow. It is the most common type of acute leukemia in adults. This type of cancer usually gets worse quickly if it is not treated. AML is also called "acute myelogenous leukemia" and "acute nonlymphocytic leukemia."

Leukemia may affect red blood cells, white blood cells, and platelets. Normally, the bone marrow makes blood stem cells (immature cells) that become mature blood cells over time. A blood stem cell may become a myeloid stem cell or a lymphoid stem cell. A lymphoid stem cell becomes a white blood cell.

A myeloid stem cell becomes one of the three types of mature blood cells:

- red blood cells that carry oxygen and other substances to all tissues of the body
- granulocytes, which are white blood cells that help fight infection and disease
- platelets that form blood clots to stop bleeding

In AML, the myeloid stem cells usually become a type of immature white blood cell called "myeloblasts" (or "myeloid blasts"). The myeloblasts in AML are abnormal and do not become healthy white blood cells. Sometimes in AML, too many stem cells become abnormal red blood cells or platelets. These abnormal white blood cells, red blood cells, or platelets are also called "leukemia cells" or "blasts." Leukemia cells can build up in the bone marrow and blood so there is less room for healthy white blood cells, red blood cells, and platelets. When this happens, infection, anemia, or easy bleeding may occur.

The leukemia cells can spread outside the blood to other parts of the body, including the central nervous system (brain and spinal cord), skin, and gums. Sometimes leukemia cells form a solid tumor called a "myeloid sarcoma." Myeloid sarcoma is also called "extramedullary myeloid tumor," "granulocytic sarcoma," or "chloroma."

Types of Acute Myeloid Leukemia

There are different subtypes of AML. Most AML subtypes are based on how mature (developed) the cancer cells are at the time of diagnosis, and how different they are from normal cells.

Acute promyelocytic leukemia (APL) is a subtype of AML. This leukemia occurs when genes on chromosome 15 switch places with some genes on chromosome 17, and an abnormal gene called "*PML::RARA*" is made. The *PML::RARA* gene sends a message that stops promyelocytes (a type of white blood cell) from maturing. Problems with severe bleeding and blood clots may occur. This is a serious health problem that needs treatment as soon as possible. APL usually occurs in middle-aged adults.

Smoking, previous chemotherapy treatment, and exposure to radiation may affect the risk of AML. Anything that increases a person's chance of getting a disease is called a "risk factor." Not every person with one or more of these risk factors will develop AML, and it can develop in people who do not have any known risk factors. Talk with your doctor if you think you may be at risk.

Risk Factors for Acute Myeloid Leukemia

Possible risk factors for AML include the following:

- being male
- older age
- smoking
- having had treatment with chemotherapy or radiation therapy in the past
- being exposed to radiation in the environment (such as nuclear radiation) or to the chemical benzene
- having a personal history of a blood disorder such as myelodysplastic syndrome
- having certain syndromes or inherited disorders

Signs and Symptoms of Acute Myeloid Leukemia

Signs and symptoms of AML include fever, feeling tired, and easy bruising or bleeding. The early signs and symptoms of AML may be like those caused by the flu or other common diseases. Check with your doctor if you have any of the following:

- weakness
- fever
- infection
- paleness or loss of normal skin color
- bleeding

Less common signs or symptoms may be caused by clusters of leukemia cells in the central nervous system (CNS) or testicles, or a tumor of myeloid cells called a "chloroma." Symptoms of acute leukemia often develop between four and six weeks before diagnosis.

How Is Acute Myeloid Leukemia Diagnosed?

Tests that examine the blood and bone marrow are used to diagnose AML. In addition to asking about your personal and family health history and doing a physical exam, your doctor may perform the following tests and procedures:

- **Complete blood count (CBC)**. A procedure in which a sample of blood is drawn and checked for the following:
  - the number of red blood cells, white blood cells, and platelets
  - the amount of hemoglobin (the protein that carries oxygen) in the red blood cells
  - the portion of the sample made up of red blood cells
- **Peripheral blood smear**. A procedure in which a sample of blood is checked for blast cells, the number and kinds of white blood cells, the number of platelets, and changes in the shape of blood cells.
- **Flow cytometry**. A laboratory test that measures the number of cells in a sample, the percentage of live cells in a sample, and certain characteristics of the cells, such as size, shape, and the presence of tumor (or other) markers on the cell surface. The cells from a sample of a patient's blood, bone marrow, or other tissue are stained with a fluorescent dye, placed in a fluid, and then passed one at a time through a beam of light. The test results are based on how the cells that were stained with the fluorescent dye react to the beam of light. This test is used to help diagnose and manage certain types of cancers, such as leukemia and lymphoma.
- **Bone marrow aspiration and biopsy**. The removal of bone marrow, blood, and a small piece of bone by inserting a hollow needle into the hipbone or breastbone. A pathologist views the bone marrow, blood, and bone under a microscope to look for signs of cancer.
- **Tumor biopsy**. A biopsy of a tumor made up of leukemia cells, also known as a "myeloid sarcoma (chloroma)," may be done.
- **Cytogenetic analysis**. A laboratory test in which the chromosomes of cells in a sample of blood or bone marrow are counted and checked for any changes, such as broken, missing, rearranged, or extra chromosomes. Changes in certain chromosomes may be a sign of cancer. Cytogenetic analysis is used to help diagnose cancer, plan treatment, or find out how well treatment is working. Other tests, such as fluorescence in situ hybridization (FISH), may also be done to look for certain changes in the chromosomes.
- **Molecular testing**. A laboratory test to check for certain genes, proteins, or other molecules in a sample of blood or bone marrow. Molecular tests also check for certain changes in a gene or chromosome that may cause or affect the chance of developing AML. A molecular test may be used to help plan treatment, find out how well treatment is working, or make a prognosis.

- **Immunophenotyping**. A laboratory test that uses antibodies to identify cancer cells based on the types of antigens or markers on the surface of the cells. This test is used to help diagnose specific types of leukemia. For example, a cytochemistry study may test the cells in a sample of tissue using chemicals (dyes) to look for certain changes in the sample. A chemical may cause a color change in one type of leukemia cell but not in another type of leukemia cell.
- **Reverse transcription-polymerase chain reaction test (RT-PCR)**. A laboratory test in which the amount of a genetic substance called "mRNA" made by a specific gene is measured. An enzyme called "reverse transcriptase" is used to convert a specific piece of RNA into a matching piece of DNA, which can be amplified (made in large numbers) by another enzyme called "DNA polymerase." The amplified DNA copies help tell whether a specific mRNA is being made by a gene. RT-PCR can be used to check the activation of certain genes that may indicate the presence of cancer cells. This test may be used to look for certain changes in a gene or chromosome, which may help diagnose cancer. This test is used to diagnose certain types of AML including acute promyelocytic leukemia (APL).

Factors Affecting Prognosis and Treatment Options

Certain factors affect prognosis (chance of recovery) and treatment options. The prognosis and treatment options depend on the following:

- the age of the patient (Older age at diagnosis may be linked to lower remission rates and more complications.)
- whether the leukemia has spread to the central nervous system
- whether the patient has a systemic infection at the time of diagnosis
- whether the patient has a very high white blood cell count at the time of diagnosis
- the subtype of AML
- whether the patient received chemotherapy or radiation therapy in the past to treat a different cancer.
- whether there is a history of a blood disorder such as myelodysplastic syndrome
- whether the cancer has been treated before or recurred (come back)

It is important that acute leukemia be treated right away.

Stages of Acute Myeloid Leukemia

Once acute myeloid leukemia (AML) has been diagnosed, tests are done to find out if the cancer has spread to other parts of the body.

The process used to find out if cancer has spread is called "staging." In AML, the subtype of AML and whether the leukemia has spread outside the blood and bone marrow are used instead of the stage to plan treatment.

The following tests and procedures may be used to determine if the leukemia has spread:

- **Lumbar puncture**. A procedure used to collect a sample of cerebrospinal fluid (CSF) from the spinal column. This is done by placing a needle between two bones in the spine and into the CSF around the spinal cord and removing a sample of the fluid. The sample of CSF is checked under a microscope for signs that leukemia cells have spread to the brain and spinal cord. This procedure is also called an "LP or spinal tap."
- **CT scan (CAT scan)**. A procedure that makes a series of detailed pictures of the abdomen, taken from different angles. The pictures are made by a computer linked to an x-ray machine. A dye may be injected into a vein or swallowed to help the organ or tissues show up more clearly. This procedure is also called "computed tomography," "computerized tomography," or "computerized axial tomography."

There is no standard staging system for AML. The disease is described as untreated, in remission, refractory, or recurrent.

Newly Diagnosed (Untreated) Acute Myeloid Leukemia

In untreated AML, the disease is newly diagnosed. It has not been treated except to relieve signs and symptoms such as fever, bleeding, or pain, and the following are true:

- the complete blood count is abnormal
- at least 20 percent of the cells in the bone marrow are blasts (leukemia cells) or there are certain gene changes
- there are signs or symptoms of leukemia

Acute Myeloid Leukemia in Remission

In AML in remission, the disease has been treated and the following are true:

- the complete blood count is normal
- less than 5 percent of the cells in the bone marrow are blasts (leukemia cells)
- there are no signs or symptoms of leukemia in the brain and spinal cord or elsewhere in the body

Refractory or Recurrent Acute Myeloid Leukemia

After treatment with chemotherapy, some patients with newly diagnosed AML will not go into remission. This is called "refractory cancer." In contrast, recurrent AML is cancer that has recurred (come back) after remission. The AML may come back in the blood or bone marrow.

Treatment Options for Acute Myeloid Leukemia

Different types of treatment are available for patients with AML. Some treatments are standard (the currently used treatment), and some are being tested in clinical trials.

A treatment clinical trial is a research study meant to help improve current treatments or obtain information on new treatments for patients with cancer. When clinical trials show that a new treatment is better than the standard treatment, the new treatment may become the standard treatment. Patients may want to think about taking part in a clinical trial. Some clinical trials are open only to patients who have not started treatment.

The treatment of AML usually has two phases. The two treatment phases of AML are as follows:

- **Remission induction therapy**. This is the first phase of treatment. The goal is to kill the leukemia cells in the blood and bone marrow. This puts the leukemia into remission.
- **Postremission therapy**. This is the second phase of treatment. It begins after the leukemia is in remission. The goal of postremission therapy is to kill any remaining leukemia cells that may not be active but could begin to regrow and cause a relapse. This phase is also called "remission continuation therapy."

Patients receive supportive care for side effects of treatment. Patients must be closely monitored during treatment of AML. Myelosuppression, a condition that results in fewer red blood cells, white blood cells, and platelets, is a side effect of both AML and treatment with chemotherapy. Supportive care during remission induction therapy may include:

- red blood cell and platelet transfusions
- antibiotics and antifungals for treatment of infections

The following types of treatment are used.

Chemotherapy

Chemotherapy is a cancer treatment that uses drugs to stop the growth of cancer cells, either by killing the cells or by stopping them from dividing. When chemotherapy is taken by mouth or injected into a vein or muscle, the drugs enter the bloodstream and can reach cancer cells throughout the body (systemic chemotherapy). When chemotherapy is placed directly into the cerebrospinal fluid (intrathecal chemotherapy), an organ, or a body cavity such as the abdomen, the drugs mainly affect cancer cells in those areas (regional chemotherapy). Intrathecal chemotherapy may be used to treat adult AML that has spread to the brain and spinal cord. Combination chemotherapy is treatment using more than one anticancer drug.

The way the chemotherapy is given depends on the subtype of AML being treated and whether leukemia cells have spread to the brain and spinal cord.

Radiation Therapy

Radiation therapy is a cancer treatment that uses high-energy x-rays or other types of radiation to kill cancer cells or keep them from growing. External radiation therapy uses a machine outside the body to send radiation toward the area of the body with cancer. Total-body irradiation sends radiation toward the whole body. It is a type of external radiation that may be used to prepare the body for a stem cell transplant when the leukemia has recurred.

Chemotherapy with Stem Cell Transplant

High doses of chemotherapy are given to kill cancer cells. Healthy cells, including blood-forming cells, are also destroyed by the cancer treatment. Stem cell transplant is a treatment to replace the blood-forming cells. Stem cells (immature blood cells) are removed from the blood or bone marrow of the patient or a donor and are frozen and stored. After the patient completes chemotherapy and/or total-body irradiation, the stored stem cells are thawed and given back to the patient through an infusion. These reinfused stem cells grow into (and restore) the body's blood cells.

Targeted Therapy

Targeted therapy is a type of treatment that uses drugs or other substances to identify and attack specific cancer cells. There are different types of targeted therapy.

- **Monoclonal antibodies**. It is an immune system proteins made in the laboratory to treat many diseases, including cancer. As a cancer treatment, these antibodies can attach to a specific target on cancer cells or other cells that may help cancer cells grow. The antibodies are able to then kill the cancer cells, block their growth, or keep them from spreading. Monoclonal antibodies are given by infusion. They may be used alone or to carry drugs, toxins, or radioactive material directly to cancer cells.
- **Gemtuzumab ozogamicin**. It is a type of antibody-drug conjugate used to treat patients with newly diagnosed or relapsed AML. It contains a monoclonal antibody that binds to CD33, which is found on some leukemia cells, and also contains a toxic substance, which may help kill cancer cells.

Other targeted therapies include:

- **Midostaurin**. A protein kinase inhibitor used with certain types of chemotherapy to treat newly diagnosed patients with AML that has a mutation in the *FLT3* gene.
- **Gilteritinib**. A tyrosine kinase inhibitor that may be used to treat patients with AML that has come back or did not get better with other treatment and has a mutation in the *FLT3* gene.

Less-intensive targeted therapies in older or frail patients who cannot receive other treatments include:

- glasdegib plus low-dose chemotherapy
- ivosidenib with or without low-dose chemotherapy for patients with AML that has a mutation in the *IDH1* gene
- enasidenib for patients with AML that has a mutation in the *IDH2* gene

Other Drug Therapies for Acute Myeloid Leukemia

Arsenic trioxide and all-trans retinoic acid (ATRA) are anticancer drugs that kill leukemia cells, stop the leukemia cells from dividing, or help the leukemia cells mature into white blood cells. These drugs are used in the treatment of a subtype of AML called "acute promyelocytic leukemia."

Clinical Trials

For some patients, taking part in a clinical trial may be the best treatment choice. Clinical trials are part of the cancer research process. Clinical trials are done to find out if new cancer treatments are safe and effective or better than the standard treatment.

Many of today's standard treatments for cancer are based on earlier clinical trials. Patients who take part in a clinical trial may receive the standard treatment or be among the first to receive a new treatment.

Patients who take part in clinical trials also help improve the way cancer will be treated in the future. Even when clinical trials do not lead to effective new treatments, they often answer important questions and help move research forward.

Patients can enter clinical trials before, during, or after starting their cancer treatment.

Some clinical trials only include patients who have not yet received treatment. Other trials test treatments for patients whose cancer has not gotten better. There are also clinical trials that test new ways to stop cancer from recurring (coming back) or reduce the side effects of cancer treatment.

Clinical trials are taking place in many parts of the country. Information about clinical trials supported by NCI can be found on NCI's clinical trials search webpage. Clinical trials supported by other organizations can be found on the ClinicalTrials.gov website.

Follow-Up Tests

Some of the tests that were done to diagnose the cancer or to find out the stage of the cancer may be repeated. Some tests will be repeated in order to see how well the treatment is working. Decisions about whether to continue, change, or stop treatment may be based on the results of these tests.

Some of the tests will continue to be done from time to time after treatment has ended. The results of these tests can show if your condition has changed or if the cancer has recurred (come back). These tests are sometimes called "follow-up tests" or "checkups."

Treatment of Untreated Acute Myeloid Leukemia

Standard treatment of untreated acute myeloid leukemia (AML) during the remission induction phase depends on the subtype of AML and may include the following:

- combination chemotherapy
- combination chemotherapy with midostaurin, for patients whose AML has a mutation (change) in the *FLT3* gene

- combination chemotherapy with gemtuzumab ozogamicin, an antibody-drug conjugate
- intrathecal chemotherapy may be used to treat central nervous system (CNS) leukemia
- supportive care

For older adults or patients too frail to receive intensive chemotherapy, the following may be continued as long as the patient benefits or until toxic effects occur:

- targeted therapy
- low-dose chemotherapy
- targeted therapy with low-dose chemotherapy
- intrathecal chemotherapy may be used to treat CNS leukemia
- supportive care

Treatment of Acute Myeloid Leukemia in Remission

Treatment of acute myeloid leukemia (AML) during the remission phase depends on the subtype of AML and may include the following:

- combination chemotherapy
- maintenance therapy with midostaurin, for patients whose AML has a mutated (changed) form of the *FLT3* gene
- maintenance therapy with chemotherapy
- high-dose chemotherapy and stem cell transplant using the patient's stem cells
- high-dose chemotherapy, with or without radiation therapy, or reduced-intensity therapy, followed by a stem cell transplant using donor stem cells

Treatment of Refractory or Recurrent Acute Myeloid Leukemia

There is no standard treatment for refractory or recurrent acute myeloid leukemia (AML). Treatment depends on the subtype of AML and may include the following:

- chemotherapy
- targeted therapy with gilteritinib, enasidenib, or ivosidenib
- gemtuzumab ozogamicin, a type of antibody-drug conjugate
- stem cell transplant using donor stem cells

Treatment of Acute Promyelocytic Leukemia

Treatment of newly diagnosed acute promyelocytic leukemia (APL) includes:

- all-trans retinoic acid (ATRA) plus arsenic trioxide (ATO) for low-risk to intermediate-risk disease
- ATRA plus combination chemotherapy followed by ATO for high-risk disease

Treatment of Recurrent Acute Promyelocytic Leukemia

Treatment of recurrent acute promyelocytic leukemia includes:

- arsenic trioxide (ATO) with or without chemotherapy
- stem cell transplant using the patient's stem cells or donor stem cells[1]

[1] "Acute Myeloid Leukemia Treatment (PDQ®)–Patient Version," National Cancer Institute (NCI), September 8, 2023. Available online. URL: www.cancer.gov/types/leukemia/patient/adult-aml-treatment-pdq. Accessed November 21, 2023.

PART 5 | OTHER HEALTH CONCERNS RELATED TO TOBACCO USE

CHAPTER 41
ANEURYSMS

What Is an Aneurysm?

An aneurysm is a bulge or "ballooning" in the wall of an artery. Arteries are blood vessels that carry oxygen-rich blood from the heart to other parts of the body. If an aneurysm grows large, it can burst and cause dangerous bleeding or even death.

Most aneurysms occur in the aorta, the main artery that runs from the heart through the chest and abdomen. Aneurysms can also happen in arteries in the brain, heart, and other parts of the body. If an aneurysm in the brain bursts, it causes a stroke.

Aneurysms can develop and become large before causing any symptoms. Often doctors can stop aneurysms from bursting if they find and treat them early. They use imaging tests to find aneurysms. Often aneurysms are found by chance during tests done for other reasons. Medicines and surgery are the two main treatments for aneurysms.[1]

Cerebral Aneurysm

What Is a Cerebral Aneurysm?

A cerebral aneurysm (also known as a "brain aneurysm") is a weak or thin spot on an artery in the brain that balloons or bulges out and fills with blood. The bulging aneurysm can put pressure on the nerves or brain tissue. It may also burst or rupture, spilling blood into the surrounding tissue (called a "hemorrhage"). A ruptured aneurysm can cause serious health problems, such as hemorrhagic stroke, brain damage, coma, and even death.

Some cerebral aneurysms, particularly those that are very small, do not bleed or cause other problems. These types of aneurysms are usually detected during imaging tests for other medical conditions. Cerebral aneurysms can occur anywhere in the brain, but most form in the major arteries along the base of the skull. All cerebral aneurysms have the potential to rupture and cause bleeding within the brain or surrounding area.

[1] MedlinePlus, "Aneurysms," National Institutes of Health (NIH), March 25, 2016. Available online. URL: https://medlineplus.gov/aneurysms.html. Accessed October 3, 2023.

Symptoms of a Cerebral Aneurysm

Unruptured Aneurysm

Most cerebral aneurysms do not show symptoms until they either become very large or rupture. Small unchanging aneurysms generally will not produce symptoms.

A larger aneurysm that is steadily growing may press on tissues and nerves causing:

- pain above and behind the eye
- numbness
- weakness
- paralysis on one side of the face
- a dilated pupil in the eye
- vision changes or double vision

Ruptured Aneurysm

When an aneurysm ruptures (bursts), one always experiences a sudden and extremely severe headache (e.g., the worst headache of one's life) and may also develop:

- double vision
- nausea
- vomiting
- stiff neck
- sensitivity to light
- seizures
- loss of consciousness (This may happen briefly or may be prolonged.)
- cardiac arrest

Leaking Aneurysm

Sometimes an aneurysm may leak a small amount of blood into the brain (called a "sentinel bleed"). Sentinel or warning headaches may result from an aneurysm that suffers a tiny leak, days or weeks prior to a significant rupture. However, only a minority of individuals have a sentinel headache prior to rupture.

If you experience a sudden, severe headache, especially when it is combined with any other symptoms, you should seek immediate medical attention.

Classifications of Cerebral Aneurysms

Type

There are three types of cerebral aneurysms:

- **Saccular aneurysm**. This type of aneurysm is a rounded sac containing blood, that is attached to a main artery or one of its branches. Also known as a "berry aneurysm" (because it resembles a berry hanging from a vine), this is the most common form of cerebral aneurysm. It is typically found in arteries at the base of the brain. Saccular aneurysms occur most often in adults.

- **Fusiform aneurysm**. This type of aneurysm balloons or bulges out on all sides of the artery.
- **Mycotic aneurysm**. This type of aneurysm occurs as the result of an infection that can sometimes affect the arteries in the brain. The infection weakens the artery wall, causing a bulging aneurysm to form.

Size

Aneurysms are also classified by size: small, large, and giant.

- **Small aneurysms**. These aneurysms are less than 11 mm in diameter (about the size of a large pencil eraser).
- **Large aneurysms**. These aneurysms are 11–25 mm (about the width of a dime).
- **Giant aneurysms**. These aneurysms are greater than 25 mm in diameter (more than the width of a quarter).

Who Is More Likely to Get a Cerebral Aneurysm?

Cerebral aneurysms form when the walls of the arteries in the brain become thin and weaken. Aneurysms typically form at branch points in arteries because these sections are the weakest. Occasionally, cerebral aneurysms may be present from birth, usually resulting from an abnormality in an artery wall.

Brain aneurysms can occur in anyone and at any age. They are most common in adults between the ages of 30 and 60 and are more common in women than in men. People with certain inherited disorders are also at higher risk.

Risk Factors for Developing an Aneurysm

Sometimes cerebral aneurysms are the result of inherited risk factors, including the following:

- genetic connective tissue disorders that weaken artery walls
- polycystic kidney disease (PKD; in which numerous cysts form in the kidneys)
- arteriovenous malformations (AVMs; snarled tangles of arteries and veins in the brain that disrupt blood flow; some AVMs develop sporadically or on their own)
- history of aneurysm in a first-degree family member (child, sibling, or parent)

Other risk factors develop over time and include the following:

- untreated high blood pressure (HBP)
- cigarette smoking
- drug abuse, especially cocaine or amphetamines (which raise blood pressure to dangerous levels; intravenous drug abuse is a cause of infectious mycotic aneurysms)
- age over 40

Less common risk factors include the following:

- head trauma
- brain tumor
- infection in the arterial wall (mycotic aneurysm)

Additionally, HBP, cigarette smoking, diabetes, and high cholesterol put one at risk of atherosclerosis (a blood vessel disease in which fats build up on the inside of artery walls), which can increase the risk of developing a fusiform aneurysm.

Risk Factors for an Aneurysm to Rupture

Not all aneurysms will rupture. Aneurysm characteristics, such as size, location, and growth during follow-up evaluation may affect the risk that an aneurysm will rupture. In addition, medical conditions may influence aneurysm rupture.

Risk factors include the following:

- **Smoking**. Smoking is linked to both the development and rupture of cerebral aneurysms. Smoking may even cause multiple aneurysms to form in the brain.
- **High blood pressure**. HBP damages and weakens arteries, making them more likely to form and to rupture.
- **Size**. The largest aneurysms are the ones most likely to rupture in a person who previously did not show symptoms.
- **Location**. Aneurysms located on the posterior communicating arteries (a pair of arteries in the back part of the brain) and possibly those on the anterior communicating artery (a single artery in the front of the brain) have a higher risk of rupturing than those at other locations in the brain.
- **Growth**. Aneurysms that grow, even if they are small, are at increased risk of rupture.
- **Family history**. A family history of aneurysm rupture suggests a higher risk of rupture for aneurysms detected in family members.

The greatest risk occurs in individuals with multiple aneurysms who have already suffered a previous rupture or sentinel bleed.

How Are Cerebral Aneurysms Diagnosed and Treated?

Diagnosing Cerebral Aneurysms

Most cerebral aneurysms go unnoticed until they rupture or are detected during medical imaging tests for another condition.

If you have experienced a severe headache or have any other symptoms related to a ruptured aneurysm, your doctor will order tests to determine if blood has leaked into the space between the skull bone and brain.

Several tests are available to diagnose brain aneurysms and determine the best treatment. These include the following:

- **Computed tomography (CT)**. This is often the first test a physician will order to determine if blood has leaked into the brain. CT uses x-rays to create two-dimensional images, or "slices," of the brain and skull. Occasionally a contrast dye is injected into the bloodstream prior to scanning to assess the arteries and look for a possible aneurysm. This process, called "CT angiography" (CTA), produces sharper, more detailed images of blood flow in the brain arteries. CTA can show the size, location, and shape of an unruptured or a ruptured aneurysm.
- **Magnetic resonance imaging (MRI)**. An MRI uses computer-generated radio waves and a magnetic field to create two- and three-dimensional detailed images of the brain and can determine if there has been bleeding into the brain. Magnetic resonance angiography (MRA) produces detailed images of the brain arteries and can show the size, location, and shape of an aneurysm.
- **Cerebral angiography**. This imaging technique can find blockages in arteries in the brain or neck. It can also identify weak spots in an artery, like an aneurysm. The test is used to determine the cause of the bleeding in the brain and the exact location, size, and shape of an aneurysm. Your doctor will pass a catheter (long, flexible tube) typically from the groin arteries to inject a small amount of contrast dye into your neck and brain arteries. The contrast dye helps the x-ray create a detailed picture of the appearance of an aneurysm and a clear picture of any blockage in the arteries.
- **Cerebrospinal fluid (CSF) analysis**. This test measures the chemicals in the fluid that cushions and protects the brain and spinal cord (CSF). Most often a doctor will collect the CSF by performing a spinal tap (lumbar puncture), in which a thin needle is inserted into the lower back (lumbar spine) and a small amount of fluid is removed and tested. The results will help detect any bleeding around the brain. If bleeding is detected, additional tests would be needed to identify the exact cause of the bleeding.

Complications of a Ruptured Cerebral Aneurysm

Aneurysms may rupture and bleed into the space between the skull and the brain (subarachnoid hemorrhage) and sometimes into the brain tissue (intracerebral hemorrhage). These are forms of stroke called "hemorrhagic stroke." The bleeding into the brain can cause a wide spectrum of symptoms, from a mild headache to permanent damage to the brain, or even death.

After an aneurysm has ruptured it may cause serious complications such as:

- **Rebleeding**. Once it has ruptured, an aneurysm may rupture again before it is treated, leading to further bleeding into the brain, and causing more damage or death.

- **Change in sodium level**. Bleeding in the brain can disrupt the balance of sodium in the blood supply and cause swelling in brain cells. This can result in permanent brain damage.
- **Hydrocephalus**. Subarachnoid hemorrhage can cause hydrocephalus. Hydrocephalus is a buildup of too much CSF in the brain, which causes pressure that can lead to permanent brain damage or death. Hydrocephalus occurs frequently after subarachnoid hemorrhage because the blood blocks the normal flow of CSF. If left untreated, increased pressure inside the head can cause coma or death.
- **Vasospasm**. This occurs frequently after subarachnoid hemorrhage when the bleeding causes the arteries in the brain to contract and limit blood flow to vital areas of the brain. This can cause strokes from lack of adequate blood flow to parts of the brain.
- **Seizures**. Aneurysm bleeding can cause seizures (convulsions), either at the time of bleed or in the immediate aftermath. While most seizures are evident, on occasion they may only be seen by sophisticated brain testing. Untreated seizures or those that do not respond to treatment can cause brain damage.

Treating Cerebral Aneurysms

Not all cerebral aneurysms require treatment. Some very small unruptured aneurysms that are not associated with any factors suggesting a higher risk of rupture may be safely left alone and monitored with MRA or CTA to detect any growth. It is important to aggressively treat any coexisting medical problems and risk factors.

Treatments for unruptured cerebral aneurysms that have not shown symptoms have some potentially serious complications and should be carefully weighed against the predicted rupture risk.

A doctor will consider a variety of factors when determining the best option for treating an unruptured aneurysm, including the following:

- type, size, and location of the aneurysm
- risk of rupture
- the person's age and health
- personal and family medical history
- risk of treatment

Individuals should also take the following steps to reduce the risk of aneurysm rupture:

- carefully control blood pressure
- stop smoking
- avoid cocaine use or other stimulant drugs

Surgery

There are a few surgical options available for treating cerebral aneurysms. These procedures carry some risk such as possible damage to other blood vessels, the potential for aneurysm recurrence and rebleeding, and a risk of stroke.

- **Microvascular clipping**. This procedure involves cutting off the flow of blood to the aneurysm and requires open brain surgery. A doctor will locate the blood vessels that feed the aneurysm and place a tiny, metal, clothespin-like clip on the aneurysm's neck to stop its blood supply. Clipping has been shown to be highly effective, depending on the location, size, and shape of the aneurysm. In general, aneurysms that are completely clipped do not recur.

Endovascular Treatment

- **Platinum coil embolization**. This is a less invasive procedure than microvascular surgical clipping. A doctor will insert a hollow plastic tube (a catheter) into an artery, usually in the groin, and thread it through the body to the brain aneurysm. Using a wire, the doctor will pass detachable coils (tiny spirals of platinum wire) through the catheter and release them into the aneurysm. The coils block the aneurysm and reduce the flow of blood into the aneurysm. The procedure may need to be performed more than once during the person's lifetime because aneurysms treated with coiling can sometimes recur.
- **Flow diversion devices**. Other endovascular treatment options include placing a small stent (flexible mesh tube) similar to those placed for heart blockages, in the artery to reduce blood flow into the aneurysm. A doctor will insert a hollow plastic tube (a catheter) into an artery, usually in the groin, and thread it through the body to the artery on which the aneurysm is located. This procedure is used to treat very large aneurysms and those that cannot be treated with surgery or platinum coil embolization.

Other Treatments

Other treatments for a ruptured cerebral aneurysm aim to control symptoms and reduce complications. These treatments include the following:

- **Anti-seizure drugs (anticonvulsants)**. It may be used to prevent seizures related to a ruptured aneurysm.
- **Calcium channel-blocking drugs**. It may reduce the risk of stroke by vasospasm.
- **Shunt**. A shunt, which funnels CSF from the brain to elsewhere in the body, may be surgically inserted into the brain following rupture if the buildup of CSF (hydrocephalus) is causing harmful pressure on surrounding brain tissue.

- **Rehabilitative therapy**. Individuals who have suffered a subarachnoid hemorrhage often need physical, speech, and occupational therapy to regain lost function and learn to cope with any permanent disability.[2]

Aortic Aneurysm

What Is an Aortic Aneurysm?

An aortic aneurysm is a balloon-like bulge in the aorta, the large artery that carries blood from the heart through the chest and torso.

Aortic aneurysms can dissect or rupture:

- The force of blood pumping can split the layers of the artery wall, allowing blood to leak in between them. This process is called a "dissection."
- The aneurysm can burst completely, causing bleeding inside the body. This is called a "rupture."
- Dissections and ruptures are the cause of most deaths from aortic aneurysms.

What Are the Types of Aortic Aneurysm?

Thoracic Aortic Aneurysm

A thoracic aortic aneurysm happens in the chest (see Figure 41.1). Men and women are equally likely to get thoracic aortic aneurysms, which become more common with increasing age.

Thoracic aortic aneurysms are usually caused by HBP or sudden injury. Sometimes people with inherited connective tissue disorders, such as Marfan syndrome and Ehlers-Danlos syndrome (EDS), get thoracic aortic aneurysms.

Signs and symptoms of thoracic aortic aneurysm can include the following:

- sharp, sudden pain in the chest or upper back
- shortness of breath
- trouble breathing or swallowing

Abdominal Aortic Aneurysm

An abdominal aortic aneurysm happens below the chest (see Figure 41.1). Abdominal aortic aneurysms happen more often than thoracic aortic aneurysms.

Abdominal aortic aneurysms are more common in men and among people age 65 and older. Abdominal aortic aneurysms are more common among White people than among Black people.

Abdominal aortic aneurysms are usually caused by atherosclerosis (hardened arteries), but infection or injury can also cause them.

[2] "Cerebral Aneurysms," National Institute of Neurological Disorders and Stroke (NINDS), March 8, 2023. Available online. URL: www.ninds.nih.gov/health-information/disorders/cerebral-aneurysms. Accessed October 3, 2023.

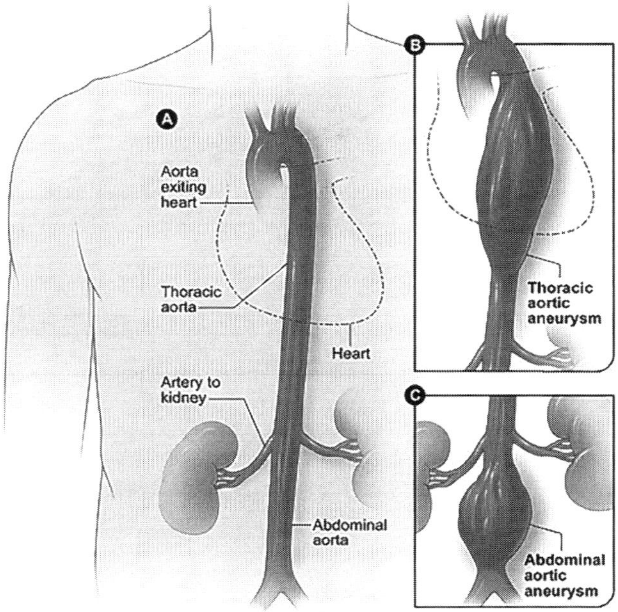

Figure 41.1. Aortic Aneurysms
National Heart, Lung, and Blood Institute (NHLBI)

Abdominal aortic aneurysms often do not have any symptoms. If an individual does have symptoms, they can include the following:

- throbbing or deep pain in the back or side
- pain in the buttocks, groin, or legs

Other Types of Aneurysms

Aneurysms can happen in other parts of your body. A ruptured aneurysm in the brain can cause a stroke. Peripheral aneurysms—those found in arteries other than the aorta—can happen in the neck, in the groin, or behind the knees. These aneurysms are less likely to rupture or dissect than aortic aneurysms, but they can form blood clots. These clots can break away and block blood flow through the artery.

Source: "Aortic Aneurysm," Centers for Disease Control and Prevention (CDC), September 27, 2021. Available online. URL: www.cdc.gov/heartdisease/aortic_aneurysm.htm. Accessed October 3, 2023.

What Are the Risk Factors for Aortic Aneurysm?

Diseases and unhealthy behaviors that damage your heart and blood vessels also increase your risk for aortic aneurysm. Smoking is the most important behavior related to aortic aneurysm.

Other factors include the following:

- HBP
- high blood cholesterol
- atherosclerosis (hardened arteries)

Some inherited connective tissue disorders, such as Marfan syndrome and EDS, can also increase your risk for aortic aneurysm. Your family may also have a history of aortic aneurysms that can increase your risk.

How Are Aortic Aneurysms Treated?

The two main treatments for aortic aneurysms are medicines and surgery. Medicines can lower blood pressure and reduce risk for an aortic aneurysm. Surgery can repair or replace the affected section of the aorta.[3]

[3] "Aortic Aneurysm," Centers for Disease Control and Prevention (CDC), September 27, 2021. Available online. URL: www.cdc.gov/heartdisease/aortic_aneurysm.htm. Accessed October 3, 2023.

CHAPTER 42
ASTHMA

What Is Asthma

Asthma is a leading chronic illness among children and adolescents in the United States. It is also one of the leading causes of school absenteeism. On average, in a classroom of 30 children, about 3 are likely to have asthma. Low-income populations, minorities, and children living in inner cities experience more emergency department visits, hospitalizations, and deaths due to asthma than the general population.

When children and adolescents are exposed to things in the environment—such as dust mites and tobacco smoke—an asthma episode can occur. These things are called "asthma triggers."[1]

What Are the Symptoms of an Asthma Attack?

- coughing
- shortness of breath or trouble breathing
- wheezing
- tightness or pain in the chest

How Is Smoking Related to Asthma?

If you have asthma, an asthma attack can occur when something irritates your airways and "triggers" an attack. Your triggers might be different from other people's triggers.

Tobacco smoke is a common trigger for asthma. Tobacco smoke—including secondhand smoke—is unhealthy for everyone, especially people with asthma. Secondhand smoke is a mixture of gases and fine particles that includes the following:

- smoke from burning tobacco products, such as cigarettes, cigars, or pipes
- smoke that has been exhaled (breathed out) by someone who smokes

Secondhand smoke contains more than 7,000 chemicals, including hundreds that are toxic and about 70 that can cause cancer.

[1] "Asthma," Centers for Disease Control and Prevention (CDC), August 18, 2022. Available online. URL: www.cdc.gov/healthyschools/asthma/index.htm. Accessed October 3, 2023.

If you have asthma, it is important that you avoid exposure to secondhand smoke.

If you are among the 21 percent of U.S. adults who have asthma and smoke, get help to quit smoking; talk to your doctor about treatments that can help you or call 800-QUIT-NOW.

How Is Asthma Treated?

There is no cure for asthma. However, to help control your asthma and avoid attacks, do the following:

- Take your medicine exactly as your doctor tells you.
- Stay away from things that can trigger an attack.

Everyone with asthma does not take the same medicine. Some medicines can be breathed in, and some can be taken as a pill. The following are the two kinds of asthma medicines:

- quick relief (can help control symptoms of an asthma attack)
- long-term control (can help you have fewer and milder attacks, but they do not help you while you are having an asthma attack)

Managing Asthma in Schools

Asthma-friendly schools are those that make the effort to create safe and supportive learning environments for students with asthma. They have policies and procedures that allow students to successfully manage their asthma. Research and case studies that looked at the following ways to best manage asthma in schools found that successful school-based asthma programs:

- Establish strong links with asthma care clinicians to ensure appropriate and ongoing medical care.
- Target students who are the most affected by asthma at school to identify and intervene with those in the greatest need.
- Get administrative buy-in and build a team of enthusiastic people, including a full-time school nurse, to support the program.
- Use a coordinated, multicomponent, and collaborative approach that includes school nursing services, asthma education for students, and professional development for school staff.
- Provide appropriate school health services for students with asthma, ensuring that students take their medicines and learn to use them when appropriate.
- Provide asthma education for students with asthma and awareness programs for students, school staff, parents, and families.
- Provide a safe and healthy school environment to reduce asthma triggers.
- Offer safe and enjoyable physical education and activities for students with asthma.
- Support evaluation of school-based programs and use adequate and appropriate outcome measures.

Source: "Asthma," Centers for Disease Control and Prevention (CDC), August 18, 2022. Available online. URL: www.cdc.gov/healthyschools/asthma/index.htm. Accessed October 3, 2023.

How Can Asthma Attacks Be Prevented?

If you or a family member has asthma, you can manage it with the help of your health-care provider (e.g., by taking your medicines exactly as your doctor tells you and by avoiding your triggers). Try to avoid asthma attacks by staying far away from tobacco smoke. Some other helpful tips are as follows:

- Do not smoke or allow others to smoke in your home or car. Opening a window does not protect you from smoke.
- If your state still allows smoking in public areas, look for restaurants and other places that do not allow smoking. "No-smoking sections" in the same restaurant with "smoking sections" do not protect adequately from secondhand smoke—even if there is a filter or ventilation system.
- Make sure your children's day care centers and schools are tobacco-free. For schools, a tobacco-free campus policy means no tobacco use or advertising on school property is allowed by anyone at any time. This includes off-campus school events.
- Teach children to stay away from secondhand smoke. Be a good role model by not smoking.[2]

[2] "Asthma and Secondhand Smoke," Centers for Disease Control and Prevention (CDC), May 5, 2022. Available online. URL: www.cdc.gov/tobacco/campaign/tips/diseases/secondhand-smoke-asthma.html. Accessed October 3, 2023.

CHAPTER 43
BLOOD CLOTS

Deep Vein Thrombosis and Pulmonary Embolism

What Is Venous Thromboembolism?

Deep vein thrombosis (DVT) and pulmonary embolism (PE) are often underdiagnosed and serious but preventable medical conditions.

DVT is a medical condition that occurs when a blood clot forms in a deep vein. These clots usually develop in the lower leg, thigh, or pelvis, but they can also occur in the arm.

It is important to know about DVT because it can happen to anybody and can cause serious illness, disability, and in some cases, death. The good news is that DVT is preventable and treatable if discovered early.

Complications of Deep Vein Thrombosis

The most serious complication of DVT happens when a part of the clot breaks off and travels through the bloodstream to the lungs, causing a blockage called "pulmonary embolism" (PE). If the clot is small, and with appropriate treatment, people can recover from PE. However, there could be some damage to the lungs. If the clot is large, it can stop blood from reaching the lungs and is fatal.

In addition, nearly one-third to one-half of people who have a DVT will have long-term complications caused by the damage the clot does to the valves in the vein called "postthrombotic syndrome" (PTS). People with PTS have symptoms such as swelling, pain, discoloration, and in severe cases, scaling or ulcers in the affected part of the body. In some cases, the symptoms can be so severe that a person becomes disabled.

For some people, DVT and PE can become a chronic illness; about 30 percent of people who have had a DVT or PE are at risk for another episode.

Risk Factors of Deep Vein Thrombosis

Almost anyone can have a DVT. However, certain factors can increase the chance of having this condition. The chance increases even more for someone who has more than one of these factors at the same time.

Following is a list of factors that increase the risk of developing DVT:

- Injury to a vein, often caused by:
  - fractures
  - severe muscle injury
  - major surgery (particularly involving the abdomen, pelvis, hip, or legs)
- Slow blood flow, often caused by:
  - confinement to bed (e.g., due to a medical condition or after surgery)
  - limited movement (e.g., a cast on a leg to help heal an injured bone)
  - sitting for a long time, especially with crossed legs
  - paralysis
- Increased estrogen, often caused by:
  - birth control pills
  - hormone replacement therapy (HRT), sometimes used after menopause
  - pregnancy, for up to three months after giving birth
- Certain chronic medical illnesses, such as:
  - heart disease
  - lung disease
  - cancer and its treatment
  - inflammatory bowel disease (IBD; Crohn's disease or ulcerative colitis)
- Other factors that increase the risk of DVT include:
  - previous DVT or PE
  - family history of DVT or PE
  - age (risk increases as age increases)
  - obesity
  - a catheter located in a central vein
  - inherited clotting disorders

Did You Know?

There are two main types of blood clots. How a clot affects the body depends on the type and location of the clot:

- A blood clot in a deep vein of the leg, pelvis, and sometimes arm is called "deep vein thrombosis" (DVT). This type of blood clot does not cause heart attack or stroke. A blood clot in an artery, usually in the heart or brain, is called "arterial thrombosis." This type of blood clot can cause heart attack or stroke.
- Both types of clots can cause serious health problems, but the causes and steps you can take to protect yourself are different.

Source: "What Is Venous Thromboembolism?" Centers for Disease Control and Prevention (CDC), June 28, 2023. Available online. URL: www.cdc.gov/ncbddd/dvt/facts.html. Accessed October 6, 2023.

Preventing Deep Vein Thrombosis

The following tips can help prevent DVT:

- Move around as soon as possible after having been confined to bed, such as after surgery, illness, or injury.
- If you are at risk for DVT, talk to your doctor about:
    - graduated compression stockings (sometimes called "medical compression stockings")
    - medication (anticoagulants) to prevent DVT
- When sitting for long periods of time, such as when traveling for more than four hours:
    - Get up and walk around every two to three hours.
    - Exercise your legs while you are sitting by:
        - raising and lowering your heels while keeping your toes on the floor
        - raising and lowering your toes while keeping your heels on the floor
        - tightening and releasing your leg muscles
    - Wear loose-fitting clothes.
- You can reduce your risk by maintaining a healthy weight, avoiding a sedentary lifestyle, and following your doctor's recommendations based on your individual risk factors.

Symptoms of Deep Vein Thrombosis and Pulmonary Embolism

Deep Vein Thrombosis

About half of people with DVT have no symptoms at all. The following are the most common symptoms of DVT that occur in the affected part of the body:

- swelling
- pain
- tenderness
- redness of the skin

If you have any of these symptoms, you should see your doctor as soon as possible.

Pulmonary Embolism

You can have a PE without any symptoms of a DVT.

Signs and symptoms of PE can include:

- difficulty breathing
- faster than normal or irregular heartbeat
- chest pain or discomfort, which usually worsens with a deep breath or coughing
- coughing up blood
- very low blood pressure, lightheadedness, or fainting

If you have any of these symptoms, you should seek medical help immediately.

Diagnosis of Deep Vein Thrombosis and Pulmonary Embolism

The diagnosis of DVT or PE requires special tests that can only be performed by a doctor. That is why it is important for you to seek medical care if you experience any of the symptoms of DVT or PE.

Treatments of Deep Vein Thrombosis and Pulmonary Embolism

Deep Vein Thrombosis

Medication is used to prevent and treat DVT. Compression stockings (also called "graduated compression stockings") are sometimes recommended to prevent DVT and relieve pain and swelling. These might need to be worn for two years or more after having DVT. In severe cases, the clot might need to be removed surgically.

Pulmonary Embolism

Immediate medical attention is necessary to treat PE. In cases of severe, life-threatening PE, there are medicines called "thrombolytics" that can dissolve the clot. Other medicines, called "anticoagulants," may be prescribed to prevent more clots from forming. Some people may need to be on medication long-term to prevent future blood clots.[1]

Buerger Disease

What Is Buerger Disease?

Buerger disease (also known as "thromboangiitis obliterans") affects blood vessels in the body, most commonly in the arms and legs. Blood vessels swell, which can prevent blood flow, causing clots to form. This can lead to pain, tissue damage, and even gangrene (the death or decay of body tissues). In some cases, amputation may be required.

The most common symptoms of Buerger disease are as follows:

- fingers or toes that appear pale, red, or bluish
- cold hands or feet
- pain in the hands and feet that may feel like burning or tingling
- pain in the legs, ankles, or feet when walking—often located in the arch of the foot
- skin changes or small painful sores on the fingers or toes

How Is Smoking Related to Buerger Disease?

The exact cause of Buerger disease is unknown; however, tobacco use is strongly linked to its development. Researchers believe that chemicals in tobacco may irritate the lining of the blood vessels, causing them to swell.

[1] "What Is Venous Thromboembolism?" Centers for Disease Control and Prevention (CDC), June 28, 2023. Available online. URL: www.cdc.gov/ncbddd/dvt/facts.html. Accessed October 6, 2023.

Almost everyone diagnosed with Buerger disease smokes cigarettes or uses other forms of tobacco, such as cigars and chewing tobacco.

If you want to prevent getting Buerger disease, do not smoke cigarettes or use any other tobacco products.

How Is Buerger Disease Treated?

There is no cure for Buerger disease. The only way to keep Buerger disease from getting worse is to stop using all tobacco products. Medicines do not usually work well to treat the disease. The best they can do is to control the symptoms.

Surgery may help restore blood flow to some areas. It may be necessary to amputate the hand or foot if infection or widespread tissue death occurs.[2]

[2] "Smoking and Buerger Disease," Centers for Disease Control and Prevention (CDC), May 5, 2022. Available online. URL: www.cdc.gov/tobacco/campaign/tips/diseases/buergers-disease.html. Accessed October 6, 2023.

CHAPTER 44

CHRONIC OBSTRUCTIVE PULMONARY DISEASE

What Is Chronic Obstructive Pulmonary Disease?

Chronic obstructive pulmonary disease (COPD) refers to a group of diseases that cause airflow blockage and breathing-related problems. COPD includes emphysema and chronic bronchitis.

With COPD, less air flows through the airways—the tubes that carry air in and out of your lungs—because of one or more of the following:

- The airways and tiny air sacs in the lungs lose their ability to stretch and shrink back.
- The walls between many of the air sacs are destroyed.
- The walls of the airways become thick and inflamed (irritated and swollen).
- The airways make more mucus than usual, which can clog them and block airflow.

In the early stages of COPD, there may be no symptoms, or you may only have mild symptoms. As COPD worsens, the symptoms may become more severe. Symptoms of COPD include the following:

- a cough that lingers for a long time and does not go away completely or a cough that produces a lot of mucus
- shortness of breath, especially with physical activity
- wheezing (a whistling sound when you breathe)
- tightness in the chest

Not everyone with these symptoms has COPD. A doctor can determine if you have COPD or another condition that has similar symptoms.

How severe your COPD symptoms are depends on how much lung damage you have. If you continue smoking, the damage will occur faster than if you stop smoking.

How Is Smoking Related to Chronic Obstructive Pulmonary Disease?

Chronic obstructive pulmonary disease is usually caused by cigarette smoking though long-term exposure to other lung irritants, such as secondhand smoke, can also contribute to COPD. As many as 1 out of 4 Americans with COPD never smoked cigarettes. However, smoking accounts for as many as 8 out of 10 COPD-related deaths, and 38 percent of the nearly 16 million U.S. adults diagnosed with COPD report smoking.

Smoking and secondhand smoke exposure during childhood and teenage years can slow lung growth and development. This can increase the risk of developing COPD in adulthood.

Does Chronic Obstructive Pulmonary Disease Raise Your Risk for Other Conditions?

Chronic obstructive pulmonary disease (COPD) may raise your risk for other health conditions that can happen because of COPD or as a result of damage to the airways. These conditions include the following:

- Frequent colds or other respiratory infections, such as the flu or influenza, often happen if you have COPD.
- Heart disease risks are higher for people who have COPD than for people who do not have COPD.
- Other health problems, such as obesity or peripheral artery disease (PAD), that are caused by similar risk factors (smoking or not getting enough physical activity) may also be present. These other health problems may, in turn, make COPD worse.

Talk to your health-care provider about your risk for other health problems and any healthy lifestyle changes you can make.

Source: "COPD—Living With," National Heart, Lung, and Blood Institute (NHLBI), October 25, 2023. Available online. URL: www.nhlbi.nih.gov/health/copd/living-with. Accessed October 27, 2023.

How Is Chronic Obstructive Pulmonary Disease Treated?

Chronic obstructive pulmonary disease treatment can alleviate symptoms, decrease the frequency and severity of exacerbations, and increase exercise tolerance. Treatment options that your physician may consider include the following:

- **Quit smoking**. For people who smoke, the most important part of treatment is smoking cessation.
- **Avoid smoke and pollutants**. Avoid tobacco smoke and other air pollutants at home and at work.
- **Ask your doctor about pulmonary rehabilitation**. Pulmonary rehabilitation is a personalized treatment program that teaches COPD management strategies to improve quality of life (QOL). Programs may include plans that teach people how to breathe better and conserve their energy, as well as provide advice on food and exercise.

- **Take medication**. Symptoms such as coughing or wheezing can be treated with medication.
- **Avoid lung infections**. Lung infections can cause serious problems in people with COPD. Certain vaccines, such as flu and pneumococcal vaccines, are especially important for people with COPD. Respiratory infections should be treated with antibiotics, if appropriate.
- **Use supplemental oxygen**. Some people may need to use a portable oxygen tank if their blood oxygen levels are low.

How Can Chronic Obstructive Pulmonary Disease Be Prevented?

The best way to prevent COPD is to never start smoking and, if you do smoke, to quit. Talk with your doctor or other health-care professional about resources that can help you quit, such as counseling and medication. Also, stay away from secondhand smoke, which is smoke from burning tobacco products, such as cigarettes, cigars, hookah, or pipes. Secondhand smoke is also smoke that has been exhaled, or breathed out, by a person smoking or that comes from the end of a lit tobacco product.[1]

[1] "Smoking and COPD," Centers for Disease Control and Prevention (CDC), May 5, 2022. Available online. URL: www.cdc.gov/tobacco/campaign/tips/diseases/copd.html. Accessed October 27, 2023.

CHAPTER 45
DIABETES

What Is Diabetes?

Diabetes is a chronic (long-lasting) health condition that affects how your body turns food into energy. Most of the food a person eats is turned into glucose (a kind of sugar) for the body's cells to use for energy. The pancreas, an organ near the stomach, makes a hormone called "insulin" that helps glucose get into the body's cells.

When you have diabetes, your body either does not make enough insulin or cannot use insulin very well. When there is not enough insulin or cells stop responding to insulin, too much sugar stays in your bloodstream. Over time, that can cause serious health problems, such as heart disease, vision loss, and kidney disease.

The following are the three types of diabetes:

- **Type 1 diabetes.** This type is thought to be caused by an autoimmune reaction (the body attacks itself by mistake) that stops your body from making insulin. Fewer people have type 1 diabetes, which is most often diagnosed in children, adolescents, or young adults.
- **Type 2 diabetes.** This type develops over many years and is usually diagnosed in adults but is increasingly being diagnosed in children, teens, and young adults. About 90–95 percent of people with diabetes have type 2. Type 2 diabetes can be prevented or delayed with healthy lifestyle changes, such as losing weight, eating healthy foods, and being active.
- **Gestational diabetes.** This type develops in pregnant women who have never had diabetes. While it usually goes away after pregnancy, gestational diabetes increases a woman's risk for type 2 diabetes later in life. The condition can also increase a baby's risk for health problems.

How Is Smoking Related to Diabetes?

We now know that smoking is one cause of type 2 diabetes. In fact, people who smoke cigarettes are 30–40 percent more likely to develop type 2 diabetes than people who do not smoke. People with diabetes who smoke are more likely than those who do not smoke to have trouble with insulin dosing and managing their condition. The more cigarettes you smoke, the higher your risk for type 2 diabetes.

No matter what type of diabetes you have, smoking makes your diabetes harder to manage. If you have diabetes and you smoke, you are more likely to have serious health problems from diabetes, including:

- heart disease
- kidney disease
- poor blood flow in the legs and feet that can lead to infections, ulcers, and possible amputation (removal of a body part by surgery, such as toes or feet)
- retinopathy (an eye disease that can cause blindness)
- peripheral neuropathy (damaged nerves in the arms and legs that cause numbness, pain, weakness, and poor coordination)

If you have diabetes and you smoke, quitting smoking will benefit your health right away. People with diabetes who quit are better able to manage their blood sugar levels.

How Smoking Can Lead to Type 2 Diabetes

- Insulin helps blood sugar enter cells, but nicotine changes cells, so they do not respond to insulin, which increases blood sugar levels.
- Chemicals in cigarettes harm cells in your body and cause inflammation. This also makes cells stop responding to insulin.
- People who smoke have a higher risk of belly fat, which increases the risk for type 2 diabetes even if they are not overweight.

Source: "Smoking and Diabetes," Centers for Disease Control and Prevention (CDC), June 20, 2022. Available online. URL: www.cdc.gov/diabetes/library/features/smoking-and-diabetes.html. Accessed October 3, 2023.

How Is Diabetes Treated?

Diabetes treatment and management can include the following:

- a healthy diet and physical activity program
- weight loss (if overweight)
- medicines to manage blood sugar by helping the body use insulin better
- insulin taken by injection or by using an insulin pump
- diabetes self-management education and support to address problem-solving and coping skills needed to help manage diabetes and its complications
- medicines to manage cholesterol and blood pressure

How Can Diabetes Be Prevented?

- Do not smoke. Smoking increases your chance of having type 2 diabetes.
- Lose weight if you are overweight.
- Stay active. Physical activity can prevent or delay type 2 diabetes in adults who are at high risk for the condition.

The National Diabetes Prevention Program (National DPP) lifestyle change program led by the Centers for Disease Control and Prevention (CDC) has been proven to help people make the changes needed to prevent or delay type 2 diabetes, improve their overall health, and build healthy habits for life. First, find out your risk by taking the one-minute prediabetes risk test.[1]

[1] "Smoking and Diabetes," Centers for Disease Control and Prevention (CDC), May 5, 2022. Available online. URL: www.cdc.gov/tobacco/campaign/tips/diseases/diabetes.html. Accessed October 3, 2023.

CHAPTER 46
DIGESTIVE DISORDERS

Smoking affects the entire body, increasing the risk of many life-threatening diseases—including lung cancer, emphysema, and heart disease. Smoking also contributes to many cancers and diseases of the digestive system. Estimates show that about one-fifth of all adults smoke, and each year at least 443,000 Americans die from diseases caused by cigarette smoking.

What Is the Digestive System?

The digestive system is made up of the gastrointestinal (GI) tract—also called the "digestive tract"—and the liver, pancreas, and gallbladder. The GI tract is a series of hollow organs joined in a long, twisting tube from the mouth to the anus. The hollow organs that make up the GI tract are the mouth, esophagus, stomach, small intestine, large intestine—which includes the colon and rectum—and anus. Food enters the mouth and passes to the anus through the hollow organs of the GI tract. The liver, pancreas, and gallbladder are the solid organs of the digestive system. The digestive system helps the body digest food, which includes breaking food down into nutrients the body needs. Nutrients are substances the body uses for energy, growth, and cell repair.

Does Smoking Increase the Risk of Cancers of the Digestive System?

Smoking has been found to increase the risk of cancers of the:

- mouth
- esophagus
- stomach
- pancreas

Research suggests that smoking may also increase the risk of cancers of the:

- liver
- colon
- rectum

What Are the Other Harmful Effects of Smoking on the Digestive System?

Smoking contributes to many common disorders of the digestive system, such as heartburn and gastroesophageal reflux disease (GERD), peptic ulcers, and some liver diseases. Smoking increases the risk of Crohn's disease, colon polyps, and pancreatitis, and it may increase the risk of gallstones.

How Does Smoking Affect Heartburn and Gastroesophageal Reflux Disease?

Smoking increases the risk of heartburn and GERD. Heartburn is a painful, burning feeling in the chest caused by reflux, or stomach contents flowing back into the esophagus—the organ that connects the mouth to the stomach. Smoking weakens the lower esophageal sphincter, the muscle between the esophagus and stomach that keeps stomach contents from flowing back into the esophagus. The stomach is naturally protected from the acids it makes to help break down food. However, the esophagus is not protected from the acids. When the lower esophageal sphincter weakens, stomach contents may reflux into the esophagus, causing heartburn and possibly damaging the lining of the esophagus.

GERD is persistent reflux that occurs more than twice a week. Chronic, or long-lasting, GERD can lead to serious health problems such as bleeding ulcers in the esophagus, narrowing of the esophagus that causes food to get stuck, and changes in esophageal cells that can lead to cancer.

How Does Smoking Affect Peptic Ulcers?

Smoking increases the risk of peptic ulcers. Peptic ulcers are sores on the inside lining of the stomach or duodenum, the first part of the small intestine. The two most common causes of peptic ulcers are infection with a bacterium called "*Helicobacter pylori*" (*H. pylori*) and long-term use of nonsteroidal antiinflammatory drugs (NSAIDs), such as aspirin and ibuprofen.

Researchers are studying how smoking contributes to peptic ulcers. Studies suggest that smoking increases the risk of *H. pylori* infection, slows the healing of peptic ulcers, and increases the likelihood that peptic ulcers will recur. The stomach and duodenum contain acids, enzymes, and other substances that help digest food. However, these substances may also harm the lining of these organs. Smoking has not been shown to increase acid production. However, smoking does increase the production of other substances that may harm the lining, such as pepsin, an enzyme made in the stomach that breaks down proteins. Smoking also decreases factors that protect or heal the lining, including the following:

- blood flow to the lining
- secretion of mucus, a clear liquid that protects the lining from acid

- production of sodium bicarbonate—a salt-like substance that neutralizes acid—by the pancreas

The increase in substances that may harm the lining and the decrease in factors that protect or heal the lining may lead to peptic ulcers.

How Does Smoking Affect Liver Disease?

Smoking may worsen some liver diseases, including the following:

- primary biliary cirrhosis, a chronic liver disease that slowly destroys the bile ducts in the liver
- nonalcoholic fatty liver disease (NAFLD) that is a condition in which fat builds up in the liver

Researchers are still studying how smoking affects primary biliary cirrhosis, NAFLD, and other liver diseases.

Liver diseases may progress to cirrhosis, a condition in which the liver slowly deteriorates and malfunctions due to chronic injury. Scar tissue then replaces healthy liver tissue, partially blocking the flow of blood through the liver and impairing liver functions.

The liver is the largest organ in the digestive system. The liver carries out many functions, such as making important blood proteins and bile, changing food into energy, and filtering alcohol and poisons from the blood. Research has shown that smoking harms the liver's ability to process medications, alcohol, and other toxins and remove them from the body. In some cases, smoking may affect the dose of medication needed to treat an illness.

How Does Smoking Affect Crohn's Disease?

Current and former smokers have a higher risk of developing Crohn's disease than people who have never smoked.

Crohn's disease is an inflammatory bowel disease (IBD) that causes irritation in the GI tract. The disease, which typically causes pain and diarrhea, most often affects the lower part of the small intestine; however, it can occur anywhere in the GI tract. The severity of symptoms varies from person to person, and the symptoms come and go. Crohn's disease may lead to complications such as blockages of the intestine and ulcers that tunnel through the affected area into surrounding tissues. Medications may control symptoms. However, many people with Crohn's disease require surgery to remove the affected portion of the intestine.

Among people with Crohn's disease, people who smoke are more likely to:

- have more severe symptoms, more frequent symptoms, and more complications
- need more medications to control their symptoms

- require surgery
- have symptoms recur after surgery

The effects of smoking are more pronounced in women with Crohn's disease than in men with the disease.

Researchers are studying why smoking increases the risk of Crohn's disease and makes the disease worse. Some researchers believe smoking might lower the intestines' defenses, decrease blood flow to the intestines, or cause immune system changes that result in inflammation. In people who inherit genes that make them susceptible to developing Crohn's disease, smoking may affect how some of these genes work.

How Does Smoking Affect Colon Polyps?

People who smoke are more likely to develop colon polyps. Colon polyps are growths on the inside surface of the colon or rectum. Some polyps are benign, or noncancerous, while some are cancerous or may become cancerous.

Among people who develop colon polyps, those who smoke have polyps that are larger, more numerous, and more likely to recur.

How Does Smoking Affect Pancreatitis?

Smoking increases the risk of developing pancreatitis. Pancreatitis is inflammation of the pancreas, which is located behind the stomach and close to the duodenum. The pancreas secretes digestive enzymes that usually do not become active until they reach the small intestine. When the pancreas is inflamed, the digestive enzymes attack the tissues of the pancreas.

How Does Smoking Affect Gallstones?

Some studies have shown that smoking may increase the risk of developing gallstones. However, research results are not consistent, and more study is needed.

Gallstones are small, hard particles that develop in the gallbladder, the organ that stores bile made by the liver. Gallstones can move into the ducts that carry digestive enzymes from the gallbladder, liver, and pancreas to the duodenum, causing inflammation, infection, and abdominal pain.

Can the Damage to the Digestive System from Smoking Be Reversed?

Quitting smoking can reverse some of the effects of smoking on the digestive system. For example, the balance between factors that harm and protect the stomach and duodenum lining returns to normal within a few hours of a person quitting smoking. The effects of smoking on how the liver handles medications also disappear when a person stops smoking. However, people who stop smoking continue to have a higher risk of some digestive diseases, such as colon polyps and pancreatitis, than people who have never smoked.

Quitting smoking can improve the symptoms of some digestive diseases or keep them from getting worse. For example, people with Crohn's disease who quit smoking have less severe symptoms than smokers with the disease.[1]

Eating, Diet, and Nutrition

Eating, diet, and nutrition can play a role in causing, preventing, and treating some of the diseases and disorders of the digestive system that are affected by smoking, including heartburn and GERD, liver diseases, Crohn's disease, colon polyps, pancreatitis, and gallstones.

Source: "Smoking and the Digestive System," National Institute of Diabetes and Digestive and Kidney Diseases (NIDDK), March 15, 2013. Available online. URL: www.niddk.nih.gov/-/media/Files/Digestive-Diseases/Smoking_Digestive_System_508.pdf. Accessed October 6, 2023.

[1] "Smoking and the Digestive System," National Institute of Diabetes and Digestive and Kidney Diseases (NIDDK), March 15, 2013. Available online. URL: www.niddk.nih.gov/-/media/Files/Digestive-Diseases/Smoking_Digestive_System_508.pdf. Accessed October 6, 2023.

CHAPTER 47
EYE DISEASE

Smoking is as bad for your eyes as it is for the rest of your body. If you smoke, you can develop serious eye conditions that can cause vision loss or blindness. Two of the greatest threats to your eyesight are as follows:

- macular degeneration (MD)
- cataracts

MD, also called "age-related macular degeneration" (AMD), is an eye disease that affects central vision. You need central vision to see objects clearly and for common tasks such as reading, recognizing faces, and driving.

The following are the two forms of AMD:

- dry AMD
- wet AMD

MD always begins in the dry form and sometimes progresses to the more advanced wet form, where vision loss can be very rapid if untreated.

Cataracts cause blurry vision that worsens over time. Without surgery, cataracts can lead to serious vision loss. The best way to protect your sight from damage linked to smoking is to quit or never start smoking.

Symptoms of Eye Diseases Related to Smoking

You may think your eyes are fine, but the only way to know for sure is by getting a full eye exam. AMD often has no early symptoms, so an eye exam is the best way to spot this eye disease early. An eye specialist will place special drops in your eyes to widen your pupils. This offers a better view of the back of your eye, where a thin layer of tissue (the retina) changes light into signals that go to the brain. The macula is a small part of the retina that you need for sharp, central vision.

When symptoms of AMD do occur, they can include the following:

- blurred vision or a blurry spot in your central vision
- the need for more light to read or do other tasks

- straight lines that look wavy
- trouble recognizing faces

Eye injections are often the preferred treatment for wet AMD. Your doctor can inject a drug to stop the growth of these blood vessels and stop further damage to your eyes. You may need injections on a regular basis to save your vision.

How Does Smoking Affect Your Eyes?

Smoking causes changes in the eyes that can lead to vision loss. If you smoke:

- you are twice as likely to develop AMD compared with people who do not smoke
- you are two to three times more likely to develop cataracts compared with people who do not smoke

How Can You Prevent Vision Loss Related to Smoking?

If you smoke, stop. Quitting may lower your risk for both AMD and cataracts.

If you already have AMD, quitting smoking may slow the disease. AMD tends to get worse over time. Quitting smoking is something within your control that may help save your sight. The following healthy habits may also help protect your eyes from cataracts and AMD:

- Exercise regularly.
- Maintain normal blood pressure and cholesterol levels.
- Eat a healthy diet rich in green, leafy vegetables and fish.
- Wear sunglasses and a hat with a brim to protect your eyes from sunlight.

How Is a Cataract Treated?

The symptoms of an early cataract may improve with new eyeglasses, brighter lighting, anti-glare sunglasses, or magnifying lenses.

When glasses and brighter lighting do not help, you may need surgery. A doctor will remove the cloudy lens and replace it with an artificial lens. This clear, plastic lens becomes a permanent part of your eye.

Help for Vision Loss

Coping with vision loss can be frightening, but there is help to make the most of the vision you have left and to continue enjoying your friends, family, and special interests. If you have already lost some sight, ask your health-care professional about low-vision counseling and devices, such as high-powered lenses, magnifiers, and talking computers.[1]

[1] "Vision Loss, Blindness, and Smoking," Centers for Disease Control and Prevention (CDC), May 5, 2022. Available online. URL: www.cdc.gov/tobacco/campaign/tips/diseases/vision-loss-blindness.html. Accessed October 3, 2023.

CHAPTER 48
HEART DISEASE AND STROKE

What Are Heart Disease and Stroke?

Heart disease and stroke are cardiovascular (heart and blood vessel) diseases (CVDs).

Heart disease includes several types of heart conditions. The most common type in the United States is coronary heart disease (also known as "coronary artery disease" (CAD)). Coronary heart disease occurs when the walls of arteries that carry blood to the heart are narrowed by plaque, a process known as "atherosclerosis." This can cause:

- chest pain
- heart attack (when blood flow to the heart becomes blocked and a section of the heart muscle is damaged or dies)
- heart failure (when the heart cannot pump enough blood and oxygen to support other organs)
- arrhythmia (when the heart beats too fast, too slow, or irregularly)

A stroke occurs when the blood supply to the brain is blocked or when a blood vessel in the brain bursts, causing parts of the brain to become damaged or die. Stroke can cause disability (such as paralysis, muscle weakness, trouble speaking, and memory loss) or death.

How Is Smoking Related to Heart Disease and Stroke?

Smoking is a major cause of CVD and causes one of every three deaths from CVD. Smoking can:

- raise triglycerides (a type of fat in your blood)
- lower "good" cholesterol
- make blood sticky and more likely to clot, which can block blood flow to the heart and brain
- damage cells that line the blood vessels
- increase the buildup of plaque (fat, cholesterol, calcium, and other substances) in blood vessels
- cause thickening and narrowing of blood vessels

How Is Breathing Secondhand Smoke Related to Heart Disease and Stroke?

Breathing secondhand smoke also harms your health. Secondhand smoke is the smoke from burning tobacco products. Secondhand smoke is also smoke breathed out by a smoker.

Breathing secondhand smoke can cause coronary heart disease and stroke. Know the following facts:

- Secondhand smoke causes nearly 34,000 early deaths from coronary heart disease each year in the United States among nonsmokers.
- Nonsmokers who breathe secondhand smoke at home or work increase their risk of developing heart disease by 25–30 percent. Secondhand smoke increases the risk of stroke by 20–30 percent.
- Each year, secondhand smoke exposure causes more than 8,000 deaths from stroke.
- Breathing secondhand smoke interferes with the normal functioning of the heart, blood, and vascular systems in ways that increase your risk of having a heart attack.
- Even briefly breathing secondhand smoke can damage the lining of blood vessels and cause your blood to become stickier. These changes can lead to a heart attack.

Can Quitting Smoking Improve Your Heart Heath?

The best way to safeguard your heart from smoking-related disease and death is to never start using cigarettes. But, if you do smoke cigarettes, the earlier you can quit, the better.

Quitting smoking benefits your heart and cardiovascular system now and in the future:

- Twenty minutes after you quit smoking, your heart rate drops.
- Just 12 hours after quitting smoking, the carbon monoxide level in your blood drops to normal, allowing more oxygen to vital organs like your heart.
- Within four years of quitting, your risk of stroke drops to that of lifetime nonsmokers.

Source: "How Smoking Affects Heart Health," U.S. Food and Drug Administration (FDA), November 9, 2021. Available online. URL: www.fda.gov/tobacco-products/health-effects-tobacco-use/how-smoking-affects-heart-health. Accessed October 6, 2023.

How Can Heart Disease and Stroke Be Prevented?

Heart disease and stroke are major causes of death and disability in the United States. Many people are at high risk for these diseases and do not know it. The good news is that many risk factors for heart disease and stroke can be prevented or controlled.

The federal government's Million Hearts® initiative aims to prevent 1 million heart attacks and strokes within five years. It is important to know your risk for heart disease and stroke and to take action to reduce that risk. A good place to start is with the ABCS of heart health:

- **Aspirin**. Aspirin may help reduce your risk for heart disease and stroke. But do not take aspirin if you think you are having a stroke. It can make some types of stroke worse. Before taking aspirin, talk to your doctor about whether aspirin is right for you.
- **Blood pressure**. Control your blood pressure.
- **Cholesterol**. Manage your cholesterol.
- **Smoking**. Quit smoking or do not start.

In addition to your ABCS, several lifestyle choices can help protect your heart and brain health. These include the following:

- Avoid breathing secondhand smoke.
- Eat fresh fruits and vegetables.
- Eat low-fat, low-salt foods most of the time.
- Maintain a healthy weight.
- Exercise regularly.
- Limit alcohol use.
- Control other health conditions (such as diabetes).[1]

[1] "Smoking and Heart Disease and Stroke," Centers for Disease Control and Prevention (CDC), March 15, 2023. Available online. URL: www.cdc.gov/tobacco/campaign/tips/diseases/heart-disease-stroke.html. Accessed October 6, 2023.

CHAPTER 49
WEAKENED IMMUNE SYSTEM

On average, compared to people who have never smoked, smokers suffer for years with more health problems due to their smoking and ultimately die earlier by a decade or more than nonsmokers.

In fact, smokers generally are much less healthy than nonsmokers.

- Smokers' overall health is worse, and they are sick more often than nonsmokers.
- Smokers need to go to the doctor more often, and they are admitted to the hospital more often than nonsmokers.
- Smokers miss more work than do nonsmokers. This costs American businesses, and American workers who smoke, billions of dollars every year.

Smoking and the Immune System

Smoking harms the immune system and can make the body less successful at fighting disease. The immune system is the body's way of protecting itself from infection and disease; it works to fight everything from cold and flu viruses to serious conditions such as cancer.

Additionally, smoking is known to compromise the equilibrium, or balance, of the immune system. This increases the risk for several immune and autoimmune disorders (conditions caused when the immune system mistakenly attacks the body's healthy cells and tissues). New evidence finds that smoking is a cause of rheumatoid arthritis (RA), an autoimmune disease in which the immune system attacks the joints and causes swelling and pain.

People with RA have a harder time getting around and doing normal daily activities. Smoking also interferes with the effectiveness of certain treatments for RA.

Chemicals and Disease

Cigarette smoke contains more than 7,000 chemical compounds. Many of them can interfere with the immune system. Diseases are able to progress when the immune system is not working effectively. Diseases that can be worsened by smoking include the following:

- viral and bacterial infections, especially of the lungs (e.g., pneumonia, influenza, tuberculosis (TB))
- periodontal or gum disease
- bacterial meningitis (a disease that attacks the protective membranes covering the brain and spinal cord)
- infections that occur after surgery
- RA
- Crohn's disease (a serious disease of the digestive system)
- cancer

Let your clients know that people who want healthy lives should not smoke. Smokers lose quality of life (QOL) as well as years of life. Smokers who want to quit can get help from their doctors.[1]

[1] "Smoking and Overall Health," Centers for Disease Control and Prevention (CDC), October 14, 2014. Available online. URL: www.cdc.gov/tobacco/sgr/50th-anniversary/pdfs/fs_smoking_overall_health_508.pdf. Accessed October 3, 2023.

CHAPTER 50
MENTAL HEALTH

People with mental health conditions smoke at rates that are at least two times higher than the general population. They may also smoke more heavily and frequently, compared to those without mental health conditions. The Centers for Disease Control and Prevention (CDC) estimates that nearly one-third (31%) of all cigarettes consumed in the United States are smoked by people with mental health conditions. The disproportionately high rates of smoking in this population are likely due to a combination of biological, psychological, and social factors that work together to create a unique vulnerability for tobacco dependence. While the underlying causal mechanisms are not yet fully understood, one thing is clear, tobacco use among persons with mental health conditions can be prevented, and those who currently smoke can quit.

Consequences of Smoking among Smokers with Mental Health Conditions

The high rates of smoking among people with mental health conditions have devastating health consequences. Smoking-related diseases, such as cardiovascular disease, lung disease, and cancer, are among the most common causes of death among adults with mental health conditions. Despite the heavy disease burden, smoking cessation interventions are not routinely offered within mental health-care settings. A U.S. national survey of mental health treatment facilities found that only about one-quarter provided services to help patients quit smoking. There is a growing recognition among health-care providers that the integration of tobacco dependence treatment into mental health care is an important part of mental health recovery and wellness. Many providers and facilities have made progress in reducing smoking in their facilities and among their patients; others are just now beginning to address tobacco use.

Smokers with Mental Health Conditions Can Quit Smoking

A common misconception among health-care providers is that smokers with mental health conditions either cannot or will not give up smoking. However, research has shown that adult smokers with mental health conditions—such as other smokers—want to quit, can quit, and benefit from proven smoking cessation treatments. In clinical studies, adults with mental health conditions are just as likely to want to quit smoking as those without such conditions. People with mental health conditions may face unique challenges in quitting smoking and may benefit from additional services, such as more intensive counseling and/or longer use or a combination of cessation medications. But, with support, they can and do quit smoking successfully.

Quitting Smoking May Benefit Mental Health Recovery

Another common misconception among some providers is that smoking has mental health benefits and helps patients cope with their psychiatric symptoms. But research suggests otherwise; smoking is not an effective mental health treatment strategy. On the contrary, smoking is associated with poor clinical outcomes, such as greater depressive symptoms, greater likelihood of psychiatric hospitalization, and increased suicidal behavior. Furthermore, smoking can complicate treatment by accelerating the metabolism of certain psychiatric medications, resulting in the need for higher doses to get the same therapeutic benefit. A large body of clinical research has shown that patients can quit without worsening their psychiatric symptoms if they are given the appropriate support (e.g., behavioral counseling, cessation medication, and monitoring). Evidence also suggests that quitting smoking is associated with mental health benefits. In several clinical and epidemiological studies, smoking cessation has been associated with significant reductions in depression and anxiety, lower rates of rehospitalization, and lower rates of suicide. A systematic review found that smoking cessation was associated with marked improvements in mental health over time, whereas continued smoking was associated with little change over the same period.

Smoking Cessation Assistance Is an Important Part of Mental Health Treatment

Providers who care for people with mental health conditions are well-positioned to help patients successfully quit tobacco use and enjoy the mental, emotional, and physical benefits of a tobacco-free life. Smoking cessation treatments work, and it is important to make them available to all people who want to quit, including people with mental health conditions. Providers can do their part by making tobacco cessation part of an overall approach to treatment and wellness.

- Ask patients if they smoke cigarettes or use other forms of tobacco; if they do, strongly advise them to quit.

- Assist patients who are ready to quit by offering proven quitting treatments, including tailored cessation assistance.
    - Refer patients interested in quitting to the "I'm Ready to Quit!" page on the Tips website, 800-QUIT-NOW (800-784-8669), www.smokefree.gov, or other resources.
    - Provide counseling, support, and stop smoking medicines.
- Monitor and adjust mental health medicines as needed in patients trying to quit smoking.[1]

[1] "Smoking and Mental Health: Five Things Every Health Care Provider Should Know," Centers for Disease Control and Prevention (CDC), November 25, 2014. Available online. URL: www.cdc.gov/tobacco/campaign/tips/resources/partners/mental-health/tips-mental-health-partners-five-things.pdf. Accessed October 9, 2023.

CHAPTER 51
PERIODONTAL DISEASE

What Is Gum Disease?

Gum (periodontal) disease is an infection of the gums and can affect the bone structure that supports your teeth. In severe cases, it can make your teeth fall out. Smoking is an important cause of severe gum disease in the United States.

Gum disease starts with bacteria (germs) on your teeth that get under your gums. If the germs stay on your teeth for too long, layers of plaque (film) and tartar (hardened plaque) develop. This buildup leads to early gum disease, called "gingivitis."

When gum disease gets worse, your gums can pull away from your teeth and form spaces that get infected. This is severe gum disease, also called "periodontitis." The bone and tissue that hold your teeth in place can break down, and your teeth may loosen and need to be pulled out.

Warning Signs and Symptoms of Gum Disease

- red or swollen gums
- tender or bleeding gums
- painful chewing
- loose teeth
- sensitive teeth
- gums that have pulled away from your teeth

How Is Smoking Related to Gum Disease?

Smoking weakens your body's infection fighters (your immune system). This makes it harder to fight off a gum infection. Once you have gum damage, smoking also makes it harder for your gums to heal.

What does this mean for you if you are a smoker?

- You have twice the risk for gum disease compared with a nonsmoker.
- The more cigarettes you smoke, the greater your risk for gum disease.

- The longer you smoke, the greater your risk for gum disease.
- Treatments for gum disease may not work as well for people who smoke.

Tobacco use in any form—cigarettes, pipes, and smokeless (spit) tobacco—raises your risk for gum disease.

How Can Gum Disease Be Prevented?

You can help avoid gum disease with good dental habits, including the following:

- Brush your teeth twice a day.
- Floss often to remove plaque.
- See a dentist regularly for checkups and professional cleanings.
- Do not smoke. If you smoke, quit.

How Is Gum Disease Treated?

Regular cleanings at your dentist's office and daily brushing and flossing can help treat early gum disease (gingivitis).

More severe gum disease may require:

- deep cleaning below the gum line
- prescription mouth rinse or medicine
- surgery to remove tartar deep under the gums
- surgery to help heal bone or gums lost to periodontitis (Your dentist may use small bits of bone to fill places where bone has been lost. Or your dentist may move tissue from one place in your mouth to cover exposed tooth roots.)

If you smoke or use spit tobacco, quitting will help your gums heal after treatment.[1]

[1] "Smoking, Gum Disease, and Tooth Loss," Centers for Disease Control and Prevention (CDC), May 5, 2022. Available online. URL: www.cdc.gov/tobacco/campaign/tips/diseases/periodontal-gum-disease.html. Accessed October 9, 2023.

CHAPTER 52
PREGNANCY AND REPRODUCTION

Most people know that smoking causes cancer and other major health problems. And smoking while you are pregnant can cause serious problems, too. Your baby could be born too early, have a birth defect, or die from sudden infant death syndrome (SIDS). Even being around cigarette smoke can cause health problems for you and your baby.

It is best to quit smoking before you get pregnant. But, if you are already pregnant, quitting can still help protect you and your baby from health problems. It is never too late to quit smoking.

If you smoked and had a healthy pregnancy in the past, there is no guarantee that your next pregnancy will be healthy. When you smoke during pregnancy, you put your health and your baby's health at risk.

How Does Smoking Affect Fertility?

Smoking can cause fertility problems for you or your partner. Women who smoke have more trouble getting pregnant than women who do not smoke. In men, smoking can damage sperm and contribute to impotence erectile dysfunction (ED). Both problems can make it harder for a man to father a baby when he and his partner are ready.

How Can Smoking Harm You and Your Baby?

- Your baby may be born too small, even after a full-term pregnancy. Smoking slows your baby's growth before birth.
- Your baby may be born too early (premature birth). Premature babies often have health problems.
- Smoking can damage your baby's developing lungs and brain. The damage can last through childhood and into the teen years.
- Smoking doubles your risk of abnormal bleeding during pregnancy and delivery. This can put both you and your baby in danger.
- Smoking raises your baby's risk for birth defects, including cleft lip, cleft palate, or both. A cleft is an opening in your baby's lip or in the roof of

his or her mouth (palate). He or she can have trouble eating properly and is likely to need surgery.
- Babies of moms who smoke during pregnancy—and babies exposed to cigarette smoke after birth—have a higher risk for SIDS.

How Can a Premature Birth Harm Your Baby?

If you smoke during pregnancy, you are more likely to give birth too early. A baby born three weeks or more before your due date is premature. Babies born too early miss important growth that happens in the womb during the final weeks and months of pregnancy.

The earlier a baby is born, the greater the chances for serious health problems or death. Premature babies can have:

- low birth weight
- feeding difficulties
- breathing problems right away
- breathing problems that last into childhood
- cerebral palsy (CP; brain damage that causes trouble with movement and muscle tone)
- developmental delays (when a baby or child is behind in language, thinking, or movement skills)
- problems with hearing or eyesight

Premature babies may need to stay at the hospital for days, weeks, or even months.

How Can Quitting Help You and Your Baby?

The best time to quit smoking is before you get pregnant, but quitting at any time during pregnancy can help your baby get a better start on life. Talk to your doctor about the best ways to quit while you are pregnant or trying to get pregnant.

When you stop smoking:

- Your baby gets more oxygen, even after just one day.
- Your baby will grow better.
- Your baby is less likely to be born too early.
- You will have more energy and breathe more easily.
- You will be less likely to develop heart disease, stroke, lung cancer, lung disease, and other smoking-related diseases.

Support for Quitting during Pregnancy

Most pregnant women who smoke want to quit, but quitting is not always easier during pregnancy. What is more, if you are pregnant and still smoking, you may feel ashamed and alone.

The right kind of support can help a pregnant woman get through the unique challenges of quitting during this phase of life. Special guidance is available for you and for the people around you.

Stay Smoke-Free for a Healthy Child

Staying smoke-free is important. Tobacco smoke contains a deadly mix of more than 7,000 chemicals. When your child is not exposed to smoke, you can expect him or her to have:

- fewer coughs and chest colds
- a lower risk for bronchitis or pneumonia (lung problems)
- fewer ear infections
- fewer asthma attacks and wheezing problems[1]

E-cigarettes and Pregnancy

- E-cigarettes are not safe to use during pregnancy.
- Nicotine is a health danger for pregnant women and developing babies and can damage a developing baby's brain and lungs.
- There is currently not enough evidence to know whether e-cigarettes increase smoking cessation.
- E-cigarettes are not currently approved by the U.S. Food and Drug Administration (FDA) as a smoking cessation aid.

Source: "Clinical Interventions to Treat Tobacco Use and Dependence Among Adults," Centers for Disease Control and Prevention (CDC), June 8, 2021. Available online. URL: www.cdc.gov/tobacco/patient-care/care-settings/clinical/index.html. Accessed October 4, 2023.

Myths: Smoking and Pregnancy

Smoking anytime during your pregnancy is dangerous. Quitting is the best thing you can do for you and your baby. Here are some common myths about quitting and pregnancy.

Quitting smoking—at any point during your pregnancy—is one of the best things you can do for your baby.

Myths versus Facts

- **Myth**: I am pregnant and have been smoking, so there is no point in stopping now.
  Fact: Quitting smoking at any stage of your pregnancy has health benefits for you and your baby. Even after just one day of not smoking, your baby will get

[1] "Smoking, Pregnancy, and Babies," Centers for Disease Control and Prevention (CDC), May 5, 2022. Available online. URL: www.cdc.gov/tobacco/campaign/tips/diseases/pregnancy.html. Accessed October 4, 2023.

more oxygen. This will help your baby's lungs develop well. Quitting now also lowers your chances of having a baby with low birth weight.

- **Myth**: Quitting smoking will be too stressful for my baby.
  Fact: Quitting smoking does not put extra stress on your baby. It is one of the best things that you can do for your health and your baby's health during pregnancy—and after the baby is born. By quitting smoking now, you will be protecting your infant from the dangers of secondhand smoke and reducing the risk of SIDS.
- **Myth**: Smoking fewer cigarettes or switching to e-cigarettes during pregnancy is okay.
  Fact: There is no safe amount of smoking. Every puff of a cigarette releases harmful chemicals that will reach your baby and affect your health too. E-cigarettes are also not harmless. Although there is still much to learn about e-cigarettes, pregnant women should not use them. The nicotine in e-cigarettes is harmful to developing babies.
- **Myth**: Smoking relaxes me, and being relaxed is better for me and my baby.
  Fact: Smoking may make you feel calmer, but it hurts your body more than it helps. The relaxed feeling is only temporary and whatever is causing your stress will likely return. Smoking speeds up your heart rate and increases your blood pressure. It also increases the carbon monoxide in your bloodstream, which means your baby gets less oxygen.
- **Myth**: There is nothing wrong with having a small baby.
  Fact: Smoking during pregnancy increases the chances of having a low birth weight baby. Babies with low birth weight are more likely to have serious health problems than normal-weight babies. These problems can affect your baby's health now, throughout their childhood, and into adulthood.
- **Myth**: The only way to quit smoking is cold turkey.
  Fact: Pregnant women have other ways to quit smoking besides cold turkey, which is quitting without any preparation or counseling. Smoke-free Women offers many resources that can help you quit. Try signing up for a text message program, like SmokefreeMom. While some smokers try medications to help them quit, the risks of using them while pregnant are not fully known. If you are having trouble quitting after trying different methods, be open with your doctor about your challenges and ask if medication may be right for you and your baby.
- **Myth**: I smoked during my last pregnancy and had a healthy baby, so this next baby will be healthy, too.
  Fact: Every time you smoke during pregnancy, you put your baby's health at risk. If you smoking but had a healthy pregnancy in the past, that does not mean your next one will be healthy, too.

- **Myth**: I smoke, so I should not breastfeed my baby.
  Fact: According to the American Academy of Pediatrics (AAP), mothers who smoke are encouraged to quit smoking but can breastfeed their baby if they continue to smoke. Breast milk is good for your baby. It provides your baby with what he or she needs for healthy growth and development. Not smoking while you are breastfeeding your baby, waiting to smoke until after you breastfeed, and making your car and home smoke-free are important ways to protect your baby from the effects of nicotine and secondhand smoke.[2]

[2] Smokefree Women, "Myths: Smoking and Pregnancy," U.S. Department of Health and Human Services (HHS), September 7, 2018. Available online. URL: https://women.smokefree.gov/pregnancy-motherhood/quitting-while-pregnant/myths-about-smoking-pregnancy. Accessed October 4, 2023.

CHAPTER 53
SLEEP DISORDERS

How Are Sleep and Tobacco Use Related?

People who use tobacco are more than twice as likely to report insufficient sleep compared to nontobacco users.

While tobacco users may report that they use tobacco to manage their sleep problems, studies show that smokers are more likely to report daytime sleepiness than nonsmokers. While the nicotine in your tobacco products may help you feel more alert during the day, it may cause and/or worsen your sleep difficulties.

What Kinds of Problems Related to Your Sleep Can Occur When You Use Tobacco?

Compared to nontobacco users, research shows that tobacco users:

- spend more time in stages 1 and 2 of sleep, which contributes to more fitful sleep
- spend less time in stage 3 of sleep, which is the period during which restful, restorative sleep occurs
- have a higher risk for sleep-disordered breathing, such as snoring and obstructive sleep apnea (OSA)

How Will Quitting Tobacco Improve Your Sleep?

While quitting tobacco can initially increase sleep problems because of nicotine withdrawal, they will decrease over time and your overall sleep quality will improve. When you quit tobacco, you:

- may fall asleep faster, have less interrupted sleep, and have longer total sleep time
- improve your mood, functioning, and quality of life (QOL) that are all associated with better sleep quality

You Want to Quit Using Tobacco. How Do You Get Started?

- Call the tobacco quitline of the U.S. Department of Veterans Affairs (VA) at 855-QUIT-VET (855-784-8838), Monday to Friday (available in English and Spanish).
- Sign up for the VA's SmokefreeVET text messaging program—text the word VET to 47848 or visit smokefree.gov/VET website (https://veterans.smokefree.gov/tools-tips-vet/smokefreevet?utm_source=vetshortlink&utm_medium=SFV&utm_campaign=Vet_SFVTXT).
- Talk to your primary care or mental health provider about tobacco cessation medications and counseling that can help you quit.
- Visit VA's Mental Health website (https://www.mentalhealth.va.gov/quit-tobacco/index.asp).[1]

How Much Sleep Do You Need?

Most adults need seven or more hours of good-quality sleep on a regular schedule each night.

Getting enough sleep is not only about total hours of sleep. It is also important to get good-quality sleep on a regular schedule, so you feel rested when you wake up.

If you often have trouble sleeping—or if you often still feel tired after sleeping—talk with your doctor.

Why Is Getting Enough Sleep Important?

Getting enough sleep has many benefits. It can help you:

- get sick less often
- stay at a healthy weight
- lower your risk for serious health problems, such as diabetes and heart disease
- reduce stress and improve your mood
- think more clearly and do better in school and at work
- get along better with people
- make good decisions and avoid injuries—for example, drowsy drivers cause thousands of car accidents every year

Source: Office of Disease Prevention and Health Promotion (ODPHP), "Get Enough Sleep," U.S. Department of Health and Human Services (HHS), August 4, 2023. Available online. URL: https://health.gov/myhealthfinder/healthy-living/mental-health-and-relationships/get-enough-sleep. Accessed October 3, 2023.

Getting Treatment

There are treatments for OSA that work well. Eric Mann, MD, PhD at the Center for Devices and Radiological Health (CRH) of the U.S. Food and Drug Administration (FDA) says, "Many FDA-approved and FDA-cleared treatments can help people with OSA wake up in the mornings feeling rested and refreshed, improving their overall health."

[1] "Sleep & Tobacco Use," U.S. Department of Veterans Affairs (VA), December 2, 2019. Available online. URL: www.mentalhealth.va.gov/quit-tobacco/docs/VAM_TH-094_Sleep_and_Tobacco_Use_One_Pager_508.pdf. Accessed October 3, 2023.

Getting treatment for OSA is key because OSA not only affects your sleep but increases your risk of serious health problems and even death. OSA may increase your risk of heart attack, stroke, type 2 diabetes, glaucoma, and some types of cancer along with other serious health conditions. Lifestyle behavior changes such as losing weight, drinking less alcohol, stopping smoking, and using devices that help you sleep in a certain position may help improve OSA but may not make it go away entirely. Taking certain medicines, such as sedatives or sleep aids, that slow or lessen breathing can also contribute to OSA. Talk to your doctor before stopping or starting any medicine.

OSA treatments can work well to manage OSA, but not every treatment is right for everyone. Some treatments work best for people with mild OSA, while others are best for people with more severe OSA. Sometimes, you must try a specific treatment before you can move on to a different treatment. Some treatments involve surgery to correct a narrow airway or a specific part of the airway that may collapse during sleep. Any type of surgery has risks, so talk with your doctor about all of your options before you decide.

The FDA evaluates the safety and effectiveness of certain medical devices before they can be marketed to the public, including the device most often used for OSA. Depending on your health status and the type of OSA you may have, your doctor may prescribe one of these OSA treatments.[2]

[2] "Always Tired? You May Have Sleep Apnea," U.S. Food and Drug Administration (FDA), July 12, 2021. Available online. URL: www.fda.gov/consumers/consumer-updates/always-tired-you-may-have-sleep-apnea. Accessed October 3, 2023.

PART 6 | TOBACCO-USE CESSATION

CHAPTER 54
WHY YOU SHOULD QUIT

There are so many great reasons to stop smoking. Understand the ways smoking affects you and your loved ones and discover the benefits of quitting. Think about why you want to be smoke-free and remind yourself of these reasons when you need some extra motivation.

Reasons to Quit

When a strong craving hits, it can be easy to lose sight of the benefits of quitting. You might lose your focus, but there is no good reason to smoke.

Remind yourself of the rewards of quitting to help yourself stay on track:

- **20 minutes**. Heart rate and blood pressure drop.
- **12 hours**. Carbon monoxide in the bloodstream drops to normal.
- **2 weeks to 3 months**. Circulation and lung function improve; heart attack risk begins to drop.
- **1–9 months**. Cough less; breathe easier.
- **1 year**. The risk of coronary heart disease is cut in half.
- **2–5 years**. The risk of cancer of the mouth, throat, esophagus, and bladder is cut in half; stroke risk is reduced to that of a nonsmoker.
- **10 years**. The chance of dying from lung cancer is less than half; risk of kidney or pancreatic cancer decreases.
- **15 years**. Risk of coronary heart disease is the same as that of nonsmokers.

Immediate Rewards

There is no safe amount of cigarette smoke. When you smoke, the chemicals in tobacco reach your lungs quickly every time you inhale. Your blood carries the toxins to every organ in your body. But, after you quit, your body begins to heal within 20 minutes of your last cigarette. The nicotine leaves your body within three days. As your body starts to repair itself, you may feel worse instead of better. Withdrawal can be difficult, but it is a sign that your body is healing.

Why Do You Want to Quit?

You are thinking of quitting smoking. Do you know the reasons you want to quit? Do you want to be healthier? Save money? Keep your family safe? All of those reasons?

If you are not sure, ask yourself the following questions:

- What do you dislike about smoking?
- What do you miss out on when you smoke?
- How is smoking affecting your health?
- What will happen to you and your family if you keep smoking?
- How will your life get better when you quit?

Once you know your reasons for quitting, remind yourself of them every day. It can inspire you to stop smoking for good.

Long-Term Rewards

Quitting can help you add years to your life. Smokers who quit before age 40 reduce their chance of dying too early from smoking-related diseases by about 90 percent. Those who quit by ages 45–54 reduce their chance of dying too early by about two-thirds. You can take control of your health by quitting and staying smoke-free. Over time, you will greatly lower your risk of death from lung cancer and other diseases, such as heart disease, stroke, chronic bronchitis, emphysema, and at least 13 other kinds of cancer.

When you quit, you will also protect your loved ones from dangerous secondhand smoke. You will set a good example and show your family that a life without cigarettes is possible.

Source: Smokefree.gov, "Reasons to Quit," U.S. Department of Health and Human Services (HHS), August 16, 2023. Available online. URL: https://smokefree.gov/quit-smoking/why-you-should-quit. Accessed October 6, 2023.

Want to Look, Feel, and Be Healthier?

Here are some more reasons to consider:

- Your chances of having cancer, heart attacks, heart disease, stroke, cataracts, and other diseases will go down.
- You will be less likely to catch colds or the flu and will be able to recover quicker if you do get sick.
- You will breathe easier and cough less.
- Your blood pressure will go down.
- Your skin will look healthier, and you will look more youthful.
- Your teeth and fingernails will not be stained.

Quitting will make you feel better and improve your health. But there are other reasons to quit that you might not have thought about.

Want a Better Lifestyle?

- You will have more money to spend.
- You can spend more time with family, catch up on work, or dive into your favorite hobby.
- You would not have to worry about when you can smoke next or where you can or cannot smoke.
- Your food will taste better.
- Your clothes will smell better.
- Your car, home, and kids would not smell like smoke.
- You will be able to smell food, flowers, and other things better.

Want a Better Family Life?

- You will set a great example for your kids; it takes a lot of strength to quit.
- Your friends, family, coworkers, and other loved ones will be proud of you.
- You will protect your friends and family from the dangers of secondhand smoke.
- Your children will be healthier.
- You will have more energy to do the things you love with friends and family.
- You will get healthy to make sure you are around to share in your family's special moments.

Make a list of all the reasons you want to become smoke-free. Keep the list in a place where you will see it often, such as your car or where you used to keep your cigarettes. When you feel the urge to smoke, take a look at the list to remind yourself why you want to quit.

Benefits of Quitting

The health benefits of quitting smoking can help most of the major parts of your body: from your brain to your DNA.

Brain

Broken Addiction Cycle

Quitting smoking can rewire your brain and help break the cycle of addiction. The large number of nicotine receptors in your brain will return to normal levels after about a month of being quit.

Head and Face

Sharp Hearing

Quitting smoking will keep your hearing sharp. Remember, even mild hearing loss can cause problems (such as not hearing directions correctly and doing a task wrong).

Better Vision

Stopping smoking will improve your night vision and help preserve your overall vision by stopping the damage that smoking does to your eyes.

Clean Mouth

Nobody likes a dirty mouth. After a few days without cigarettes, your smile will be brighter. Not smoking now will keep your mouth healthy for years to come.

Clear Skin

Quitting smoking is better than antiaging lotion. Quitting can help clear up blemishes and protect your skin from premature aging and wrinkling.

Heart

Decreased Heart Risks

Smoking is the leading cause of heart attacks and heart disease. But many of these heart risks can be reversed simply by quitting smoking. Quitting can lower your blood pressure and heart rate almost immediately. Your risk of a heart attack declines within 24 hours.

Thin Blood

Another effect of quitting smoking is that your blood will become thinner and less likely to form dangerous blood clots. Your heart will also have less work to do because it will be able to move the blood around your body more easily.

Lower Cholesterol

Quitting smoking will not get rid of the fatty deposits that are already there. But it will lower the levels of cholesterol and fats circulating in your blood, which will help slow the buildup of new fatty deposits in your arteries.

Lungs

Stop Lung Damage

Scarring of the lungs is not reversible. That is why it is important to quit smoking before you do permanent damage to your lungs. Within two weeks of quitting, you might notice it is easier to walk up the stairs because you may be less short of breath. Do not wait until later; quit today!

Prevent Emphysema

There is no cure for emphysema. But quitting when you are young, before you have done years of damage to the delicate air sacs in your lungs, will help protect you from developing emphysema later.

Return of Cilia

Cilia start to regrow and regain normal function very quickly after you quit smoking. They are one of the first things in your body to heal. People sometimes notice that they cough more than usual when they first quit smoking. This is a sign that the cilia are coming back to life. But you are more likely to fight off colds and infections when your cilia are working properly.

DNA

Lower Cancer Risk

Quitting smoking will prevent DNA damage from happening and can even help repair the damage that has already been done. Quitting smoking immediately is the best way to lower your risk of getting cancer.

Stomach and Hormones

Smaller Belly

Quitting smoking will reduce your belly fat and lower your risk of diabetes. If you already have diabetes, quitting can help you keep your blood sugar levels in check.

Normal Estrogen Levels

If you are a woman, your estrogen levels will gradually return to normal after you quit smoking. And if you hope to have children someday, quitting smoking right now will increase your chances of a healthy pregnancy in the future.

Erectile Dysfunction

Sexual Healing

If you quit smoking now, you can lower your chances of erectile dysfunction and improve your chances of having a healthy sexual life.

Blood and the Immune System

Normal White Blood Cell Count

When you quit smoking, your body will begin to heal from the injuries that smoking causes. Eventually, your white blood cell counts will return to normal and will no longer be on the defensive.

Proper Healing

Quitting smoking will improve blood flow to wounds, allowing important nutrients, minerals, and oxygen to reach the wound and help it heal properly.

Stronger Immune System

When you quit smoking, your immune system is no longer exposed to tar and nicotine. It will become stronger, and you will be less likely to get sick.

Muscles and Bones

Strong Muscles

Quitting smoking will help increase the availability of oxygen in your blood, and your muscles will become stronger and healthier.

Stronger Bones

Quitting smoking can reduce your risk of fractures, both now and later in life. Keep your bones strong and healthy by quitting now.

How Smoking Affects Your Workout

When you smoke, you harm your ability to exercise and be physically fit. Smoking hurts your athletic performance in several ways.

Blood

The nicotine and carbon monoxide from smoking may make your blood "sticky," and your arteries may become narrow. Narrow arteries reduce the flow of blood to your heart, muscles, and other body organs, making exercise harder. During exercise, blood flow helps boost the oxygen supply to your muscles. If your muscles do not get oxygen fast enough, your body cannot work as well.

Heart

Smoking increases your resting heart rate. Your resting heart rate is how many beats per minute your heart produces when you are not being active. When you smoke, this number is increased because of the extra work your heart has to do to keep your body going. Your heart rate could possibly rise to dangerous levels to perform the physical activities you are asking your heart to do. A higher-than-normal resting heart rate can increase the risk of death.

Lungs

You are able to exercise better when your lung capacity is good and your lungs work well. Smoking hurts your lung capacity. The tar in cigarette smoke coats your lungs and makes the air sacs less elastic. Smoking also produces phlegm that can make your lungs congested. Smoking even a few cigarettes a day can decrease your body's ability to use oxygen effectively.

Use Exercise to Help You Quit

Exercise can be an important part of your plan to quit smoking. Exercise reduces cravings, helps you manage other withdrawal symptoms, and reduces stress. Plus, when you quit, your heart rate will decrease; your blood circulation will increase; and your lung function will improve—making your workout performance better, too.

Secondhand Smoke

Smoking harms both you and the ones you love. Quitting smoking will benefit you plus help you protect the people in your life.

Quitting will make the people you care about happier and healthier. This may be one of your reasons for quitting.

Dangers of Secondhand Smoke

The main way smoking hurts nonsmokers is through secondhand smoke. Secondhand smoke is the combination of smoke that comes from a cigarette and smoke breathed out by a smoker. When a nonsmoker is around someone smoking, they breathe in secondhand smoke.

Secondhand smoke is dangerous to anyone who breathes it in. It can stay in the air for several hours after somebody smokes. Breathing secondhand smoke for even a short time can hurt your body.

Health Effects of Secondhand Smoke

Over time, secondhand smoke has been associated with serious health problems in nonsmokers:

- lung cancer in people who have never smoked
- more likely that someone will get heart disease, have a heart attack, and die early
- breathing problems, such as coughing, extra phlegm, wheezing, and shortness of breath

Secondhand smoke is especially dangerous for children, babies, and women who are pregnant:

- Mothers who breathe secondhand smoke while pregnant are more likely to have babies with low birth weight.
- Babies who breathe secondhand smoke after birth have more lung infections than other babies.
- Secondhand smoke causes kids who already have asthma to have more frequent and severe attacks.
- Children exposed to secondhand smoke are more likely to develop bronchitis, pneumonia, and ear infections and are at increased risk for sudden infant death syndrome (SIDS).

The only way to fully protect nonsmokers from the dangers of secondhand smoke is to not allow smoking indoors. Separating smokers from nonsmokers (such as "no smoking" sections in restaurants), cleaning the air, and airing out buildings do not get rid of secondhand smoke.

Other Ways Smoking Affects Others

Smoking affects the people in your life in other ways, beyond their health. When you smoke, you may miss out on:

- spending time with family and friends
- having more money to spend on the people you love
- setting a good example for your children (Children who are raised by smokers are more likely to become smokers themselves.)

Steps You Can Take to Protect Your Loved Ones

The best thing you can do to protect your family from secondhand smoke is to quit smoking. Right away, you get rid of their exposure to secondhand smoke in your home and car and reduce it anywhere else you go together.

Make sure your house and car remain smoke-free. Kids breathe in secondhand smoke at home more than any other place. The same goes for many adults. Do not allow anyone to smoke in your home or car. Setting this rule will:

- reduce the amount of secondhand smoke your family breathes in
- help you quit smoking and stay smoke-free
- lower the chance of your child becoming a smoker

When you are on the go, you can still protect your family from secondhand smoke:

- Make sure caretakers, such as nannies, babysitters, and day care staff do not smoke.
- Eat at smoke-free restaurants.
- Avoid indoor public places that allow smoking.
- Teach your children to stay away from secondhand smoke.[1]

[1] Smokefree.gov, "Reasons to Quit," U.S. Department of Health and Human Services (HHS), August 16, 2023. Available online. URL: https://smokefree.gov/quit-smoking/why-you-should-quit. Accessed October 6, 2023.

CHAPTER 55
BEHAVIORAL THERAPIES FOR TOBACCO DEPENDENCE

Behavioral counseling is typically provided by specialists in smoking cessation for four to eight sessions. Both in-person and telephone counseling have been found beneficial for patients who are also using cessation medications. A variety of approaches to smoking cessation counseling are available.

Cognitive Behavioral Therapy

Cognitive behavioral therapy (CBT) helps patients identify triggers—the people, places, and things that spur behavior—and teaches them relapse-prevention skills (e.g., relaxation techniques) and effective coping strategies to avoid smoking in the face of stressful situations and triggers. A study that compared CBT and basic health education observed that both interventions reduced nicotine dependence. However, another study found that among smokers trying to quit with the nicotine replacement therapy (NRT) patch, patients who participated in six sessions of intensive group CBT had better quit rates than those who received six sessions of general health education.

Motivational Interviewing

In motivational interviewing (MI), counselors help patients explore and resolve their ambivalence about quitting smoking and enhance their motivation to make healthy changes. MI is patient-focused and nonconfrontational, and providers point out discrepancies between patients' goals or values and their current behaviors. They adjust to patients, resistance to change, and support self-efficacy and optimism. Studies of MI suggest that this intervention results in higher quit rates than brief advice to stop smoking or usual care.

Mindfulness

In mindfulness-based smoking cessation treatments, patients learn to increase awareness of and detachment from sensations, thoughts, and cravings that may lead to relapse. In this therapy, patients purposely attend to the thoughts that trigger cravings and urges for tobacco and cognitively reframe them as expected and tolerable. Patients learn techniques that help them tolerate negative emotions—including stress and cravings—without returning to tobacco use or other unhealthy behaviors. Interest in mindfulness-based treatments has increased during the past decade, and studies show that this approach benefits overall mental health and can help prevent relapse to smoking. However, well-controlled clinical trials are needed.

Smoking Cessation for Pregnant Women

Given the risks associated with smoking during pregnancy but also the challenges faced by all smokers when trying to quit, researchers have studied an array of approaches to improve cessation rates for this population. Many women are motivated to quit during pregnancy, but like other smokers, most will need assistance.

Studies show that behavioral treatments are effective, whereas pharmacotherapies have only marginal success. A combination of incentives and behavioral counseling is most effective for pregnant women. Adding vouchers to routine care (which included free NRT for 10 weeks and four weekly support phone calls) more than doubled cessation rates during pregnancy. Pooled results of behavioral intervention studies indicate that treatment reduced preterm births and the proportion of infants born with low birth weight, compared with usual care. This finding is supported by an analysis of pooled results from studies with economically disadvantaged pregnant smokers, which found that voucher-based incentives improved sonographically estimated fetal growth, birth weight, percentage of low-birth-weight deliveries, and breastfeeding duration.

Source: "What Are Treatments for Tobacco Dependence," National Institute on Drug Abuse (NIDA), May 2022. Available online. URL: https://nida.nih.gov/publications/research-reports/tobacco-nicotine-e-cigarettes/what-are-treatments-tobacco-dependence. Accessed October 6, 2023.

Telephone Support and Quitlines

As part of tobacco control efforts, all states offer toll-free telephone numbers (or quitlines) with smoking cessation counselors who provide information and support (800-QUIT-NOW or 800-784-8669). Studies of quitline interventions indicate that smokers who call quitlines benefit from these services, 179 particularly when a counselor calls them back for multiple sessions. There is limited evidence on the optimal number of calls needed, but smokers who participated in three or more calls had a greater likelihood of quitting, compared with those who only received educational materials, brief advice, or pharmacotherapy alone. Quitlines have also been shown to help smokeless tobacco cessation. The U.S. Department of Health and Human Services (HHS) provides a smoking quitline (877-44U-QUIT or 877-448-7848), as well as more information and tools for quitting (including text messages and other telephone-based support) at https://smokefree.gov.

Text Messaging, Web-Based Services, and Social Media Support

Technology, including mobile phones, the Internet, and social media platforms can be used to provide smoking cessation interventions. These technologies have the power to increase access to care by extending the work of counselors and overcoming the geographical barriers that may deter people from entering treatment.

A review of the literature on technology-based smoking cessation interventions (Internet, personal computer, and mobile telephone) found that these supports can increase the likelihood of adults quitting, compared with no intervention or self-help information, and they can be a cost-effective adjunct to other treatments. Technology does not necessarily have to be recent or highly sophisticated to help boost cessation rates. For example, studies suggest that adults who receive encouragement, advice, and quitting tips via text message—a capability on even the most basic mobile devices—show improved quit rates compared with control programs.

Among adult tobacco users who called a "state quitline," most selected an integrated phone/web cessation program in favor of a web-only intervention. Participants who chose the web-only option tended to be younger and healthier smokers, with a higher socioeconomic status. These participants tended to interact intensely with the site once but did not reengage as much as those who opted for the phone/web combination. A review of Internet-based smoking cessation programs for adults suggested that interactive Internet-based interventions that are tailored to individual needs can help people quit for six months or longer. Future research should determine the effectiveness of different technologies for smoking cessation support among populations that may be hard to reach, including those of low socioeconomic status and adults older than age 50.

Technology-based cessation interventions are particularly relevant to young adults aged 18–25—about 3.2 million of whom smoked daily in 2016. A systematic review and meta-analysis of published randomized trials of technology-based interventions—including computer programs, Internet, telephone, and text messaging—for smoking cessation among this population found that they increased abstinence by 1.5 times that of comparison subjects. Researchers recommend embedding cessation interventions in commonly used social networking platforms, and there has been some exploratory work in this area. Results of a trial with a relatively small number of participants suggested that Facebook was an accessible, low-cost platform for engaging young adults considering cessation. However, the study pointed to challenges in maintaining participation, retaining young people in the program, and the need for gender-specific features. A randomized controlled trial (RCT) has been designed to test a stage-based smoking cessation intervention on Facebook tailored for smokers aged 18–25. Participants will be recruited online, will be randomly assigned to a Facebook group according to their readiness to quit, and will receive tailored daily messages and weekly counseling. The study will assess the intervention's effect on abstinence from smoking 3, 6, and 12 months after treatment; number of cigarettes smoked; quit attempts lasting 24 hours or more; and commitment to abstinence.[1]

[1] "What Are Treatments for Tobacco Dependence," National Institute on Drug Abuse (NIDA), May 2022. Available online. URL: https://nida.nih.gov/publications/research-reports/tobacco-nicotine-e-cigarettes/what-are-treatments-tobacco-dependence. Accessed October 6, 2023.

CHAPTER 56

PHARMACOLOGICAL TREATMENTS FOR TOBACCO DEPENDENCE

There are effective treatments that support tobacco cessation, including both behavioral therapies and U.S. Food and Drug Administration (FDA)-approved medications. The FDA-approved pharmacotherapies include various forms of nicotine replacement therapy (NRT) as well as bupropion and varenicline. Research indicates that smokers who receive a combination of behavioral treatment and cessation medications quit at higher rates than those who receive minimal intervention. Interventions, such as brief advice from a health-care worker, telephone helplines, automated text messaging, and printed self-help materials can also facilitate smoking cessation. Cessation interventions utilizing mobile devices and social media also show promise in boosting tobacco cessation. It is important for cessation treatment to be as personalized as possible, as some people smoke to avoid the negative effects of withdrawal while others are more driven by the rewarding aspects of smoking.

The prevalence of tobacco use and dependence among adolescents—as well as the neurobiological effect and medical consequences of nicotine exposure—suggest that pediatric primary care settings should deliver tobacco cessation treatments to both youth and parents who use tobacco. Clinical guidance does not recommend medications for adolescent tobacco cessation because of a lack of high-quality studies; however, a combination of behavioral treatments—such as motivational enhancement and cognitive behavioral therapy (CBT)—has shown promise for helping adolescents quit tobacco. More well-designed smoking cessation studies need to be conducted with adolescent smokers, particularly in the area of pharmacologic treatments for nicotine dependence.

Medications

Nicotine replacement therapy—A variety of formulations of nicotine NRTs are available over the counter (OTC)—including the transdermal patch, spray, gum, and lozenges—and are equally effective for cessation. NRTs stimulate the brain receptors targeted by nicotine, helping relieve nicotine withdrawal symptoms and cravings that lead to relapse. Many people use NRT to help them get through the early stages of cessation, and those with more severe nicotine addiction can benefit from longer-term treatment. The use of NRT improves smoking cessation outcomes, and adding behavioral therapies further increases quit rates. A combination of continual nicotine delivery through the transdermal patch and one other form of nicotine taken as needed (e.g., lozenge, gum, nasal spray, inhaler) has been found to be more effective at relieving withdrawal symptoms and cravings than a single type of NRT. Researchers estimate that NRT increases quit rates by 50–70 percent. Using the patch for up to 24 weeks has been shown to be safe.

Bupropion

Bupropion (immediate-release and extended-release) was originally approved as an antidepressant. It works by inhibiting the reuptake of the brain chemicals norepinephrine and dopamine as well as stimulating their release. Bupropion has been found to increase quit rates compared with placebo in both short- and long-term follow-up studies and is indicated for smoking cessation. It is equally effective as NRT.

Varenicline

Varenicline helps reduce nicotine cravings by stimulating the alpha-4 beta-2 nicotinic receptor but to a lesser degree than nicotine. Varenicline boosts the odds of successfully quitting, compared with unassisted attempts. Varenicline increased the likelihood of quitting compared with placebo, and some studies find that it is more effective than single forms of NRT, and bupropion. In a primary care setting, 44 percent of patients on varenicline, either alone or combined with counseling, were abstinent at the two-year follow-up. Patients who participated in group therapy and adhered to the medication were more likely to remain abstinent. Research also suggests that this medication may be more effective than bupropion.

Medication Combinations

Some studies suggest that combining NRT with other medications may facilitate cessation. For example, a meta-analysis found that a combination of varenicline and NRT (especially, providing a nicotine patch prior to cessation) was more effective than varenicline alone. Similarly, adding bupropion to NRT also improved cessation rates. For smokers who could not cut down significantly by using the NRT patch, combining extended-release bupropion and varenicline was more effective than placebo, particularly for men and those who were severely nicotine dependent.

Other Antidepressants

In addition to bupropion, some other antidepressant medications have also been found effective for smoking cessation, independent of their antidepressant effects, and are considered second-line treatments. A few small studies suggest that nortriptyline is equally effective as NRT. Although nortriptyline may have side effects in some patients, the small studies on its use in smoking cessation have not reported any. Researchers have not observed any effect of selective serotonin reuptake inhibitors (SSRIs) (e.g., fluoxetine, paroxetine, and sertraline) on smoking, either alone or in combination with NRT.

Precision Medicine

Researchers have been examining ways to personalize treatment-based on important individual biological differences, including genetic differences. The field of pharmacogenetics examines how genes influence therapeutic response to medications, providing critical information to help tailor pharmacotherapies to the individual for maximum benefit. For example, people metabolize nicotine at different rates because of variations in several genes. Individuals who metabolize nicotine quickly smoke more, show greater dependence, and have more difficulty quitting. Such genetic variation influences the therapeutic responses to NRT and other cessation medications. A study compared rates of abstinence one week after treatment for slow, normal, and fast metabolizers of nicotine who were randomly assigned to either placebo, NRT, or varenicline. Results indicated that varenicline worked best for normal nicotine metabolizers, whereas NRT patches were most effective for slow metabolizers.

Promising Medications and Ongoing Research

The National Institute on Drug Abuse (NIDA) supports research to develop new and improve treatment options for smoking cessation based on a growing understanding of the neurobiology of addiction. In the area of medications, research is focusing on the receptors targeted by nicotine and the brain circuits and regions known to influence nicotine consumption. Newer brain targets—including the orexin and glutamate signaling systems—have also shown promise for medication treatment. Repurposing medications already on the market for other indications may also prove useful in the search for new smoking cessation therapies. This approach has been successful in the past, as bupropion was an established antidepressant before the FDA approved it as a smoking cessation medication. One current candidate is N-acetylcysteine, a medication for acetaminophen overdose, which has shown promise as a treatment for various substance use disorders—including nicotine dependence. Another approach that could prevent relapse and that has shown promise in early studies is a nicotine vaccine, which would generate antibodies that keep nicotine from reaching the brain.

Transcranial Magnetic Stimulation

Transcranial magnetic stimulation (TMS) is a relatively new approach being tested to treat addiction. It is a physiological intervention that noninvasively stimulates neural activity in targeted areas of the brain using magnetic fields. Multiple TMS pulses given consecutively are referred to as "repetitive TMS" (rTMS). The FDA has approved two rTMS devices for depression treatment in adults.

Research on rTMS as a treatment for smoking cessation is in the early stages but has shown promise. Among adult smokers who had not been able to quit using other treatments, high-frequency TMS treatment significantly reduced the number of cigarettes smoked. Combining high-frequency TMS with exposure to smoking cues improved effectiveness and boosted the overall abstinence rate to 44 percent at the end of the treatment. Six months after treatment, 33 percent of participants remained abstinent from cigarettes. Future randomized controlled clinical trials with large numbers of patients will be needed to establish its efficacy for smoking cessation.[1]

[1] "What Are Treatments for Tobacco Dependence," National Institute on Drug Abuse (NIDA), May 2022. Available online. URL: https://nida.nih.gov/publications/research-reports/tobacco-nicotine-e-cigarettes/what-are-treatments-tobacco-dependence. Accessed October 6, 2023.

CHAPTER 57
NICOTINE REPLACEMENT THERAPY

Many people use quit smoking medications to help reduce withdrawal feelings and cigarette cravings. Quit smoking medications can double your chances of quitting for good.

Nicotine replacement therapy (NRT) is the most commonly used family of quit smoking medications. NRT reduces withdrawal feelings by giving you a small controlled amount of nicotine but none of the other dangerous chemicals found in cigarettes. This small amount of nicotine helps satisfy your craving for nicotine and reduces the urge to smoke.

Doctors and other medical experts think NRT is one of the most helpful tools smokers can use to quit. Some smokers have mild-to-moderate side effects. However, research shows that NRT is safe and effective. NRT can be an important part of almost every smoker's quit smoking strategy.

The NRT comes in a variety of forms that are used in different ways (see Table 57.1). You can choose which forms you like best. Some NRT products work better than others for some people. Some people might prefer certain NRT products instead of others.

Combining Nicotine Replacement Therapy with Other Strategies

The NRT cannot do all the work. It can help with withdrawal and cravings, but it would not completely take away the urge to smoke. Even if you use NRT to help you stop smoking, quitting can still be hard. Combining NRT with other strategies can improve your chances of quitting and staying quit. To give yourself the best chance for success, explore other quit methods you can combine with medication. Also, think about:

- developing a quit plan
- using quit programs, such as SmokefreeTXT (sign up online or text QUIT to 47848)
- calling a quitline
- using the QuitGuide app for tips and inspiration to help you be smoke-free[1]

---

[1] Smokefree.gov, "Using Nicotine Replacement Therapy," U.S. Department of Health and Human Services (HHS), May 28, 2016. Available online. URL: https://smokefree.gov/tools-tips/how-to-quit/using-nicotine-replacement-therapy. Accessed October 6, 2023.

Table 57.1. Types of Nicotine Replacement Therapy

NRT Types	How to Get Them	How to Use Them
Patch	Over the counter	• Place on the skin. • It gives a small and steady amount of nicotine.
Gum	Over the counter	• Chew to release nicotine. • Chew until you get a tingling feeling, then place between cheek and gums.
Lozenge	Over the counter	• Place in the mouth like hard candy. • It releases nicotine as it slowly dissolves in the mouth.
Inhaler	Prescription	• A cartridge is attached to a mouthpiece. • Inhaling through the mouthpiece gives a specific amount of nicotine.
Nasal spray	Prescription	• Pump bottle containing nicotine. • Put into the nose and spray.

Busting Nicotine Replacement Therapy Myths

- **Myth**: NRT does not work.
  Truth: NRT works. NRT can double a smoker's chances of quitting smoking for good.
  Many smokers find NRT helpful for quitting. Every person is different. It might be worth trying NRT to see if it is right for you. Even if you tried NRT before, it might be worth trying again. NRT will help you the most if you follow directions carefully. Use enough and use it for the recommended time. Other medications and strategies are also available to help you quit smoking.
- **Myth**: If I use NRT, I would not have withdrawal symptoms or cravings from quitting smoking.
  Truth: You may still have withdrawal symptoms or cravings while using NRT. Try to be patient. Most people find withdrawal symptoms especially difficult the first week or two after quitting. Most smokers find withdrawal symptoms less intense when using NRT. If withdrawal symptoms continue a few days after you start using NRT, talk to your doctor or pharmacist about different NRT products that can help.
  Follow NRT product directions carefully. Some NRT products (gum, lozenge, and inhaler) work better if they are not used at the same time as high-acid drinks, such as sodas and fruit juices. It is safe to continue using NRT even if you slip and smoke one or two cigarettes. Staying on NRT increases your chances of getting back on track for quitting.
- **Myth**: If I use one NRT product, I cannot use others.
  Truth: NRT products can be used safely together. For example, you might use long-acting NRT such as the patch with short-acting NRT such as a lozenge. Some people find both a long-acting patch and short-acting gum to be useful when cravings are high to handle withdrawal symptoms and fight off cravings.

- **Myth**: NRT is too expensive.
  Truth: Many states in the United States offer free NRT through their state quitlines. The North American Quitline Consortium has a quitline map to help you find free quit smoking support and other resources near you.
  People eligible for Medicare or Medicaid may also be eligible for free NRT. In recent years, insurance coverage for NRT has expanded under many private insurance plans. Check your insurance plan to learn if you are eligible for coverage.
  Even if NRT is not covered through your insurance or state quitline, the cost of NRT for several weeks will still be less than the cost of buying cigarettes.
- **Myth**: Some people should not use NRT.
  Truth: NRT has been available for more than 30 years. A great deal of research has been done on NRT. The research shows that NRT is safe and effective for almost all adults for quitting smoking. For most people, there is no need to talk to a doctor or health-care provider before using NRT.
  Pregnant women, teens, and people with serious health issues should talk to their doctor before using NRT. Serious health issues can include lung disease and heart problems. People with these problems might still be able to use NRT but should talk to their doctor first.[2]

[2] Smokefree.gov, "Busting NRT Myths," U.S. Department of Health and Human Services (HHS), May 28, 2016. Available online. URL: https://smokefree.gov/tools-tips/how-to-quit/busting-nrt-myths. Accessed October 6, 2023.

CHAPTER 58

UNDERSTANDING AND MANAGING NICOTINE WITHDRAWAL

Nicotine withdrawal is challenging for most smokers. The good news is that the worst withdrawal symptoms usually last less than two weeks, but that time can be really tough. Know what to expect when going through nicotine withdrawal and get ideas for easing your symptoms.[1]

Managing Your Nicotine Withdrawal Symptoms

Some days may be a breeze, while others are harder to handle after you quit smoking. Over time, the cravings and other symptoms will fade as long as you stay smoke-free. Quit smoking medications can help reduce symptoms of nicotine withdrawal and make quitting easier. Noticing your symptoms, finding strategies to address them that work for you, or trying a quit smoking medication can ease these uncomfortable feelings.

Common Nicotine Withdrawal Symptoms and What You Can Do about Them

- **Having cravings for cigarettes**. Most people experience cravings after they quit. These thoughts and feelings can range from mild to intense or even overwhelming. When cravings are tough to handle, it is important to remember that quitting smoking is the best action you can take for your health. Plan ahead for how you will get through cravings to help you manage them more successfully. The good news is that every craving will pass if you give it time.
    - **Make a quit plan**. Think ahead about ways you will manage your cravings to help you get through them when they happen.

[1] Smokefree.gov, "Nicotine Withdrawal," U.S. Department of Health and Human Services (HHS), September 5, 2023. Available online. URL: https://smokefree.gov/challenges-when-quitting/withdrawal. Accessed October 3, 2023.

    - **Distract yourself**. Do things to distract yourself, practice mindfulness, and remember your reasons for why you want to quit to keep you focused on your goal.
    - **Know your triggers**. Cravings and thoughts about smoking can be triggered by the people you spend time with, the places you go, and the situations you encounter. Avoid your triggers, at least temporarily, after you quit to help lessen your cravings and give you time to build confidence and skills for remaining smoke-free, even when you do encounter triggers.
    - **Get text message support**. Text the keyword CRAVE to 47848 to get 24/7 immediate support whenever you have a craving or text QUIT to 47848 to sign up for SmokefreeTXT, a six-to-eight-week program of daily text message support, tips, and encouragement.
    - **Try a quit smoking medication**. If nicotine withdrawal symptoms are difficult for you, nicotine replacement therapy or prescription quit smoking medications can make these symptoms easier to handle. Talk to a health-care provider about what medications might work best for you.
    - **Use a free Smokefree.gov app**. Track your cravings and understand your smoking patterns with one of the Smokefree.gov apps.
- **Feeling irritable or grouchy**. Change is often hard and can make people feel out of sorts. Remember that you are doing a very good thing for yourself by quitting smoking. Stick with your commitment to quit now, and it will help your withdrawal symptoms get easier more quickly.
- **Having trouble sleeping**. Getting good quality sleep is important, especially when you quit smoking. When you are tired, you are less resilient and may be more likely to slip and return to smoking. Try the following steps to help:
    - Go to bed and wake up at the same time every day.
    - Keep your phone, television, and other screens out of your bedroom.
    - Limit caffeine, alcohol, and big meals close to bedtime.
    - Ask your heath-care provider for advice if you use quit smoking medications and they are affecting your sleep.
- **Having trouble thinking clearly or concentrating**. Some people notice that it is harder to concentrate or that their brain feels foggy in the days after they quit. If you feel this way, know that this too shall pass. If you are not currently using a quit smoking medication, consider trying one to help ease your symptoms.
- **Feeling restless or jumpy**. If you have restless energy or feel on edge, try getting some physical activity to release the tension. You do not have to be an athlete or even get to a gym. Just going for a walk or doing yard work or chores can be helpful. If you drink coffee, tea, or other caffeinated drinks, try to cut back for a while to lessen the symptoms.
- **Feeling sad, anxious, or depressed**. People who smoke are more likely to have anxiety or depression than people who do not smoke. And some people feel

increased anxiety, sadness, or depression after they quit smoking. Watch out for this, especially if you have ever had these symptoms before. Take a quick quiz to find out if you have signs of depression. There are resources available to help you:

- If you feel down or sad, do something positive such as participating in hobbies or activities that make you feel good, exercising, or reaching out to supportive people in your life. You can also:
    - call a trained tobacco counselor at 800-QUIT-NOW (800-784-8669)
    - reach out to other people trying to quit smoking on our Smokefree.gov social media channels
    - chat with a trained quit smoking counselor (LiveHelp is available Monday through Friday, 9:00 a.m. to 9:00 p.m. Eastern time.)
- If your feelings worsen or do not go away, tell a friend or family member and talk to a health-care professional. If you or someone you know is in distress or having suicidal thoughts, get help now. Call or text 988 or chat online to receive 24-hour, free, confidential support from trained counselors.

- **Feeling hungrier**. As your body adjusts to a new and healthier normal after quitting, you may find that you feel hungrier. Keep a stash of healthy snacks handy. Crunchy snacks such as carrots or raw nuts can also help combat cravings by keeping your hands and mouth busy. You may also be worried about weight gain after quitting. For those who do gain weight, it can be disappointing, but it is important to remember that quitting smoking adds years to your life and reduces your risk for serious diseases and poor health outcomes.[2]

[2] Smokefree.gov, "Managing Nicotine Withdrawal," U.S. Department of Health and Human Services (HHS), March 9, 2023. Available online. URL: https://smokefree.gov/challenges-when-quitting/withdrawal/managing-nicotine-withdrawal. Accessed October 3, 2023.

CHAPTER 59
MANAGING TOBACCO CRAVINGS

Understanding the Triggers

Triggers are the things that make you want to smoke. Different people have different triggers, such as a stressful situation, sipping coffee, going to a party, or smelling cigarette smoke.

Most triggers fall into one of the following four categories:

- emotional
- pattern
- social
- withdrawal

Knowing your triggers and understanding the best way to deal with them is your first line of defense.

Emotional Triggers

Many people smoke when they have intense emotions. An emotional trigger reminds you how you felt when you used smoking to enhance a good mood or escape a bad one, such as when you were:

- stressed
- anxious
- excited
- bored
- down
- happy
- lonely
- satisfied
- cooled off after a fight

How to Deal with Emotional Triggers

You can learn how to cope with your feelings without leaning on cigarettes. Try the following ways to deal with emotional triggers:

- **Talk about your emotions**. Telling a friend or family member how you feel can help.
- **Take some slow, deep breaths**. Deep breathing will slow down your body, quiet your mind, and reduce cravings. This is also a great way to manage stress and anxiety.
- **Exercise**. Physical activity is a great way to handle emotions. When you exercise, your brain releases endorphins. Endorphins are chemicals in the brain that make you feel good.
- **Listen to calming music**. Music can relax you by slowing your heart rate, lowering blood pressure, and decreasing stress hormones.

> **Feeling Irritated, Grouchy, or Upset**
>
> It is very common to feel irritated or grouchy when you quit. Even many people who have never smoked know this is part of quitting. Knowing this is normal can be helpful.
>
> **Ways to Manage**
>
> Remind yourself that you likely feel this way because your body is getting used to being without nicotine. Take a few deep breaths and remind yourself why you are quitting.
>
> *Source:* "7 Common Withdrawal Symptoms," Centers for Disease Control and Prevention (CDC), December 12, 2022. Available online. URL: www.cdc.gov/tobacco/campaign/tips/quit-smoking/7-common-withdrawal-symptoms/index.html. Accessed October 9, 2023.

Pattern Triggers

A pattern trigger is an activity that you connect with smoking. Some examples of these activities are as follows:

- talking on the phone
- drinking alcohol
- watching TV
- driving
- finishing a meal
- drinking coffee
- taking a work break
- after having sex
- before going to bed

How to Deal with Pattern Triggers

One way to beat pattern triggers is to break the association with the trigger and transfer the feeling to another activity.

- **Find a replacement**. Chew gum. Eat sugar-free candy. Suck on a straw.
- **Try activities that keep your hands busy**. Squeeze a handball. Do beading or needlework. Hold on to a silver dollar or "worry stone."
- **Get moving**. Go for a walk. Ride a bike. Go swimming. Exercising can distract you from smoking.
- **Change your routine**. For example, try drinking your coffee at a different time or brushing your teeth right after you eat a meal.

Social Triggers

Social triggers are occasions that usually include other people who smoke. Here are some examples:

- going to a bar
- going to a party or other social event
- going to a concert
- seeing someone else smoke
- being with friends who smoke
- celebrating a big event

How to Deal with Social Triggers

Once you have made the decision to quit, it is best to avoid places where people smoke and ask your friends not to smoke around you. Over time, it will get easier. Tell your friends and family that you have quit. Ask them for their support.

Withdrawal Triggers

If you have been a longtime smoker, your body is used to getting a regular dose of nicotine. When you quit, withdrawal symptoms will produce cravings for nicotine. Withdrawal triggers include:

- craving the taste of a cigarette
- smelling cigarette smoke
- handling cigarettes, lighters, and matches
- needing to do something with your hands or mouth
- feeling restless or having other withdrawal symptoms

How to Deal with Withdrawal Triggers

- **Distract yourself**. Find something to take your mind off the craving. See if nicotine replacement therapy (NRT) is right for you—it can reduce withdrawal symptoms. Teens, women who are pregnant, and people with severe medical conditions should talk to their doctor before using NRT.

- **Understand triggers**. Identify the ones that you want to control and make a plan to manage your cravings.[1]

How to Manage Cravings

You would not be able to avoid all of your triggers. And learning how to deal with triggers takes practice. So, when a craving is triggered, it is important to have a plan to beat that urge to smoke.

Cravings are uncomfortable, but they do not last forever. Having a list of strategies can help you get through it. Here are a few to try.

Get Support

- **Call or text someone**. You do not have to do this alone. Learn how to lean on people you trust.
- **Try SmokefreeTXT**. Sign up online or text QUIT to 47848 to get 24/7 support sent right to your phone.
- **Download a smartphone app**. The free apps help you track cravings and understand your smoking patterns.
- **Visit Smokefree on social media**. Grow your support network and stay connected.
- **Talk to an expert at a quitline**. Call the National Cancer Institute (NCI) Quitline at 877-44U-QUIT (877-448-7848), Monday through Friday, from 9:00 a.m. to 9:00 p.m. or find your state's quitline by calling 800-QUIT-NOW (800-784-8669).
- **Chat with a counselor**. Get real-time help from the NCI's LiveHelp online chat.

Think about Your Reasons for Quitting

- **Review your reasons**. Remind yourself why you want to quit. This can be a powerful motivator to keep you smoke-free.
- **Calculate your savings**. Cigarettes are expensive. Add up the money you will save and decide what to do with it. This is a great way to stay motivated and kill time while you let a craving pass.

Stay Busy

- **Keep your mouth busy**. Chew a stick of gum instead of picking up a cigarette. Keep hard candy with you. Drink more water.
- **Do something else**. When a craving hits, stop what you are doing immediately and switch to doing something different. Simply changing your routine might help you shake off a craving.
- **Go for a walk or jog**. Or go up and down the stairs a few times. Physical activity, even in short bursts, can help boost your energy and beat a craving.

[1] Smokefree.gov, "Know Your Triggers," U.S. Department of Health and Human Services (HHS), May 9, 2016. Available online. URL: www.smokefree.gov/challenges-when-quitting/cravings-triggers/know-your-triggers. Accessed October 9, 2023.

- **Take slow, deep breaths**. Breathe through your craving. Inhale through your nose and exhale through your mouth. Repeat this 10 times or until you are feeling more relaxed.

Go to a Smoke-Free Zone

- **Visit a public place**. Most public places do not allow smoking. Go to a movie, a store, or another place where you cannot smoke.
- **Practice what you already do**. What have you done before when you found yourself in a smoke-free place? Tap into that same approach when your next craving comes along.

Try Nicotine Replacement Therapy

Even if you use NRT, you might have a craving that is difficult to deal with. Think about trying a short-acting NRT, such as a lozenge or gum, plus a long-acting NRT, such as the patch, to get past the craving.

Do a Good Deed

Try distracting yourself for a few minutes by being helpful to a friend, family member, or coworker. This takes the focus off yourself and how you are feeling and instead allows you to think of another person's needs. It can be a helpful way to cope with a craving until it passes. Plus, doing good deeds can have positive effects on your health, such as reducing stress. Managing stress can be a key part of quitting smoking.

Use of the Four Ds Can Help You Cope with Cravings

- **Drink water**. Drink six to eight glasses of water every day.
- **Take a deep breath**. Try a few deep breaths when you get the urge to smoke.
- **Delay smoking**. Most urges to smoke only last a few minutes at a time. Try this meditation to help resist the immediate urge to smoke.
- **Distract yourself**. Do anything to keep yourself from smoking. Here are a few suggestions:
  - Read a magazine or complete a crossword puzzle.
  - Change your routines. Sit in a different chair or take a walk after meals and on work breaks. Small changes in routine can be a big help.
  - Keep smoking substitutes handy. Try carrots, sugarless gum, flavored toothpicks, or breath mints.
  - Exercise. Even a short walk will help.
  - Visit with a good friend, eat a meal out, see a movie, play with a pet, buy flowers, or read to a child.
  - Spend time in places where smoking is not allowed—libraries, museums, theaters, stores, places of worship, or nonsmoking places at work.

Source: Smokefree.gov, "Dealing with Withdrawal," U.S. Department of Health and Human Services (HHS), August 21, 2020. Available online. URL: www.60plus.smokefree.gov/quit-smoking-60plus/dealing-with-withdrawal. Accessed October 9, 2023.

Do Not Give Up

Do whatever it takes to beat the urge to smoke. Keep trying different things until you find what works for you. Just do not smoke, not even one puff.[2]

[2] Smokefree.gov, "How to Manage Cravings," U.S. Department of Health and Human Services (HHS), June 29, 2016. Available online. URL: www.smokefree.gov/challenges-when-quitting/cravings-triggers/know-your-triggers. Accessed October 9, 2023.

CHAPTER 60
FIGHTING CRAVINGS WITH EXERCISE

Having cravings for a cigarette is one of the most common symptoms of nicotine withdrawal when you quit smoking. It helps have a plan to manage cravings when they hit. Including exercise in your plan can help you get past cravings. Exercise can distract you and keep you busy until the craving passes.

Exercise has other benefits too:

- Studies show that even short periods of physical activity, especially aerobic exercise, reduce the urge to smoke. Aerobic exercise is a physical activity that makes you sweat, causes you to breathe harder, and gets your heart beating faster. It strengthens your heart and lungs. Walking, swimming, running, dancing, cycling, and boxing are a few types of aerobic exercise.
- Withdrawal symptoms and cravings for cigarettes decrease during exercise and up to 50 minutes after exercising.
- Exercise decreases appetite and helps limit the weight gain some people have when they quit smoking.
- Exercise helps you cope with stress and have more energy.
- Exercise can improve your mood. If you are feeling low, take a walk, jump rope, or run up and down the stairs.

Get Physical

Here are some tips to get you started with exercise and help you ride out cravings:

- Try to set aside a regular time for exercise that works with your schedule.
- Try for 30 minutes of physical activity most days of the week. Do not have 30 minutes? Studies show that exercising for 10 minutes three times a day gives the same benefits as 30 minutes of nonstop exercise.
- Do activities you enjoy. Walking is one way of getting more physical activity. You might also think about biking, swimming, dancing, or yoga. Even housework or gardening can provide exercise benefits. Playing music while you clean out your closets will help you step up the pace.

- Build exercise into other activities. Take the stairs at work instead of the elevator. At the mall, use the stairs instead of the escalator. Wherever you go, park your car farther away and walk to your destination.
- Plan activities with family, friends, or coworkers that include physical activity, maybe a hike or a volleyball game.
- Change your exercise routine or try a new activity from time to time, so you do not get bored.[1]

Ten-Minute Workout

Getting at least 10 minutes of continuous, moderate activity three times a day can give you the same health benefits as 30 minutes of nonstop exercise. Here are some ways to squeeze in 10-minute workouts:

- Walk up and down the stairs at work for 10 minutes.
- Start your day with 10 minutes of stretches or strengthening exercises, such as lunges and bicep curls.
- Search YouTube for short workout videos. You will find many quick routines for a variety of skill levels from beginner to advanced.
- Work off some of the stress of the day by exercising or dancing to your favorite music for 10 minutes.
- If you are on a long phone call, do 10 minutes of squats or calf raises to strengthen lower-body muscles.

Source: Smokefree Women, "Get Moving," U.S. Department of Health and Human Services (HHS), September 7, 2018. Available online. URL: https://women.smokefree.gov/live-healthier/care-for-your-body/get-moving. Accessed October 9, 2023.

Health Benefits of Exercising

No matter how old you are, regular physical activity can help you look younger and stay more fit than people who are not active. Regular exercise can also be good medicine in your fight to stay off cigarettes. You will sleep better, be less likely to gain weight, and have more energy.

Physical activity also helps:

- reduce high blood pressure (HBP)
- reduce the risk for type 2 diabetes, heart attack, stroke, and several forms of cancer
- reduce arthritis pain and related disability
- reduce the risk for brittle bones and falls
- reduce feelings of depression and anxiety

[1] Smokefree.gov, "Fight Cravings with Exercise," U.S. Department of Health and Human Services (HHS), September 7, 2016. Available online. URL: www.smokefree.gov/challenges-when-quitting/cravings-triggers/fight-cravings-exercise. Accessed October 9, 2023.

Should You Talk with Your Health-Care Provider before Doing Physical Activity?

Most people do not need to check with their health-care provider before doing physical activity. However, you may want to talk with your health-care provider if you are not used to energetic activity, and you want to start a vigorous exercise program or significantly increase your physical activity. Ask your health-care provider how physical activity can help you, whether you should avoid certain activities, and how to modify exercises to fit your situation.

If you already have a fitness routine, keep it up! If you have not started one yet, here are five steps to help you kick-start your new exercise routine.

The following are the five steps to help kick-start your new exercise routine:

- **Start moving**. Go for a walk. Walking is great for people of any age. It builds fitness, burns calories, and keeps your muscles and bones strong. Even small amounts of exercise can boost your health and your ability to quit smoking.
- **Try smaller goals first**. Starting with smaller goals can help you gain the confidence you need to develop an exercise routine you can stick with. Try going for a 10-minute walk two or three days a week or doing three or four strength-training exercises one day a week. As you reach your goals and you feel stronger, you can set new goals.
- **Alternate and try new activities**. Alternate your workout routine by doing strength-training exercises one day and cardiovascular exercises another day. Or try out new ways of exercising that sound like fun—such as finding a new hiking trail or checking out a water aerobics class. Invite a friend to join you. Mixing up your workouts allows your muscles to recover in between and keeps it fun!
- **Routine and consistency will help you stick with it**. Plan ahead. It is easy for exercise to take a back seat when you have so many other demands on your time and energy. Whether you like to exercise at the same time of the day or on the same days of the week or find that you need to be more flexible to fit exercise into your life, having a weekly plan will help you stick with it.
- **Track your activity**. Write down your physical activity goals and track your progress.[2]

[2] Smokefree.gov, "Stay Fit after You Quit," U.S. Department of Health and Human Services (HHS), August 21, 2020. Available online. URL: https://60plus.smokefree.gov/healthier-lifestyle/stay-fit-after-quit. Accessed October 9, 2023.

CHAPTER 61

MANAGING STRESS: A KEY PART OF QUITTING SMOKING

Causes of Stress

Smokers often deal with stress by smoking. Stress can be caused by anything from major life events to daily hassles that add up over time.

Facing a problem, trying to get a task done in a short time, or changing the way you live are just some challenges that might cause stress. The causes of stress are different for everybody.

Major Life Events

Stress can happen when life presents challenges. Big events or changes—such as serious illness, death of a family member, divorce, or losing your job—can cause stress. Even happy events—such as weddings, graduations, or the birth of a child—can be stressful.

Daily Hassles

Car trouble, fights with your partner, deadlines at work, traffic jams, bad weather, and home repairs are hassles that can happen on a regular basis. Dealing with many hassles can weigh you down and wear you out as much as one large stressor.

Knowing your stressors is an important step in finding ways to deal with them. Take a quick stress quiz to help you learn the stressors in your life. Explore ways to deal with stress without smoking.

Stress and Smoking

Some people smoke when they feel stressed. They use smoking as a way to cope. There are many problems with using cigarettes as a way to cope with stress or other unpleasant feelings.

- Smoking is not a long-term stress reliever. In the time it takes to smoke a cigarette, you could do something else that is more effective—such as taking a short walk or trying a relaxation exercise.
- Smoking does not solve the problem that is giving you stress. Your stress will return.
- Nicotine addiction causes stress. Cravings for nicotine feel stressful because your body begins to go through withdrawal.

Some smokers find it hard to give up cigarettes as a way to cope with stress. It is important to find healthy ways to handle stress and take care of yourself without smoking. There are many other ways to cope with stress that do not involve smoking.

Everyday Mindfulness

Practicing mindfulness involves breathing methods and other techniques, such as guided imagery, to relax the body and mind. Guided imagery allows you to use all your senses to direct your imagination to a relaxed, focused state. Mindfulness is a skill you can practice in all areas of your life. Mindfulness can:

- help you manage nicotine cravings or feelings of withdrawal when you are quitting smoking
- reduce stress, anxiety, and depression
- increase positive emotions and enjoyment in daily life
- encourage healthier eating habits
- improve relationships

If you have a busy schedule, it can be hard to slow down and notice the little things. A great way to start practicing mindfulness is to set aside time every day to slow down, pay attention to your breathing, and "reset" yourself. Setting aside even one minute, or several times a day, can have a big effect.

Source: Smokefree.gov, "Practice Mindfulness," U.S. Department of Health and Human Services (HHS), May 18, 2017. Available online. URL: https://smokefree.gov/challenges-when-quitting/stress/practice-mindfulness. Accessed October 10, 2023.

Handling Stress

Some people smoke to try to deal with stress. When they quit smoking, they may replace it with other unhealthy behaviors that do not address the source of stress and may even make stress worse. This can make quitting harder. Understand the connection between stress and smoking and plan ahead to find better ways to deal with stress while quitting and after.

Coping with Stress without Smoking

Stress is a normal part of life—in moderation, it can help you reach your goals, but too much stress creates more problems. Managing stress is a key part of quitting smoking.

You may have learned to deal with stress by smoking. But there are ways to handle stress without smoking. Here are a few ideas you might find helpful. Some of these tips may take practice, but others you can do right away. Try one or more to learn what works for you.

Relax

Our bodies respond to stress by releasing hormones that increase your heart rate and raise your blood pressure. Practicing relaxation techniques, such as the ones that follow, may improve your health and help you handle your stress in positive ways.

Breathe

Take a few slow, deep breaths in through your nose and out through your mouth. You will feel your body start to relax.

Locate Your Stress

Take a minute to figure out how stress affects your body. Where do you feel the tension in your body? Finding ways to reduce that tension will also help your mental stress. A warm bath, a massage, or stretching can help you release built-up tension.

Visualize

Think of a place where you feel safe, comfortable, and relaxed. Picture it as clearly as you can, including imagining what you would feel, hear, and maybe even smell if you were in that relaxing place. Let yourself enjoy being there for a few minutes.

Exercise

Being active sends out natural chemicals that help your mood and reduce your stress. Sometimes, a short walk is all it takes to relieve stress. And walking is free.

Talk

You do not have to deal with stress alone. Share your feelings with friends, family, and other important people in your life who are able to support you in staying smoke-free.

Focus

Life can sometimes be overwhelming. Try not to get caught up in worrying about what is next. Instead, try to focus on what is happening now, not what you might have to deal with in the future.

Care

Make an extra effort to take care of yourself. This includes basic things such as eating a balanced diet, drinking lots of water, and getting enough sleep.

Do Good

Doing something nice for others can make your day a little better, too. Being caring toward others helps you reduce your own stress.

Decaffeinate

Caffeine can help you stay awake, but it can also make you feel tense, jittery, and stressed. Cutting back or even doing away with caffeine can help reduce your feelings of stress. Switching to herbal tea or even hot water with lemon gives you a chance to enjoy a hot beverage but without the caffeine.

Accept

Life is full of twists and turns. You will always have some stress in your life. Acceptance helps understand that there will be good days and bad days.[1]

[1] Smokefree.gov, "Causes of Stress," U.S. Department of Health and Human Services (HHS), June 29, 2016. Available online. URL: www.smokefree.gov/challenges-when-quitting/stress/causes-of-stress. Accessed October 10, 2023.

CHAPTER 62
MANAGING MOOD SWINGS TO STAY QUIT

Managing Your Mood

Some smokers do not feel like themselves when they quit smoking. Cravings and nicotine withdrawal can affect your mood and make you feel sad, irritable, or anxious. Prepare yourself for mood changes. Learn smoke-free ways to cope with bad moods and how to recognize when a bad mood may be a sign of something more serious.

Smoking and Depression

Smokers are more likely to have depression than nonsmokers. Nobody knows for sure why this is. People who have depression might smoke to feel better. Or smokers might get depression more easily because they smoke. No matter what the cause, there are treatments that work for both depression and smoking.

Mood Changes

Mood changes are common after quitting smoking. Some people feel increased sadness. You might be irritable, restless, or feel down or blue. Changes in mood from quitting smoking may be part of withdrawal. Withdrawal is your body getting used to not having nicotine. Mood changes from nicotine withdrawal usually get better in a week or two. If mood changes do not get better in a couple of weeks, you should talk to your doctor. Something else, such as depression, could be the reason.

Smoking may seem to help you with depression. You might feel better at the moment. But there are many problems with using cigarettes to cope with depression. There are other things you can try to lift your mood:

- **Exercise**. Being physically active can help. Start small and build up over time. This can be hard to do when you are depressed. But your efforts will pay off.
- **Structure your day**. Make a plan to stay busy. Get out of the house if you can.

- **Be with other people**. Many people who are depressed are cut off from other people. Being in touch or talking with others every day can help your mood.
- **Reward yourself**. Do things you enjoy. Even small things add up and help you feel better.

Boosting Your Mood

Mood changes are common after quitting smoking. You might be irritable, restless, or feel down or blue. If you have these feelings after quitting smoking, there are things you can do to help lift your mood.

Stay Active

Any kind of exercise can help—taking a walk, going to the gym, and joining a team sport are a few you might try. If you need to, start small and build up over time. This can be hard to do when you are feeling down, but making the effort can pay off.

Structure Your Day

Create a plan to stay busy. Try to get out of the house whenever you can.

Do Things with Other People

Some people who are feeling down are cut off from others. Having regular contact with other people can help your mood. Try to connect with people regularly, whether it is in person, over the phone, or via text message.

Build Rewards into Your Life

For many people who are sad, rewards and fun activities are missing from their lives. Finding ways to reward yourself can help lift your mood. Even small things, such as reading a magazine or listening to music, can add up and help you feel better.

Do What Used to Be Fun

One of the common signs of depression is not wanting to do activities that used to be fun. It may be hard, but you might try doing fun activities again to help improve your mood. Try making a list of activities or events that you enjoy and plan to do one a day.

Get Support

You do not have to deal with negative moods alone. Your friends, family, and others who are important to you can support you. Let them know what they can do to help.

Doing Good to Feel Good

When you do a good deed for someone, you make their day a little better. Research shows that doing something nice for others can make your day a little better too.

Learn New Skills and Behaviors

Try new activities to replace smoking.

- Instead of smoking after a meal, take a brisk walk in your neighborhood or around your office building.
- Take up knitting, carpentry, or other hobbies and activities that keep your hands busy.
- Avoid other people who smoke. Ask those you cannot avoid respecting your effort to stop smoking and not smoke around you.
- Remove cigarettes, ashtrays, and lighters from your home, office, and car.
- Do not smoke at all—not even one puff.
- Try to avoid alcohol and caffeine. People who drink alcohol are more likely to start smoking again after quitting.
- You can help control your weight gain from quitting smoking, which is on average 10 pounds or less, by following a heart-healthy lifestyle and being physically active.
- Each step you take to remove smoking from your life improves the health of your heart and blood vessels.
- Remember to celebrate the small wins you achieve as you work toward becoming smoke-free.

Source: "Strategies to Quit Smoking," National Heart, Lung, and Blood Institute (NHLBI), March 24, 2022. Available online. URL: www.nhlbi.nih.gov/health/heart/smoking/tips-to-quit. Accessed October 11, 2023.

Random Acts of Kindness

When a craving hits, try distracting yourself for a few minutes by being helpful to a friend, family member, coworker, or complete stranger. Put your neighbor's newspaper on the porch when you are out walking your dog. Make a kind comment to the grocery store checkout person, whose last customer was grumpy. Hold the door for someone with their hands full. Actions like these let you focus on another person's needs. This makes it easier to focus less on your own for a moment and cope with a craving until it passes. Good deeds such as these take very little time, cost you nothing, and help both of you feel good. Plus, good deeds can have benefits beyond helping you beat the urge to smoke.

Doing a good deed helps you focus your thoughts outward toward others. It helps you take a step outside your own world for a little while. Performing good deeds can have positive effects on your health, such as reducing stress. Managing stress can be a key part of quitting smoking. Being caring toward others helps you reduce your own stress and may even help you live longer. That makes being kind to others a great smoke-free way to deal with stress.

Plan to Do Good

Good deeds are done on purpose. That is different from not doing something you might normally do, such as not screaming at another driver who cuts you off. That does not count as a good deed. Some good deeds take planning. Planning helps you pay attention and be mindful of the good deeds you are doing. It also helps you be mindful of the other person's needs. You might help friends or family members by running errands or helping with child care. Make some cookies for a person who did you a favor. Clean the house or cook dinner for an older friend or relative. Good deeds like these take some planning and help you understand what makes the other person happy.

You can also do good deeds for total strangers to make their lives a little better. Or giving up some of your free time to volunteer, whether it is serving at a soup kitchen, cleaning up litter, or taking elderly people to the grocery store.

Studies show that one good deed leads to another. If you perform a generous or kind act, you are likely to be happier. The happier you feel, the more likely you are to do another kind act.[1]

[1] Smokefree.gov, "Manage Your Mood," U.S. Department of Health and Human Services (HHS), June 8, 2016. Available online. URL: www.smokefree.gov/challenges-when-quitting/mood. Accessed October 11, 2023.

CHAPTER 63
NUTRITION AND APPETITE WHILE QUITTING

It is common for smokers to have bigger appetites and slower metabolisms after quitting smoking. Sometimes, this leads to overeating and weight gain—but it does not have to. Understand what happens to your body after becoming nicotine-free and get tips for managing your weight after quitting.

Quitting and Appetite

It is normal for your appetite to increase and your sense of taste to change after quitting smoking. Avoid overeating, weight gain, and poor nutrition by staying in control of your food choices.

Increased appetite is a common withdrawal symptom after quitting. It tends to last longer than other symptoms. When you quit smoking, your senses of taste and smell improve and return to normal. Food is more enjoyable. This may also increase your appetite.

After quitting, your food likes and dislikes might change. It is common for people to say that before quitting they did not have a sweet tooth, but now eat sweet foods. Studies show that people want more sweet and fatty foods after quitting. Sweet and fatty foods are usually high in calories.

Snack Smart

Eating or snacking is like the action of smoking. This need to have something in your mouth goes away over time. Try to keep your hands and mouth busy with a toothpick or straw. Or you can chew on healthy foods, such as carrots and celery, or even sugar-free mints.

Eat Mindfully

Research shows that people tend to use food in the same ways they used cigarettes. They use food to deal with stress or boredom, reward themselves, pass time, or help them be social. It is important to know why you eat even when you are not hungry. You can eat mindfully by eating slower. Eating slower is healthier, too. Take time to enjoy your food. You are more likely to notice when you are full. Try turning off the TV and shutting off your phone while you eat. Going gadget-free helps you pay attention to the details of your food. You might notice flavors and textures you otherwise would have missed.

Control Weight

Changes in your diet or eating more food might cause you to gain weight. It is possible to reduce the chance you will gain weight after you quit smoking. If you have a plan to deal with appetite and nutrition changes, you can manage your weight. Exercise can be an important part of that plan to help you reduce cravings, reduce your appetite, and handle stress.

Set Healthy Eating Goals

You do not have to change your whole diet at once. Think of changes that are reachable, positive, under your control, and specific. Here are a few other goals that might work for you or give you ideas for your own:

- Make half your plate a variety of different colored fruits and vegetables.
- Make half the grains you eat whole grains.
- Choose a variety of lean protein foods.
- Eat smaller portions.
- Drink water instead of sugary drinks.
- Eat some seafood every week.
- Prepare meals at home that consist of whole (unprocessed) foods.

Reward yourself when you reach each goal. It will give you something to look forward to. Avoid using food as a reward. Treat yourself with extra time spent with a friend, a hobby you have wanted to try, or an activity that gets you moving. Or combine rewards, such as taking a yoga class or going for a bike ride with a friend.

Source: Smokefree Women, "Healthy Eating," U.S. Department of Health and Human Services (HHS), September 6, 2018. Available online. URL: www.women.smokefree.gov/live-healthier/care-for-your-body/healthy-eating. Accessed October 3, 2023.

Manage Weight Gain after Quitting

Many people delay quitting smoking because they are worried about weight gain. While many smokers gain some weight after they quit, it is better for your health if you quit as soon as possible.

Once you quit, you can begin to build healthy habits for exercise, nutrition, and—if necessary—weight loss.

How to Control Weight Gain after Quitting

- **Control your appetite**. Smoking cigarettes makes you feel less hungry. When you quit smoking, you might feel hungrier and eat more than you used to eat. Portion control can help you prevent overeating. And make sure you stay hydrated. It will keep you from eating when you are actually thirsty.

- **Start exercising regularly**. Smoking cigarettes increases your metabolism, so you burn more calories. When you stop smoking, you may burn fewer calories, which can lead to weight gain. Regular exercise can help you continue to burn those calories. Just 10 minutes of exercise a day can make a difference.
- **Learn how to eat mindfully**. Eating can become a substitute for smoking. It does not have to. Mindful eating means preparing, choosing, and eating with awareness. Here are some tips to help you eat healthier and enjoy your food more:
    - Avoid distractions. Turn off the phone, TV, and computer.
    - Eat at your dinner table, so you can focus on eating.
    - Think carefully about your portion sizes. Consider starting with a smaller portion.
    - Avoid serving food family style. If you still feel hungry, you will have to get up from the table for seconds.
    - Do a belly check. Are you really hungry or eating for some other reason?
- **Learn to cope with emotions without cigarettes**. When you stop smoking, you may want to turn to eating when you feel bad or life is stressful. But you can learn other ways to cope without smoking.[1]

[1] Smokefree.gov, "Weight Gain & Appetite," U.S. Department of Health and Human Services (HHS), May 19, 2018. Available online. URL: https://smokefree.gov/challenges-when-quitting/weight-gain-appetite. Accessed October 3, 2023.

CHAPTER 64
SLIPS AND RELAPSES

Many people try quitting smoking often before they finally succeed. Slips are a common part of quitting.

A slip is one or two cigarettes after you quit. For most people, even "just one puff" counts. If you have a slip ("I will have just one"), it could be harder for you to stay smoke-free. But a slip is different from a relapse. A relapse means going back to smoking regularly.

You can learn from slips. Remind yourself that you have had a temporary setback. You have not failed, and you are not back to square one. A slip does not make you a smoker again. It also is not an excuse to relapse and go back to smoking regularly.

Prepare yourself to recover from slips and avoid a relapse. Think about how you will avoid or handle your triggers and deal with cravings.

Slips Happen

Quitting smoking is a process. It may take time. During that time, you might get frustrated. There is a chance you might slip at some point and smoke a cigarette. Slips happen to a lot of people who quit smoking.

Slips often happen in the first three months after quitting, but they can happen at any time. Many people need several tries before they quit for good.

It is possible to get back on track. Think about all you have accomplished. Try to stay positive and remind yourself that a slip is just one bump in the road on your smoke-free journey.

Knowing your triggers can help you understand what led to the slip. Find ways to avoid your triggers along the way. And having a plan to deal with cravings can help you get past them.

Use the QuitGuide app to track your smoke-free progress, cravings, triggers, and smoking slips. You can tag the times and places that make it hard for you to stay smoke-free. The app will give you extra support when you need it most.

Tips for Slips

Many smokers slip and smoke a cigarette while they are quitting smoking. You are not alone. Do not use a slip as an excuse to start smoking again.

If you slip, you might try the following ways to get back on track:

- Slips are common, so do not be too hard on yourself. A slip does not make you a failure or does not mean you are relapsing. It does not mean you cannot quit for good.
- Feel proud of the time you went without smoking cigarettes. Think about ways you avoided your triggers and beat cravings. Try to use those ways to cope again.
- It is important to restart quitting right away—today or tomorrow at the latest. Do not give up on your goal of no cigarettes at all.
- If quitting forever seems too hard right now, try a text message program to help you prepare to quit in the future. These programs help you build skills for dealing with cravings, triggers, and stressful situations. You can try a Practice Quit for a few days or do a week of Daily Challenges without quitting. Sign up online or by texting GO to 47848.
- Use nicotine replacement therapy (NRT). You do not need to stop using NRT after you slip and smoke one or two cigarettes. Using NRT increases your chances of staying smoke-free for good.
- Get support. If you slip, talk to family or friends. Ask them for help to stay smoke-free. You do not have to do it alone.
- Think about what you learned when you were not smoking. What helped you stay smoke-free and what caused you to have a slip? What can you do differently now to help yourself be smoke-free again?

Source: Smokefree.gov, "Tips for Slips," U.S. Department of Health and Human Services (HHS), June 9, 2016. Available online. URL: www.smokefree.gov/challenges-when-quitting/stick-with-it/tips-for-slips. Accessed October 11, 2023.

How to Stay Smoke-Free

Quitting smoking is hard. It is a process that may take time. Using NRT can help. But it can be just as tough to stay smoke-free.

There are steps you can take to help you stay smoke-free, both now and long-term.

Understand Your Triggers

Certain people, places, things, and situations can trigger an urge to smoke, even years after quitting. Triggers are the things that make you want to smoke. They can affect you no matter how long it is been since you have quit. Knowing your triggers can help you be prepared and fight off cravings.

Beat Cravings

It is difficult to stay smoke-free when cravings hit. But the longer you go without smoking, the more these urges will fade. Fighting cravings can be easier if you have a plan. Prepare by making a list of things you can try when you have the urge to smoke. Take a walk, practice deep breathing, or do whatever works for you to get past cravings. Keep your list handy.

Be Positive

The first hours, days, and weeks without cigarettes can be hard. Quitting is a process: take it one day at a time. Keeping a positive outlook can help you get through. There are ways to deal with stress and other strong emotions without cigarettes.

Celebrate You

Staying smoke-free is a big accomplishment. Treat yourself regularly. Now that you are not buying cigarettes, you might have extra money to buy yourself something special. But your rewards do not have to cost anything. Enjoy an outdoor hike now that you can breathe easier. Or invite a friend over for a movie night. If you have already built your quit plan, remind yourself of the rewards you chose. If you have not made a quit plan, it is never too late.

Get Support

Controlling your triggers and managing cravings can be hard, even after you have been smoke-free for a while. Getting support from the people around you can help. Talk to the people who supported you when you first quit smoking. Friends and family members can play a big role in helping you stay smoke-free. Let them know you are in it for the long haul and what they can do to help.[1]

[1] Smokefree.gov, "Slips and Relapses," U.S. Department of Health and Human Services (HHS), June 9, 2016. Available online. URL: www.smokefree.gov/challenges-when-quitting/stick-with-it/slips-relapses. Accessed October 11, 2023.

CHAPTER 65
HELPING OTHERS QUIT

For Loved Ones

Quitting smoking is hard, but your support can be an important part of a loved one's smoking cessation experience. Not sure how to help? Want tips for being a more effective part of your quitter's support system? Understand what smokers go through when they quit and how you can be there for them throughout the process.

How to Support Your Quitter

Someone who feels supported is more likely to quit smoking for good. That is why friends, family members, and significant others can play a big part in helping a person become smoke-free.

It Is Hard to Quit

Smoking cigarettes is not a bad habit. It is a serious and complicated addiction. That makes quitting smoking one of the biggest challenges many smokers will ever face.

Deciding to quit does not mean thoughts of smoking go away at once. It takes time for cravings to fade, and it can take a person more than one try to successfully quit. Most people who quit do not do it on their own. They get a lot of help and support from friends, family, and significant others.

Know Your Relationship Style

The way you deal with smoking can have an effect on a person who is trying to quit. It helps become aware of your relationship style. Your style affects their smoking, their quitting, their health, and yours. Ask yourself the following questions:

- Do you mind that they smoke around you?
- Do you argue about smoking?
- Do you avoid talking about smoking?
- Has a health problem changed the way you deal with smoking?

Understanding your relationship style can help you understand what both of you may have to change to better deal with their smoking and quitting. For example, you may need to:

- recognize your friend or family member's small successes when quitting
- avoid criticizing them if they slip and have a cigarette
- decide it is time for you to quit smoking, too

Start the Conversation

It can be hard to get someone to talk about quitting smoking. To get a conversation started, look for an opening. Respond positively when someone says the following:

- "I am thinking about quitting smoking."
- "My doctor told me that I should quit smoking."
- "I am pregnant. I should probably quit smoking."
- "My wife is pregnant. I should probably quit smoking for her."
- "My kids are asking me about my cigarettes. I should probably quit smoking for them."

Let them know you think it is great they are considering quitting and that you are ready to help. If you are an ex-smoker, you can draw from your own experience of quitting. Let them know how much better you feel now that you are smoke-free. You might say the following:

- "I am so proud of you for trying to quit smoking. I will help with whatever you need to make it happen."
- "Quitting smoking will be hard, but I know you can do it. Have you set a quit date?"
- "You are not in this alone. Even if it gets tough, I will be here for you."
- "Quitting smoking is the best thing I ever did! Let me know if you need any tips."

Create an Opening

If someone does not give you an opening, create one. Ask them whether they have thought about quitting. Or you could try a different approach. You might say the following:

- "I heard on the news that taxes on cigarettes might go up soon. Sounds expensive. What do you think?"
- "I saw a commercial last night that showed an ex-smoker who lost teeth from gum disease caused by smoking. I did not know that could happen. Did you?"

Ask Questions

Asking open-ended questions can help you understand what a smoker who is quitting is going through. You might ask the following questions:

- "What made you want to start smoking?"
- "What things make you crave a cigarette?"

- "What made you decide to quit smoking?"
- "What things have been stressing you out lately?"
- "What could I do to help make quitting easier for you?"

Listen

Quitting smoking is about them—not you. Listen to what they have to say. If you ask a question, be quiet and give them time to answer. Resist the urge to insert your own comments.

Do Not Lecture

Lectures, nagging, and scolding will not help your friend or family member quit smoking. It might just put you on their bad side, and they may not come to you for help when they really need it.

Here are some things to avoid when you are trying to help someone quit smoking:

- nagging them about why smoking is bad
- counting the number of cigarettes they smoked
- asking them if they smoked today
- arguing with them about being irritable when they are going through withdrawal
- giving them a hard time if they have a bigger appetite from withdrawal
- getting upset if they slip and smoke a cigarette

Offer Distractions

Lend support to your friend or family member by helping them plan smoke-free activities. If you are still smoking, avoid smoking around them, especially if you call an activity "smoke-free."

Here are a few activities you could suggest:

- Go to the movies (and let them choose the show).
- Take a walk.
- Plan a game night with a group of friends.
- Make dinner.
- Go out to eat at their favorite restaurant.
- Sign up for a class, such as photography, painting, or cooking.
- Go to a concert.
- Go to a basketball, baseball, or football game where smoking is not allowed.

Triggers and cravings are a normal part of the quitting process. Help your friend or family member plan ahead by thinking of ways to handle these urges until they go away. Some people find that distracting themselves by texting or checking their social media helps pass the time until the craving is gone, while other people are helped by a change of scenery or routine. Talk about it and plan for different situations.

Here are some ideas:

- Chew gum or slowly eat hard candy.
- Play a game on your cell phone.
- Put a straw or toothpick in your mouth.
- Switch tasks for a change of scenery.
- Play with a rubber band.
- Munch on some carrot sticks, nuts, or celery.
- Squeeze a stress ball.
- Take deep breaths and try to relax.
- Drink lots of water.

Put together a smoke-free quit kit with a few of these items for your friend or family member to help them be ready to deal with cravings at the moment.

Be Patient and Positive

Supporting someone who is trying to quit smoking can be frustrating and exhausting. Focus on staying upbeat. Do not give up on them. Your support is important.

The withdrawal that can come from quitting smoking may make a person moody and irritable. Avoid:

- taking their moods personally
- telling them it was easier to put up with their moods when they were smoking
- suggesting it would be easier for them to just go back to smoking

The cravings a person might face can be hard to deal with. Do not let them lose confidence in quitting. Check in on them and let them know you support them. You might say the following:

- "I can tell this is hard on you, but I am proud of you for sticking with it. Let's do something fun to celebrate how far you have come!"
- "It sounds like you are having a rough day. How about I take care of dinner tonight/watch the kids/mow the lawn, so you can have some time for yourself? You deserve it."

Do Not Be Too Hard on Them If They Slip

Your friend or family member may slip at some point and smoke a cigarette. They will probably feel guilty, so getting angry with them will not help. Instead, you could:

- tell them you know they can still quit and remind them of all the progress they have made
- help them figure out what triggered the craving that led to the slip
- help them come up with a plan for dealing with the craving if it happens again
- ask if there is anything else you can do to help

Here are some ways you could respond to a slip:

- "Slips happen. Do not beat yourself up over it. Like anything tough, you learn as you go. Use right now as a time to restart and get back on track."
- "So you slipped. Quitting is not easy, and many people need several tries before they quit for good. You have got this, and I am here for you."
- "Let's talk about what is triggering you to smoke. That will help you stay on track this time. Just do not smoke that next cigarette."

Celebrate Successes Big and Small

Recognize your friend or family member's smoke-free successes and milestones. Staying smoke-free for one day, one week, or one year are all reasons to celebrate. So are throwing out all of the ashtrays in the house, ditching any reminder of cigarettes, and passing on an after-dinner cigarette. Help your friend or family member celebrate by:

- sending flowers or a card
- surprising them with tickets to a concert or show
- giving them a gift card to their favorite store
- making a home-cooked dinner

A compliment can go a long way to recognize the positive changes they have made:

- "The smoke-free life works well for you—you look great!"
- "You make quitting smoking look easy. You should be proud of yourself. I am."

Help Them De-stress

Quitting smoking can create a lot of stress, which may cause someone to reach for a cigarette. If you notice they are stressed, help them break the cycle by finding healthier ways to de-stress. If you smoke, remember not to agree to have a cigarette together—that will set them back.

Consider suggesting one of the following smoke-free stress relievers:

- Close your eyes and take a few deep breaths.
- Play with a pet.
- Take a walk.
- Make a nice dinner.
- Read the Sunday comics.
- Try yoga or a spin class.
- Go to a comedy club or watch a funny TV show.
- Do a fun home project.
- Watch a sunset or sunrise.
- Do a crossword puzzle.
- Meet a friend at a cafe to chat.

- Take a nap.
- Take a bath or long shower.

Be There for the Long Haul

The challenges of quitting smoking do not end when a person puts down their last cigarette. Cravings can pop up weeks, or even months, later. It is not uncommon for ex-smokers to start smoking again within the first three months of quitting.

Let your friend or family member know you are there for the long haul. Keep celebrating their smoke-free anniversaries and offer distractions to help them deal with cravings. Your ongoing support could be all they need to make this quit attempt their last.[1]

[1] Smokefree.gov, "Help Others Quit," U.S. Department of Health and Human Services (HHS), July 21, 2016. Available online. URL: https://smokefree.gov/help-others-quit. Accessed October 11, 2023.

CHAPTER 66
FREE QUITLINE SERVICES

What Is a Quitline?

Quitlines are effective, evidence-based tobacco cessation interventions that help tobacco users quit through a variety of service offerings, including counseling, practical information on how to quit, referral to other cessation resources, and mailed self-help materials.

Quitlines:

- are free
- can be easily accessed by calling 800-QUIT-NOW (800-784-8669)
- are confidential
- overcome some of the barriers to seeking tobacco treatment, such as transportation, childcare, and financial or geographical barriers
- tailor their help to meet the needs of individual callers
- increase a tobacco user's chances of successfully quitting (the 2008 update to the Public Health Service's Clinical Practice Guideline Treating Tobacco Use and Dependence determined that quitlines increased the odds of six-month abstinence by approximately 60%)
- are staffed by counselors who are highly trained health-care professionals

Quitlines may offer a variety of other services, such as web-assisted tobacco interventions and text messaging. They also offer information and support for family, friends, and health-care professionals who want to help tobacco users quit.

Some state quitlines offer free cessation medications or provide tobacco users with vouchers or discounts to receive these medications at reduced cost. Most quitlines also offer counseling protocols and materials designed for specific populations, such as pregnant women or smokers with chronic diseases.

Are Quitlines Effective in Helping People to Quit?

Quitlines are effective, evidence-based treatments for smoking cessation. The evidence base for tobacco cessation quitlines was established through numerous clinical trials and meta-analyses. After an exhaustive review of the randomized clinical trial (RCT) research literature, the 2008 update to the Public Health Service's Clinical Practice Guideline Treating Tobacco Use and Dependence concluded that quitlines increase six-month smoking cessation quit rates compared with no intervention (the guideline reported quit rates among quitline users of 12.7% for counseling alone and 28.1% for counseling plus medication) and therefore recommended the use of quitlines to help tobacco users quit. Quitlines have been shown to be a cost-effective intervention.

Are Quitline Services Available in Every State?

All 50 U.S. states, the District of Columbia, Puerto Rico, and Guam operate quitlines can be accessed through the 800-QUIT-NOW quitline (operated by the National Cancer Institute (NCI)). This toll-free number automatically transfers callers to their state quitline. This easy-to-remember number allows for national promotion of quitline services. Health-care professionals can refer patients who are interested in quitting to 800-QUIT-NOW.

What Happens When Your Patient Calls 800-QUIT-NOW?

When patients call the quitline, they will be asked about their tobacco use, previous quit attempts, how they heard about the quitline, and some basic demographic questions, including gender, age, race/ethnicity, and education level. Citizenship documentation is not asked. This initial process usually takes about 10 minutes. All information collected is kept strictly confidential and is treated as protected health information.

Callers then receive information about the services the quitline offers. If a caller is interested in receiving mailed self-help materials, an address is taken, and materials are typically shipped within 24 hours. If a caller would like referrals to local cessation services or information on web-based cessation help, that information is provided. If a caller is interested in receiving cessation counseling, he/she is typically transferred to a tobacco cessation counselor. Cessation counselors are highly trained professionals who are skilled in motivational interviewing and delivering client-centered interventions. The counseling session may focus on creating a tailored quit plan, providing medication or decision support in choosing medications, and discussing tips and tools for overcoming everyday urges to smoke.

It is important to note that during times of heavy call volume (especially during national media campaigns that promote 800-QUIT-NOW), a cessation counselor may not be immediately available. In these cases, the quitline will schedule an appropriate callback time with the caller.

Who Is Eligible for Quitline Services?

The majority of states do not have eligibility criteria for providing quitline counseling beyond being a state resident. Many states also require that callers be interested in quitting tobacco in the next 30 days. However, some states may have more detailed eligibility criteria or may prioritize multiple call services or free medications for those meeting specific criteria (e.g., uninsured, Medicaid insured, etc.). For specific details on your state quitline's eligibility criteria, visit the North American Quitline Consortium (NAQC) Quitline Map (https://map.naquitline.org/default.aspx). Click on your state to view the quitline profile page.

How Do You Refer a Patient to the Quitline?

After asking if a patient uses tobacco and advising them to quit if they do, you will need to determine if they are ready to quit. For those patients who are not ready to quit, remind them that you have resources to help them quit when they are ready.

If a patient is ready to quit, you can refer them to your state quitline in one of two ways:

- Provide your patient with the 800-QUIT-NOW number and briefly explain what will happen when they call. This referral method requires your patient to make the initial call to the quitline. For example, you might say: "I am happy to hear you are ready to quit, and I want you to know that help is available. Our state has a telephone-based tobacco quitline that is free and offers help to people who want to quit. When you call, you will be asked a few questions about yourself and your tobacco use and then you will have the opportunity to talk to a person who has been trained to help you develop a quit plan."
- Use your state quitline's proactive referral system. This referral method prompts the quitline to call your patient directly to start services. In most states, health-care providers can send a referral with the patient's contact information to the state quitline through a fax or an electronic health record (EHR). This typically involves briefly explaining to the patient what will happen when the quitline calls, obtaining the patient's written consent to be contacted by the quitline, and faxing or electronically submitting the referral form. Many quitline referral programs offer feedback to referring providers to track patients' progress.

How Are State Quitlines Funded?

The majority of funding for state quitlines comes from state Master Settlement Agreement (MSA) funds, state general funds, and state tobacco taxes. In addition, some quitlines have partnerships with health insurance plans and/or employers to offer qualifying callers with expanded quitline and cessation services.[1]

[1] "Quitlines and Other Cessation Support Resources," Centers for Disease Control and Prevention (CDC), February 27, 2023. Available online. URL: www.cdc.gov/tobacco/patient-care/quitlines-other/index.html. Accessed October 4, 2023.

What If You Prefer to Speak to Someone in a Language Other Than English?

Most quitlines can arrange for a translator if you or someone you know who wants to quit speaks a different language.

Will the Coaches Make You Feel Bad about Smoking?

Absolutely not. Quitline coaches are hired and trained based on their ability to help you. Many used to smoke themselves, so they understand what you are going through. Your success is theirs, too.

What If You Are Not Sure You Are Ready to Quit?

You do not have to be ready to quit today to call the quitline. Your quit coach can help you explore your worries and doubts about quitting and help you identify solutions. The coaches have helped many people who smoke to successfully quit, and they can help you too.

What If You Use Other Kinds of Tobacco Products?

Quitline coaches can help you if you are using smokeless tobacco, cigars, hookah, e-cigarettes, or other tobacco products, in addition to cigarettes.

What If You Do Not Smoke, but You Want to Help a Friend or Family Member Who Does?

It can be a real challenge to know how best to help a friend or relative who smokes to quit. Maybe they do not want to quit, but their smoking is affecting you. Maybe they smoke inside, and it bothers you. Or maybe you are even worried about their health and the diseases that smoking causes. Maybe they want to quit, and you support them, but you do not know how to help. Quit coaches can help you come up with a plan to help them quit.

How Do You Know Using a Quitline Will Help?

Many studies have been done over the past 25 years on the advantages of quitlines. These studies report that people who call a quitline are more likely to quit and stay quit. Combining counseling and quit smoking medications such as patches can double or triple your chances of success.

What If You Do Not Like to Talk on the Phone?

There are other ways to quit. Quitlines can help you find out about other quit smoking services, such as apps and texting programs.

Will the Coaches Ask You Personal Information?

To provide callers with the best care, you will be asked to provide some information about yourself. You may be asked for your contact information during your initial call so that you can be reached for follow-up coaching. In addition, you will be asked about your smoking status and history, as well as past attempts at quitting and what caused you to continue smoking. You may also be asked your age, sex, and race. If you do not feel comfortable answering a question, you can always choose not to answer. All of the information you provide will be kept confidential.

Will It Cost Anything?

Quitline services are free to callers.

How Can You Learn More about Quitlines?

Call 800-QUIT-NOW (800-784-8669) and ask questions.[2]

Five Reasons Why Calling a Quitline Can Be Key to Your Success

- You can get help to stop smoking—free, with no judgment.
- Quit coaches help create a plan that can work for you.
- Quit coaches can help you get quit-smoking medicines.
- You can get helpful tips on managing cravings and avoiding triggers.
- And the best reason of all to use a quitline—you are more likely to stay quit!

Source: "Five Reasons Why Calling a Quitline Can Be Key to Your Success," Centers for Disease Control and Prevention (CDC), November 21, 2022. Available online. URL: www.cdc.gov/tobacco/campaign/tips/quit-smoking/quitline/index.html. Accessed October 4, 2023.

[2] "Top 10 Questions People Ask about Quitlines," Centers for Disease Control and Prevention (CDC), November 21, 2022. Available online. URL: www.cdc.gov/tobacco/campaign/tips/quit-smoking/quitline/top-10-questions-people-ask-about-quitlines.html. Accessed October 4, 2023.

PART 7 | IF YOU NEED MORE HELP OR INFORMATION

CHAPTER 67

WHERE TO GET HELP WHEN YOU DECIDE TO QUIT SMOKING

Which Health-Care Professionals Can Help You Quit Smoking?

Many health-care professionals can be good sources of information about the health risks of smoking and the benefits of quitting. Talk to your doctor, dentist, pharmacist, or other health-care provider about the proper use and potential side effects of nicotine replacement products and other medicines. They can also help you find local resources for assistance in quitting smoking.

Here are some things you should not do:

- Do not send quit smoking materials to smokers unless they ask for them.
- Do not blame or criticize the smoker for their addiction to tobacco.
- Do not criticize, nag, or remind the smoker about past failures.

Source: "Where to Get Help When You Decide to Quit Smoking," National Cancer Institute (NCI), October 28, 2010. Available online. URL: www.cancer.gov/about-cancer/causes-prevention/risk/tobacco/help-quitting-fact-sheet. Accessed October 6, 2023.

How Can You Find Out about National and Local Resources to Help You Quit Smoking?

Smokefree.gov of the National Cancer Institutes (NCI) offers science-driven tools, information, and support that have helped smokers quit. You will find state and national resources, free materials, and quitting advice from the NCI.

Smokefree.gov was established by the Tobacco Control Research Branch (TCRB) of the NCI, a component of the National Institutes of Health (NIH), in collaboration with the Centers for Disease Control and Prevention (CDC) and other organizations.

Publications available from the Smokefree.gov website include the following:

- Clearing the Air: Quit Smoking Today for smokers interested in quitting
- Clear Horizons for smokers over age 50

The NCI's Smoking Quitline at 877-44U-QUIT (877-448-7848) offers a wide range of services, including individualized counseling, printed information, referrals to other resources, and recorded messages. Smoking cessation counselors are available to answer smoking-related questions in English or Spanish, Monday through Friday, from 9:00 a.m. to 9:00 p.m., Eastern time. Smoking cessation counselors are also available through LiveHelp, an online instant messaging service. LiveHelp is available Monday through Friday, from 9:00 a.m. to 9:00 p.m., Eastern time.

Your state has a toll-free telephone quitline. Call 800-QUIT-NOW (800-784-8669) to get one-on-one help with quitting, support and coping strategies, and referrals to resources and local cessation programs. The toll-free number routes callers to state-run quitlines, which provide free cessation assistance and resource information to all tobacco users in the United States. This initiative was created by the Department of Health and Human Services (HHS). For more information about quitlines, speak to an expert on the Smokefree.gov website.[1]

[1] "Where to Get Help When You Decide to Quit Smoking," National Cancer Institute (NCI), October 28, 2010. Available online. URL: www.cancer.gov/about-cancer/causes-prevention/risk/tobacco/help-quitting-fact-sheet. Accessed October 6, 2023.

CHAPTER 68
DIRECTORY OF RESOURCES

Resources in this chapter were compiled from several sources deemed reliable; all contact information was verified and updated in January 2024.

Government Organizations

Agency for Healthcare Research and Quality (AHRQ)

5600 Fishers Ln.
7th Fl.
Rockville, MD 20857
Phone: 301-427-1364
Website: www.ahrq.gov

Centers for Disease Control and Prevention (CDC)

1600 Clifton Rd.
Atlanta, GA 30329-4027
Toll-Free: 800-CDC-INFO (800-232-4636)
Phone: 404-639-3311
Toll-Free TTY: 888-232-6348
Website: www.cdc.gov
Email: cdcinfo@cdc.gov

Centers for Medicare & Medicaid Services (CMS)

7500 Security Blvd.
Baltimore, MD 21244
Toll-Free: 877-267-2323
Phone: 410-786-3000
TTY: 410-786-0727
Toll-Free TTY: 866-226-1819
Website: www.cms.gov
Email: omh@cms.hhs.gov

Federal Trade Commission (FTC)
600 Pennsylvania Ave., N.W.
Washington, DC 20580
Toll-Free: 877-FTC-HELP (877-382-4357)
Phone: 202-326-2222
Website: www.ftc.gov

MedlinePlus
8600 Rockville Pike
Bethesda, MD 20894
Toll-Free: 888-FIND-NLM (888-346-3656)
Phone: 301-594-5983
Website: medlineplus.gov

National Cancer Institute (NCI)
9609 Medical Center Dr.
Rockville, MD 20850
Toll-Free: 800-4-CANCER (800-422-6237)
Website: www.cancer.gov
Email: NCIinfo@nih.gov

National Heart, Lung, and Blood Institute (NHLBI)
31 Center Dr.
Bldg. 31
Bethesda, MD 20892
Toll-Free: 877-NHLBI4U (877-645-2448)
Website: www.nhlbi.nih.gov
Email: nhlbiinfo@nhlbi.nih.gov

National Institute of Dental and Craniofacial Research (NIDCR)
Toll-Free: 866-232-4528
Website: www.nidcr.nih.gov
Email: nidcrinfo@mail.nih.gov

National Institute of Mental Health (NIMH)
6001 Executive Blvd.
MSC 9663
Bethesda, MD 20892-9663
Toll-Free: 866-615-6464
Website: www.nimh.nih.gov
Email: nimhinfo@nih.gov

National Institute on Drug Abuse (NIDA)

16071 Industrial Dr.
3WFN, MSC 6024
Gaithersburg, MD 20892
Phone: 301-443-6441
Website: https://nida.nih.gov

Office of the Surgeon General (OSG)

200 Independence Ave., S.W.
Humphrey Bldg., Ste. 701H
Washington, DC 20201
Toll-Free: 877-696-6775
Phone: 202-401-7529
Website: www.hhs.gov/surgeongeneral/index.html
Email: surgeongeneral@hhs.gov

Smokefree.gov

9609 Medical Center Dr.
BG 9609, MSC 9760
Bethesda, MD 20892-9760
Phone: 301-496-8584
Fax: 301-496-8675
Website: www.smokefree.gov
Email: NCISmokeFreeTeam@mail.nih.gov

Substance Abuse and Mental Health Services Administration (SAMHSA)

5600 Fishers Ln.
Rockville, MD 20857
Toll-Free: 877-SAMHSA-7 (877-726-4727)
Toll-Free TTY: 800-487-4889
Website: www.samhsa.gov
Email: SAMHSAInfo@samhsa.hhs.gov

U.S. Bureau of Alcohol, Tobacco, Firearms, and Explosives (ATF)

99 New York Ave., N.E.
Washington, DC 20226
Phone: 202-648-8410
Website: www.atf.gov
Email: ATFTips@atf.gov

U.S. Department of Health and Human Services (HHS)

200 Independence Ave., S.W.
Hubert H. Humphrey Bldg.
Washington, DC 20201
Toll-Free: 877-696-6775
Website: www.hhs.gov

U.S. Environmental Protection Agency (EPA)

1200 Pennsylvania Ave., N.W.
Washington, DC 20460
Phone: 202-564-4700
Website: www.epa.gov

U.S. Food and Drug Administration (FDA)

10903 New Hampshire Ave.
Silver Spring, MD 20993-0002
Toll-Free: 888-INFO-FDA (888-463-6332)
Website: www.fda.gov

Private Organizations

Action on Smoking and Health (ASH)

1250 Connecticut Ave., N.W.
7th Fl.
Washington, DC 20036
Phone: 202-659-4310
Website: www.ash.org
Email: info@ash.org

American Academy of Family Physicians (AAFP)

11400 Tomahawk Creek Pkwy.
Leawood, KS 66211-2680
Toll-Free: 800-274-2237
Phone: 913-906-6000
Fax: 913-906-6075
Website: www.aafp.org
Email: aafp@aafp.org

American Cancer Society, Inc. (ACS)

3380 Chastain Meadows Pkwy., N.W., Ste. 200
Kennesaw, GA 30144
Toll-Free: 800-227-2345
Website: www.cancer.org

American College of Chest Physicians (CHEST)

2595 Patriot Blvd.
Glenview, IL 60026
Toll-Free: 800-343-2227
Phone: 224-521-9800
Fax: 224-521-9801
Website: www.chestnet.org
Email: HelpTeam@chestnet.org

American Council on Science and Health (ACSH)

Phone: 212-362-7044
Website: www.acsh.org
Email: acsh@acsh.org

American Dental Hygienists' Association (ADHA)

444 N. Michigan Ave., Ste. 400
Chicago, IL 60611
Phone: 312-440-8900
Website: www.adha.org
Email: mail@adha.net

American Heart Association, Inc. (AHA)

7272 Greenville Ave.
Dallas, TX 75231
Toll-Free: 800-AHA-USA-1 (800-242-8721)
Phone: 214-570-5943
Website: www.heart.org

American Lung Association (ALA)

55 W. Wacker Dr., Ste. 1150
Chicago, IL 60601
Toll-Free: 800-LUNGUSA (800-586-4872)
Website: www.lung.org
Email: info@lung.org

American Public Health Association (APHA)

800 I St., N.W.
Washington, DC 20001
Phone: 202-777-2742
TTY: 202-777-2500
Fax: 202-777-2534
Website: www.apha.org
Email: comments@apha.org

Bureau of Tobacco Free Florida (BTFF)
4052 Bald Cypress Way
Bin C-23
Tallahassee, FL 32399-1743
Phone: 850-245-4144
Website: tobaccofreeflorida.com
Email: contact@tobaccofreeflorida.com

Campaign for Tobacco-Free Kids
1400 I St., N.W., Ste. 1200
Washington, DC 20005
Phone: 202-296-5469
Fax: 202-296-5427
Website: www.tobaccofreekids.org
Email: info@tobaccofreekids.org

CancerCare®
275 7th Ave., 22nd Fl.
New York, NY 10001
Toll-Free: 800-813-HOPE (800-813-4673)
Phone: 212-712-8400
Fax: 212-712-8495
Website: www.cancercare.org
Email: info@cancercare.org

The Center for Social Gerontology (TCSG)
2307 Shelby Ave.
Ann Arbor, MI 48103
Phone: 734-665-1126
Fax: 734-665-2071
Website: www.tcsg.org
Email: tcsg@tcsg.org

Foundation for a Smoke-Free World
420 Lexington Ave., Ste. 300
New York, NY 10170
Website: www.smokefreeworld.org
Email: smokefreeworld@smokefreeworld.org

Fred Hutchinson Cancer Center

1100 Fairview Ave., N.
P.O. Box 19024
Seattle, WA 98109-1024
Toll-Free: 855-557-0555
Phone: 206-667-5000
Fax: 206-606-1025
Website: www.fredhutch.org
Email: helpdesk@fredhutch.org

The Ohio State University Wexner Medical Center (OSUMC)

410 W. 10th Ave.
Columbus, OH 43210
Phone: 614-293-8000
Website: wexnermedical.osu.edu
Email: OSUCareConnection@osumc.edu

Partnership to End Addiction

711 3rd Ave., Ste. 500
5th Fl.
New York, NY 10017
Phone: 212-841-5200
Website: www.drugfree.org
Email: contact@toendaddiction.org

Prevention for ME

11 State House Stn.
Key Bank Plz., 4th Fl.
Augusta, ME 04330-0011
Website: preventionforme.org
Email: tsup.dhhs@maine.gov

Public Health Law Center

875 Summit Ave.
St. Paul, MN 55105
Phone: 651-290-7506
Fax: 651-290-7515
Website: www.publichealthlawcenter.org
Email: publichealthlawcenter@mitchellhamline.edu

Robert Wood Johnson Foundation (RWJF)

50 College Rd., E.
Princeton, NJ 08540-6614
Toll-Free: 877-843-7953
Phone: 609-627-6000
Website: www.rwjf.org

Society for Research on Nicotine and Tobacco (SRNT)

2424 American Ln.
Madison, WI 53704
Phone: 608-443-2462
Fax: 608-333-0310
Website: www.srnt.org
Email: info@srnt.org

Tobacco Free Allegheny

1501 Reedsdale St., Ste. 2006
The Cardello Bldg.
Pittsburgh, PA 15233
Phone: 412-322-8321
Fax: 412-322-8323
Website: www.tobaccofreeallegheny.org

Tobaccofree Earth

8117 W. Manchester Ave., Ste. 500
Playa del Rey, CA 90293-8745
Phone: 310-577-9828
Website: tobaccofree.org

Truth Initiative

900 G St., N.W.
4th Fl.
Washington, DC 20001
Phone: 202-454-5555
Fax: 202-454-5773
Website: https://truthinitiative.org
Email: comms@truthinitiative.org

University of Wisconsin Center for Tobacco Research and Intervention (UW-CTRI)

1930 Monroe St., Ste. 200
Madison, WI 53711
Phone: 608-262-8673
Website: ctri.wisc.edu
Email: infoctri@ctri.wisc.edu

Virginia Smoke Free Association (VSFA)

10104 Chester Rd.
Chester, VA 23831
Phone: 804-318-9183
Website: www.virginiasmokefree.org
Email: info@virginiasmokefree.org

INDEX

INDEX

Page numbers followed by "n" refer to citation information; by "b" refer to information contained in boxes; by "t" indicate tables; and by "f" indicate figures.

A

B

C

D

E

F

G

H

I

J

K

L

M

N

O

P

Q

R

S

T

U

V

W

X